Advances in Oligosaccharides and Polysaccharide Modifications in Marine Bioresources

Advances in Oligosaccharides and Polysaccharide Modifications in Marine Bioresources

Editors

Yuya Kumagai
Hideki Kishimura
Benwei Zhu

MDPI • Basel • Beijing • Wuhan • Barcelona • Belgrade • Manchester • Tokyo • Cluj • Tianjin

Editors
Yuya Kumagai
Hokkaido University
Hakodate, Japan

Hideki Kishimura
Hokkaido University
Hakodate, Japan

Benwei Zhu
Nanjing Tech University
Nanjing, China

Editorial Office
MDPI
St. Alban-Anlage 66
4052 Basel, Switzerland

This is a reprint of articles from the Special Issue published online in the open access journal *Marine Drugs* (ISSN 1660-3397) (available at: https://www.mdpi.com/journal/marinedrugs/special_issues/Advances_Oligosaccharides_Polysaccharide_Modifications_Marine_Bioresources).

For citation purposes, cite each article independently as indicated on the article page online and as indicated below:

LastName, A.A.; LastName, B.B.; LastName, C.C. Article Title. *Journal Name* **Year**, *Volume Number*, Page Range.

ISBN 978-3-0365-8364-8 (Hbk)
ISBN 978-3-0365-8365-5 (PDF)

Contents

About the Editors vii

Preface to "Advances in Oligosaccharides and Polysaccharide Modifications in Marine Bioresources" ix

Peng He, Deling Shi, Yunran Li, Ke Xia, Seon Beom Kim, Rohini Dwivedi and et al.
SPR Sensor-Based Analysis of the Inhibition of Marine Sulfated Glycans on Interactions between Monkeypox Virus Proteins and Glycosaminoglycans
Reprinted from: *Marine Drugs* **2023**, *21*, 264, doi:10.3390/md21050264 1

Blessing Mabate, Chantal Désirée Daub, Brett Ivan Pletschke and Adrienne Lesley Edkins
Comparative Analyses of Fucoidans from South African Brown Seaweeds That Inhibit Adhesion, Migration, and Long-Term Survival of Colorectal Cancer Cells
Reprinted from: *Marine Drugs* **2023**, *21*, 203, doi:10.3390/md21040203 11

Cheng Yang, Rongrong Yang, Ming Gu, Jiejie Hao, Shixin Wang and Chunxia Li
Chitooligosaccharides Derivatives Protect ARPE-19 Cells against Acrolein-Induced Oxidative Injury
Reprinted from: *Marine Drugs* **2023**, *21*, 137, doi:10.3390/md21030137 31

Chengying Yin, Jiaxia Sun, Hainan Wang, Wengong Yu and Feng Han
Identification and Characterization of a New Cold-Adapted and Alkaline Alginate Lyase TsAly7A from *Thalassomonas* sp. LD5 Produces Alginate Oligosaccharides with High Degree of Polymerization
Reprinted from: *Marine Drugs* **2023**, *21*, 6, doi:10.3390/md21010006 47

Juanjuan Wang, Zebin Liu, Xiaowei Pan, Ning Wang, Legong Li, Yuguang Du and et al.
Structural and Biochemical Analysis Reveals Catalytic Mechanism of Fucoidan Lyase from *Flavobacterium* sp. SA-0082
Reprinted from: *Marine Drugs* **2022**, *20*, 533, doi:10.3390/md20080533 57

Shengsheng Cao, Li Li, Benwei Zhu and Zhong Yao
Biochemical Characterization and Elucidation of the Hybrid Action Mode of a New Psychrophilic and Cold-Tolerant Alginate Lyase for Efficient Preparation of Alginate Oligosaccharides
Reprinted from: *Marine Drugs* **2022**, *20*, 506, doi:10.3390/md20080506 77

Lei Wang, Jun-Geon Je, Caoxing Huang, Jae-Young Oh, Xiaoting Fu, Kaiqiang Wang and et al.
Anti-Inflammatory Effect of Sulfated Polysaccharides Isolated from *Codium fragile* In Vitro in RAW 264.7 Macrophages and In Vivo in Zebrafish
Reprinted from: *Marine Drugs* **2022**, *20*, 391, doi:10.3390/md20060391 93

Sora Yu, So Young Park, Dong Hyun Kim, Eun Ju Yun and Kyoung Heon Kim
Multi-Step Enzymatic Production and Purification of 2-Keto-3-Deoxy-Galactonate from Red-Macroalgae-Derived Agarose
Reprinted from: *Marine Drugs* **2022**, *20*, 288, doi:10.3390/md20050288 101

Yuya Kumagai, Hideki Kishimura, Weeranuch Lang, Takayoshi Tagami, Masayuki Okuyama and Atsuo Kimura
Characterization of an Unknown Region Linked to the Glycoside Hydrolase Family 17 β-1,3-Glucanase of *Vibrio vulnificus* Reveals a Novel Glucan-Binding Domain
Reprinted from: *Marine Drugs* **2022**, *20*, 250, doi:10.3390/md20040250 113

Xue-Bing Ren, Yan-Ru Dang, Sha-Sha Liu, Ke-Xuan Huang, Qi-Long Qin, Xiu-Lan Chen and et al.
Identification and Characterization of Three Chitinases with Potential in Direct Conversion of Crystalline Chitin into *N,N′*-diacetylchitobiose
Reprinted from: *Marine Drugs* **2022**, *20*, 165, doi:10.3390/md20030165 . . . . **127**

Limin Ning, Zhong Yao and Benwei Zhu
Ulva (*Enteromorpha*) Polysaccharides and Oligosaccharides: A Potential Functional Food Source from Green-Tide-Forming Macroalgae
Reprinted from: *Marine Drugs* **2022**, *20*, 202, doi:10.3390/md20030202 . . . . **147**

About the Editors

Yuya Kumagai

Dr. Yuya Kumagai received B.S., M.S., and Ph.D. degrees in Fisheries Science from the Hokkaido University, Hakodate, Japan in 2005, 2008, and 2010, respectively. He is currently an Associate Professor of Faculty of Fisheries Science with Hokkaido University, Hakodate, Japan. His research interests include Marine Biology and Biochemistry, the characterization of functional materials from seaweed, enzymes, and the modification of them.

Hideki Kishimura

Dr. Hideki Kishimura is a Professor of Fisheries Sciences, Hokkaido University in Hokkaido, Japan. His research fields are the "purification of biochemical compounds from fisheries by-products and underused marine organisms" and the "determination of their structures and investigation of their health benefits". He is a society board member of the Japanese Society for Marine Biotechnology and a secretary board member of the Hokkaido Branch of the Japanese Society of Fisheries Science and serves on the Editorial Board of Marine Drugs.

Benwei Zhu

Dr. Benwei Zhu is a Professor at College of Food Science and Light Industry, Nanjing Tech University in Nanjing, China. He was also a Visiting Researcher in Prof. Kishimura's laboratory in 2020-2021. His research interests include the discovery and enzymatic and structural characterization of new marine polysaccharide-degrading enzymes.

Preface to "Advances in Oligosaccharides and Polysaccharide Modifications in Marine Bioresources"

Oligosaccharides and polysaccharides derived from marine bioresources are sustainable materials that are synthesized via seaweed photosynthesis. These are widely used by aquatic organisms and human beings as valuable foodstuffs and industrial raw materials, respectively. Seaweed polysaccharides have various structures depending on their origin, such as red algae, green algae, and brown algae. They exhibit various functionalities depending on small structural differences. This Special Issue includes content that will deepen our understanding of marine polysaccharides and oligosaccharides, e.g., the functional analysis of enzymes, the production of specific structural saccharides using specific enzymes, and the elucidation of their new functionality. We hope that this book will facilitate the achievement of a sustainable society by providing modified sustainable resources.

Yuya Kumagai, Hideki Kishimura, and Benwei Zhu
Editors

marine drugs

MDPI

Article

SPR Sensor-Based Analysis of the Inhibition of Marine Sulfated Glycans on Interactions between Monkeypox Virus Proteins and Glycosaminoglycans

Peng He [1,2], Deling Shi [1,2], Yunran Li [1,3], Ke Xia [1,2], Seon Beom Kim [4,5], Rohini Dwivedi [4], Marwa Farrag [4], Vitor H. Pomin [4], Robert J. Linhardt [1,2,3,6], Jonathan S. Dordick [1,6,*] and Fuming Zhang [1,6,*]

1 Center for Biotechnology and Interdisciplinary Studies, Rensselaer Polytechnic Institute, Troy, NY 12180, USA; hep3@rpi.edu (P.H.); shid2@rpi.edu (D.S.); liy77@rpi.edu (Y.L.); xiak@rpi.edu (K.X.); linhar@rpi.edu (R.J.L.)
2 Department of Chemistry and Chemical Biology, Rensselaer Polytechnic Institute, Troy, NY 12180, USA
3 Department of Biomedical Engineering, Rensselaer Polytechnic Institute, Troy, NY 12180, USA
4 Department of BioMolecular Sciences, Research Institute of Pharmaceutical Sciences, The University of Mississippi, Oxford, MS 38677, USA; rdwived1@olemiss.edu (R.D.); mmmoham1@go.olemiss.edu (M.F.); vpomin@olemiss.edu (V.H.P.)
5 Department of Food Science & Technology, College of Natural Resources and Life Science, Pusan National University, Miryang 46241, Republic of Korea
6 Departments of Chemical and Biological Engineering, Rensselaer Polytechnic Institute, Troy, NY 12180, USA
* Correspondence: dordick@rpi.edu (J.S.D.); zhangf2@rpi.edu (F.Z.)

Abstract: Sulfated glycans from marine organisms are excellent sources of naturally occurring glycosaminoglycan (GAG) mimetics that demonstrate therapeutic activities, such as antiviral/microbial infection, anticoagulant, anticancer, and anti-inflammation activities. Many viruses use the heparan sulfate (HS) GAG on the surface of host cells as co-receptors for attachment and initiating cell entry. Therefore, virion–HS interactions have been targeted to develop broad-spectrum antiviral therapeutics. Here we report the potential anti-monkeypox virus (MPXV) activities of eight defined marine sulfated glycans, three fucosylated chondroitin sulfates, and three sulfated fucans extracted from the sea cucumber species *Isostichopus badionotus*, *Holothuria floridana*, and *Pentacta pygmaea*, and the sea urchin *Lytechinus variegatus*, as well as two chemically desulfated derivatives. The inhibitions of these marine sulfated glycans on MPXV A29 and A35 protein–heparin interactions were evaluated using surface plasmon resonance (SPR). These results demonstrated that the viral surface proteins of MPXV A29 and A35 bound to heparin, which is a highly sulfated HS, and sulfated glycans from sea cucumbers showed strong inhibition of MPXV A29 and A35 interactions. The study of molecular interactions between viral proteins and host cell GAGs is important in developing therapeutics for the prevention and treatment of MPXV.

Keywords: monkeypox virus; protein A29; protein A35; heparin; sea cucumbers; marine sulfated glycans; surface plasmon resonance

Citation: He, P.; Shi, D.; Li, Y.; Xia, K.; Kim, S.B.; Dwivedi, R.; Farrag, M.; Pomin, V.H.; Linhardt, R.J.; Dordick, J.S.; et al. SPR Sensor-Based Analysis of the Inhibition of Marine Sulfated Glycans on Interactions between Monkeypox Virus Proteins and Glycosaminoglycans. *Mar. Drugs* **2023**, *21*, 264. https://doi.org/10.3390/md21050264

Academic Editors: Yuya Kumagai, Hideki Kishimura and Benwei Zhu

Received: 15 March 2023
Revised: 20 April 2023
Accepted: 23 April 2023
Published: 25 April 2023

1. Introduction

Monkeypox was first found in a colony of cynomolgus monkeys that had smallpox-like symptoms in 1958 [1]. Over the next ten years, several outbreaks among captive monkeys were reported in both the Netherlands and the United States, but no human cases were reported [2]. In 1970 the first human case was diagnosed in a baby boy from the Democratic Republic of Congo (DRC), then the monkeypox virus spread to other African countries and became endemic in Africa [3]. Human monkeypox cases were limited in Africa until 2003, which was when the first monkeypox case was reported in the United States because of the importation of rats from Africa [4]. More imported cases were then sporadically reported in the United Kingdom, Israel, Singapore, and the United States. In May 2022, a monkeypox outbreak in humans started in the UK that then spread across the world. According to the

World Health Organization (WHO), by March 2023, 86,391 confirmed cases and 111 deaths were reported, and 110 countries were impacted worldwide [5].

Monkeypox is caused by the monkeypox virus (MPXV), which is a double-stranded DNA virus with a genome of nearly 197 kb and around 190 nonoverlapping ORFs [6]. This zoonotic virus [7] belongs to the family *Poxviridae*, subfamily genus *Orthopoxvirus* (smallpox virus, variola virus, camelpox virus, and cowpox virus all belong to this genus). Monkeypox is genetically divided into two groups: the West African clade (clade I) and the Congo Basin clade (clade II, including clade IIa and clade IIb). The MPXV outbreak nowadays belongs to clade IIb. Unlike the large and quick mutations of single-stranded RNA viruses, such as influenza virus and SARS-CoV-2, the double-stranded DNA structure limited MPXV's mutations. However, in 2022, MPXV had more than 50 mutations in DNA compared with its 2018 version, and this mutation rate was much higher than before and makes the MPXV a globally concerning infectious disease [8]. Although the smallpox vaccine offers 78% protection against monkeypox [9], there remains a high demand to develop new anti-monkeypox drugs due to the large jump in the viral mutation rate.

The central portion of the genome in different *Orthopoxviruses* is highly conserved, and their proteins are highly homologous. The MPXV has a set of highly conserved *Orthopoxvirus* surface proteins, which can be targeted to block the viral infection [6]. Among these surface proteins, MPXV A29 and M1 are involved in the cellular entry into the intracellular mature virion, while proteins B6 and A35 play important roles in the transmission on the surface of extracellular enveloped virion [10]. The poxvirus A35 protein is reported to be an important virulence factor of poxviruses. A 1000-fold virulence attenuation was detected when the poxvirus lost its A35 proteins. We previously reported that MPXV A29 protein shows high binding affinity to the GAGs, including heparin, chondroitin sulfate (CS), and dermatan sulfate (DS) [11]. We proposed the following three-step model of MPXV host cell entry in which (i) MPXV virions attach to the host cell surface by binding to heparan sulfate proteoglycan (HSPG), (ii) host cell surface proteases initiate viral–host cell membrane fusion, and (iii) virions finally enter the host cell. It is a promising therapeutic target to develop drugs that can bind to A29 to stop the viral entry or binding to the A35 protein, reducing the virulence of the MPXV.

Our previous study found that the sulfated glycans pentosan polysulfate and mucopolysaccharide polysulfate showed strong inhibition of MPXV A29 binding to heparin. Marine-sourced sulfated glycans attracted much attention due to their antiviral activities against the influenza virus, respiratory syncytial virus, cytomegalovirus, and dengue virus. Recently, we reported a series of marine sulfated glycans that showed strong inhibitory activity against SARS-CoV-2 by binding with the viral surface S-protein [12–15]. In this study, a small library of marine echinoderm sulfated glycans (fucosylated chondroitin sulfates and sulfate fucans; see the structures in Figure 1) derived from three sea cucumbers and one sea urchin were prepared and evaluated for the inhibition activity on the MPXV A29 and A35 protein–heparin interactions using surface plasmon resonance (SPR). Our results demonstrated that MPXV A29 and A35 bind to heparin and the tested sulfated glycans from sea cucumbers showed strong inhibition of the interaction between heparin and A29/A35.

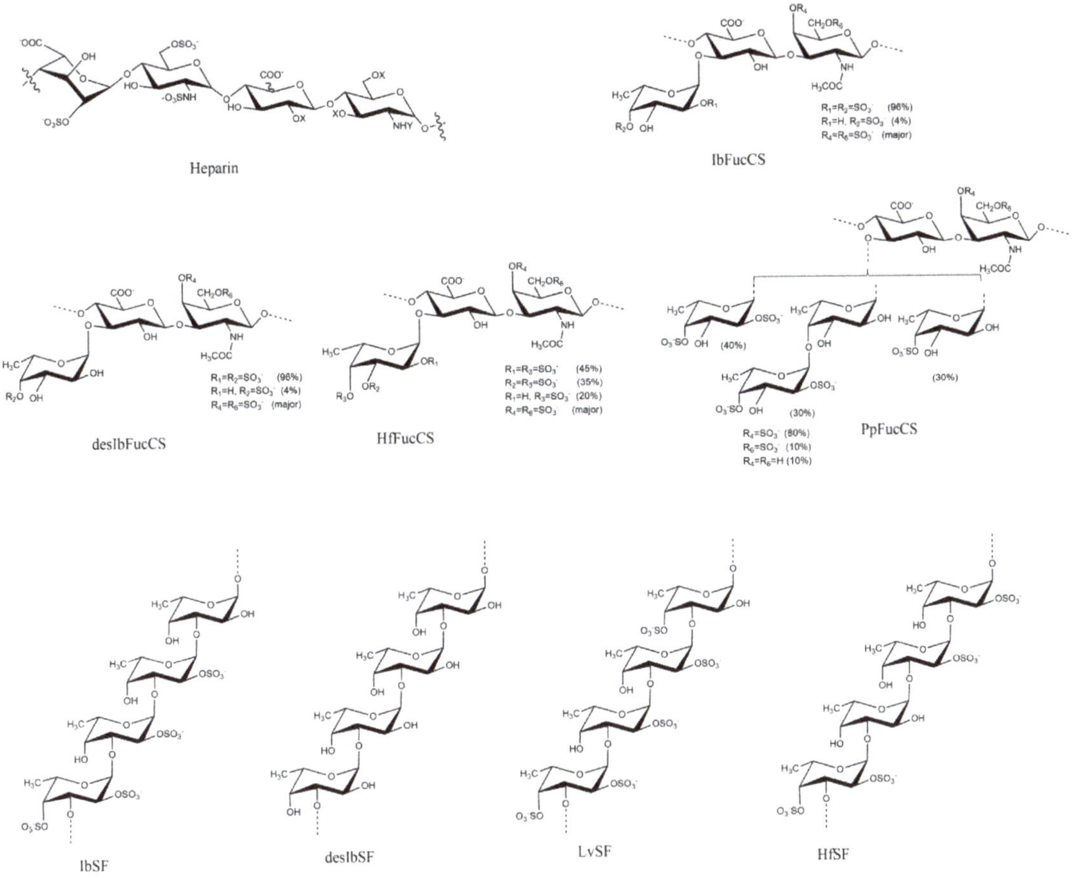

Figure 1. Chemical structures of heparin and marine sulfated glycans.

2. Results and Discussion

2.1. Binding Affinity and Kinetics Measurement of Heparin–MPXV Protein Interactions

Smallpox vaccines based on the vaccinia virus (VACV), such as ACAM2000 and MVA-BN, were shown to be effective in preventing and controlling MPXV by WHO and the CDC [16]. Eight well-studied VACV proteins were applied as immunogenic proteins to neutralize antibodies in humans: A33R, A28L, A27L, A17L, H3, D8L, L1R, and B5R. Among these, MPXV A35 proteins and VACV A33R proteins have a 95.5% genetic similarity [17]. The A35 protein is an extracellular enveloped virus (EEV) that envelops glycoprotein, which is an important component of actin-containing microvilli and plays critical roles in cell-to-cell spread. Heparin is a naturally occurring linear anionic GAG, which is structurally like HS, with a wide distribution in chain molecular weight and sulfation density. Heparin interacts with multiple proteins, endowing heparin with a variety of pharmacological activities, such as anticoagulation, antithrombosis, and anti-inflammation. Many publications demonstrate that many viruses, including SARS-CoV-2, the herpes simplex virus, the influenza virus, and the Zika virus, can infect the host by binding HS on the cell surface [18,19]. HS, as part of the glycocalyx on host cells, facilitates the attachment of viruses to host cells, usually constituting the initial step of viral infection. Heparin and HS also exhibit antiviral activity by blocking viral receptors, thereby inhibiting viruses from engaging with host cells. Recently, three models for how viruses involve HS or therapeutic sulfated GAGs were proposed [20]: (i) viruses use HS as a primary receptor required for infection, such as HSV-1 and HSV-2; (ii) HS serves as a co-receptor that provides localization of the virus on the cell surface by increasing viral concentration and carrying the virus closer to the more specific receptors for viral entry, such as SARS-CoV-2, using HS to facilitate its binding the receptor angiotensin-converting enzyme 2 (ACE2); and (iii) HS can also serve as a protector of the host cell from viral engagement by shielding key receptors. Heparin, which is an HS mimetic, can competitively inhibit the binding of viral proteins to HS on the host cell surface. Here, a heparin chip, as well as CS and DS (GAGs also present on the cell surface) chips, were prepared to evaluate their binding activities with MPXV A35 proteins. Unlike protein A29 binding to the CS and DS [11], neither CS nor DS showed binding to MPXV A35 protein (data not shown). Sensorgrams of interactions of heparin with MPXV A29 and A35 are shown in Figure 2.

AA sequence of A29:

^{1}MDGTLFPGDDDLAIPATEFFSTKAAKNPET
KREAIVKAYGDDNEETLKQRLTNLEKKITN
ITTKFEQIEKCCKHNDEVLFRLENHAETLR
AAMISLA^{97}

AA sequence of A35:

^{1}MMTPENDEEQTSVFSATVYGDKIQGKNKRKRVIGLCI
RISMVISLLSMITMSAFLIVRLNQCMSANEAAITDSAVA
VAAASSTHRKVASSTTQYDHKESCNGLYYQGSCYILHSD
YKSFEDAKANCAAESSTLPN^{137}

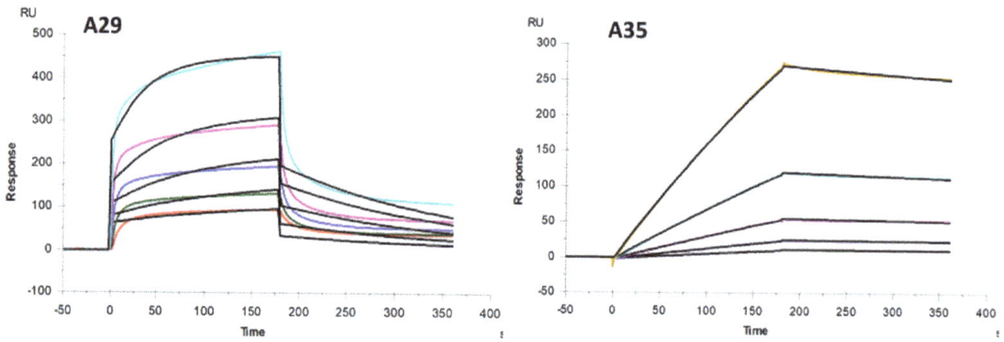

Figure 2. Amino acid sequence of MPXV A29 and A35 proteins (positively charged amino acids histidine (H), lysine (K), and arginine (R) are in red) and SPR sensorgrams of MPXV A29 and A35 protein binding with heparin. Concentrations of A35 protein were 1000, 500, 250, 125, 62.5 and 31.3 nM (from top to bottom, respectively).

Both the binding kinetics and affinity (*ka*, association rate constant; *kd*, dissociation rate constant; and K_D (*ka*/*kd*), binding equilibrium dissociation constant) were obtained through globally fitting the entire association and dissociation phases by employing a 1:1 Langmuir binding model. Table 1 shows the kinetic parameters of the interaction between the MPXV A29 and A35 proteins with heparin. The binding affinity of the MPXV A35 protein with heparin was 220 nM and showed a strong binding affinity between heparin and A35 protein. The binding activities of heparin with MPXV A29 protein were also tested as a comparison. The binding kinetic results indicated (i) a similar binding affinity (K_D) for heparin interaction with A29 and A35: K_D = 250 nM for the heparin–A29 interaction and K_D = 220 nM for the heparin–A35 interaction; (ii) the A29 protein showed a quick association rate and a quick disassociation rate, while the A35 protein showed a slow association rate and a slow disassociation rate. The interactions between these proteins and heparin were primarily of an electrostatic nature: negatively charged GAGs interacted with positively charged amino acids, including lysine, arginine, and histidine. Based on the sequences of A29 and A35 (Figure 2), some positively charged amino acid clusters served as the heparin-binding domain.

Table 1. Kinetic data of the interaction of the MPXV A29 and A35 proteins with heparin.

	k (M^{-1}S^{-1})	K_d (S^{-1})	K_D (M)
A29 protein	2.0×10^4 (±190) *	5.1×10^{-3} (±4.1×10^{-5}) *	2.5×10^{-7}
A35 protein	1.8×10^3 (±14) *	4.0×10^{-4} (±1.6×10^{-6}) *	2.2×10^{-7}

* The data with (±) in parentheses are the standard deviations (SDs) from the global fitting of five injections.

2.2. SPR Solution Competition between Surface-Immobilized Heparin and Marine Sulfated Glycans

The sulfated glycans studied were the sulfated fucan (IbSF) and the fucosylated chondroitin sulfate (IbSFucCS) isolated from the sea cucumber *Isostichopus badionotus*, along with their chemical fully desulfated derivatives desIbSF (polymer of fucose) and desIbFucCS (Figure 1) [21,22]. IbSF has a structure of [→3)-α-Fuc2,4S-(1→3)-α-Fuc2S-(1→3)-α-Fuc2S-(1→3)-α-Fuc-(1→]$_n$. IbFucCS has a structure of [→3)-β-GalNAc4,6S-(1→4)β-GlcA-[(3→1)Y]-(1→]$_n$, where Y = α-Fuc2,4S (96%) or α-Fuc4S (4%). Both IbSF and IbFucCS showed excellent inhibitory activity against SARS-CoV-2 wild-type and Delta (B.1.617.2) strains by thoroughly disrupting the S-protein interaction with HS on the host cell surface. Fully desulfated IbSF (desIbSF) and IbFucCs (desIbFucCS) were obtained via chemical desulfation using solvolysis after conversion to their pyridinium salt derivatives [23].

Solution/surface competition experiments were performed using SPR to study the ability of *I. badionotus* (Ib)-sourced glycans IbSF, IbFucCS, desIbSF, and desIbFucCS to inhibit the interaction between heparin with MPXV A29 and A35 proteins. The same concentration of Ib glycan (100 μg/mL) was individually mixed in the MPXV A29 or A35 proteins (250 nM). Solution competition studies between heparin and IB glycans are shown in Figure 3. All the Ib glycans inhibited the binding of both the MPXV A29 protein and A35 protein to the surface-immobilized heparin. Soluble heparin inhibited the binding of MPXV A29 and A35 to surface-immobilized heparin by 60% and 72%, respectively. IbSF and IbFucCS showed slightly better results in the inhibitions of A35 binding to surface-immobilized heparin, with 75.8% and 79.9%, respectively. Surprisingly, both IbSF and IbFucCS showed very strong competitive inhibitions, with 95% and 91.5%, respectively. After full desulfation, both desIbSF and desIbFucCS showed a reduced competitive ability to inhibit heparin binding to both the A29 and A35 proteins. This observation indicated that sulfation in the marine sulfated glycans is a key structural element for interactions with MPXV A29 and A35 proteins and, therefore, anti-monkeypox activity.

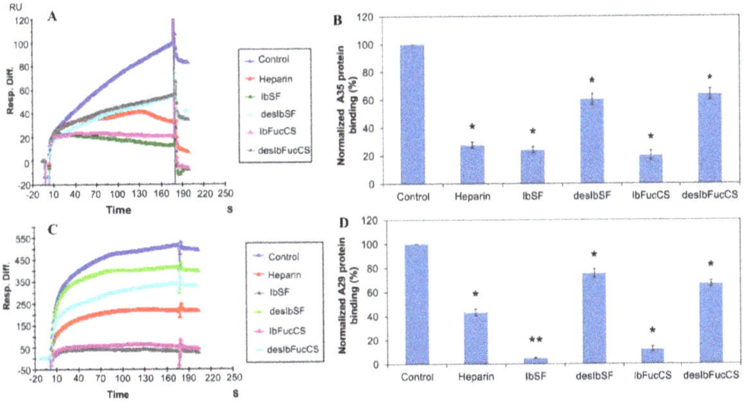

Figure 3. Solution competition between heparin and heparin Ib glycans. (**A**) SPR sensorgrams of the MPXV A35 protein–heparin interaction competing with different Ib glycans. The concentration of the MPXV A35 protein was 250 nM mixed with 100 μg/mL of different Ib glycans. (**B**) Bar graphs (based

on triplicate experiments with standard deviation) of normalized MPXV A35 protein binding preference to surface heparin by competing with different Ib glycans. (**C**) SPR sensorgrams of the MPXV A29 protein–heparin interaction competing with different Ib glycans. The concentration of the MPXV A29 protein was 250 nM mixed with 100 µg/mL of different Ib glycans. (**D**) Bar graphs (based on triplicate experiments with standard deviations) of the normalized MPXV A29 protein binding preference to surface heparin by competing with different Ib glycans. Statistical analysis was performed using an unpaired two-tailed *t*-test (*: $p \leq 0.05$ compared with the control, **: $p \leq 0.01$ compared with the control).

2.3. SPR Solution Competition between Surface-Immobilized Heparin and Holothuria-floridana-Sourced Sulfated Glycans HfSF and HfFucCS

HfSF is a sulfated fucan derived from the sea cucumber *Holothuria floridana* (Hf) with a structure of [→3)-α-Fuc2,4S-(1→3)-α-Fuc-(1→3)-α-Fuc2S-(1→3)-α-Fuc2S-(1→]$_n$, while HfFucCS is a fucosylated chondroitin sulfate with a structure of [→3)-β-GalNAc4,6S-(1→4)-β-GlcA-[(3→1)Y]-(1→]$_n$, where Y = αFuc2,4S (45%), α-Fuc3,4S (35%), or α-Fuc4S (20%) [24] (Figure 1). These two Hf glycans were found to be good inhibitors of both wild-type and Delta SARS-CoV-2 [13].

Solution/surface competition experiments were performed using SPR to study the ability of HfSF and HfFucCS to inhibit the interactions between heparin with the MPXV A29 and A35 proteins. The same concentration of Hf glycan (100 µg/mL) was individually mixed in the MPXV A29 or A35 proteins (250 nM). Solution competition study results between heparin and Hf glycans are shown in Figure 4. Heparin inhibited the binding of MPXV A29 and A35 binding to surface-immobilized heparin by 60% and 72%, respectively. IbSF and IbFucCS showed slightly better results for the inhibitions of A35 binding to surface-immobilized heparin, with 77.4% and 77%, respectively. However, IbSF and IbFucCS showed strong competitive inhibition results, with 92.4% and 86.1%, respectively.

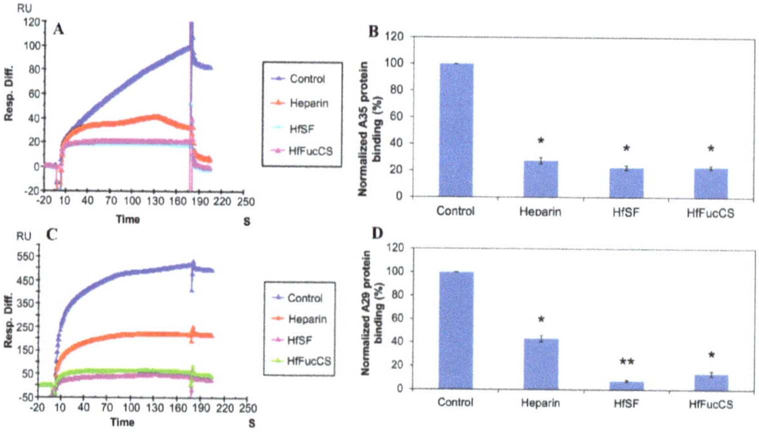

Figure 4. Solution competition between heparin and Hf glycans. (**A**) SPR sensorgrams of the MPXV A35 protein–heparin interaction competing with different Hf glycans. The concentration of the MPXV A35 protein was 250 nM mixed with 100 µg/mL of different Hf glycans. (**B**) Bar graphs (based on triplicate experiments with standard deviations) of the normalized MPXV A35 protein binding preference to surface heparin by competing with different Hf glycans. (**C**) SPR sensorgrams of the MPXV A29 protein–heparin interaction competing with different Hf glycans. The concentration of the MPXV A29 protein was 250 nM mixed with 100 µg/mL of different Hf glycans. (**D**) Bar graphs (based on triplicate experiments with standard deviations) of the normalized MPXV A29 protein binding preference to surface heparin by competing with different Hf glycans. Statistical analysis was performed using an unpaired two-tailed *t*-test (*: $p \leq 0.05$ compared with the control, **: $p \leq 0.01$ compared with the control).

2.4. SPR Solution Competition between Surface-Immobilized Heparin and two Marine-Soured Sulfated Glycans LvSF and PpFucCS

LvSF is a sulfated fucan isolated from the sea urchin *Lytechinus variegatus* and has a structure of [→3)-α-Fuc2,4S-(1→3)-αFuc2S-(1→3)-α-Fuc2S-(1→3)-α-Fuc4S-(1→]$_n$ [14], while PpFucCS is the fucosylated chondroitin sulfate isolated from the sea cucumber *Pentacta pygmaea* and has a structure of [→3)-β-GalNAcX(1→4)-β-GlcA-[(3→1)Y]-(1→]$_n$, where X = 4S (80%), 6S (10%), or non-sulfated (10%), and Y = α-Fuc2,4S (40%), αFuc2,4S-(1→4)-α-Fuc (30%), or α-Fuc4S (30%) [15] (Figure 1).

Solution/surface competition experiments were performed using SPR to study the inhibition of LvSF and PpFucCS for the interaction between heparin with MPXV A29 and A35 proteins. The same concentration of Hf glycan (100 μg/mL) was individually mixed in the MPXV A29 or A35 proteins (250 nM). The solution competition study results between heparin and sulfated glycans are shown in Figure 5. Heparin inhibited the binding of MPXV A29 and A35 to surface-immobilized heparin by 60% and 72%, respectively. LvSF and PpFucCS showed a better result of the inhibition of A35′s binding to surface-immobilized heparin, with 83.1% and 89%, respectively. LvSF and PpSFucCS showed strong competitive inhibition results, with 76.4% and 87%, respectively.

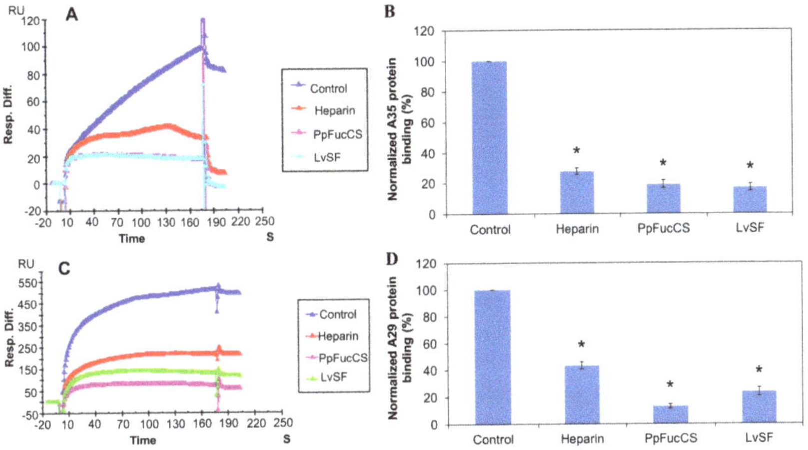

Figure 5. Solution competition between heparin and LvSF and PpFucCS glycans. (**A**) SPR sensorgrams of the MPXV A35 protein–heparin interaction competition with different LvSF and PpFucCS glycans. The concentration of the MPXV A35 protein was 250 nM mixed with 100 μg/mL of different LvSF and PpFucCS glycans. (**B**) Bar graphs (based on triplicate experiments with standard deviations) of the normalized MPXV A35 protein binding preference to surface heparin by competing with different LvSF and PpFucCS glycans. (**C**) SPR sensorgrams of the MPXV A29 protein–heparin interaction competing with different LvSF and PpFucCS glycans. The concentration of the MPXV A29 protein was 250 nM mixed with 100 μg/mL of different LvSF and PpFucCS glycans. (**D**) Bar graphs (based on triplicate experiments with standard deviations) of the normalized MPXV A29 protein binding preference to surface heparin by competing with different LvSF and PpFucCS glycans. Statistical analysis was performed using an unpaired two-tailed *t*-test (*: $p \leq 0.05$ compared with the control).

All six natural marine-derived sulfated glycans (IbSF, IbFucCS, HfSF, HfFucCS, PpFucCS, LvSF) showed the ability to inhibit the interactions between monkeypox virus proteins (both A29 and A35) and surface-immobilized heparin. However, both desulfated glycans, desIbSF and desIbFucCS showed significantly reduced binding properties of both viral proteins to surface-immobilized heparin (Table 2). This dataset indicates that sulfation is a key structural element for the inhibition activity of marine sulfated glycans. All six natural marine sulfated glycans exhibited remarkable inhibition activity against surface-immobilized heparin binding with the MPXV A29 protein. Among the three kinds of fucosylated chondroitin sulfates, IbFucCS had the highest sulfation level (96% branching disulfated fucoses) and exhibited the best inhibitory property. HfFucCS (80% branching disulfated fucoses) and PpFucCS (70% branching disulfated fucoses) showed similar inhibitory activity despite the lower sulfation content in PpFucCS. Although IbSF, LvSF, and HfSF are all tetrasaccharide-repeating sulfated fucans, IbSF and HfSF are tetrasulfated per tetrasaccharide building blocks, while LvSF is pentasulfated per tetrasaccharide building blocks. IbSF and HfSF showed very similar inhibitory activities and, interestingly, higher action than LvSF despite the higher sulfation content of the latter. This indicates that the sulfation pattern can play a more significant role in the interactions with the monkeypox proteins than the sulfation content. Although all tested sulfated glycans showed strong inhibitory activity against both viral proteins in the SPR-based binding to the heparin surface, no clear correlations between the structural features of these glycans and binding properties could be drawn. Similar results were observed in our previous study on the inhibitory activity of these sulfated glycans against evolving SARS-CoV-2 strains [13].

Table 2. Summary of solution competition between heparin and eight marine-derived glycans binding to MPXV proteins [a].

	Control [b]	Heparin	IbSF	desIbSF	IbFucCS	desIbFucCS	HfSF	HfFucCS	PpFucCS	LvSF
Normalized A29 protein binding (%)	100	43.3 *	5.0 **	75.4 *	7.6 *	66.8 *	8.5 **	13.9 *	13.0 *	23.6 *
Normalized A35 protein binding (%)	100	27.7 *	24.3 *	60.4 *	20.1 *	63.9 *	23.9 *	23.0 *	19.0 *	16.9 *

[a] SPR sensorgrams of MPXV A29/A35 protein–heparin interaction competing with eight different marine-derived glycans. The concentration of proteins was 250 nM mixed with 100 µg/mL of different glycans. [b] The control had the same concentration of A29/A35 protein (125 nM) without any mixed glycans. Statistical analysis was performed using an unpaired two-tailed t-test (*: $p \leq 0.05$ compared with the control, **: $p \leq 0.01$ compared with the control).

3. Materials and Methods

3.1. Materials

Eight marine sulfated glycans (IbSF, desIbSF, IbFucCS, desIbFucCS, PpFucCS, LvSF, HfSF, HfFucCS) from the sea cucumbers *I. badionotus* and *P. pygmaea*, sea urchin *L. variegatus*, and the Florida sea cucumber *Holothuria floridana* were purified [19,21] in Dr. Pomin's lab at the University of Mississippi. MPXV A29 and A35 proteins were purchased from Sino Biological Inc. (Wayne, PA, USA). The recombinant MPXV protein A29 consists of 97 amino acids and has a predicted molecular mass of 11.36 kDa. The recombinant MPXV protein A35 consists of 135 amino acids and has a predicted molecular mass of 15.12 kDa (see the amino acid sequences in Figure 2). Porcine intestinal heparin was purchased from Celsus Laboratories (Cincinnati, OH, USA) with an average molecular weight of 15 kDa and polydispersity of 1.4. Sensor SA chips were purchased from Cytiva (Uppsala, Sweden). SPR measurements were performed on a BIAcore 3000 or T200 SPR (Uppsala, Sweden), which was operated using Biaevaluation software (version 4.0.1 or 3.2).

3.2. Preparation of Heparin Biochips

The biotinylated heparin was prepared using the following method: 1 mg of heparin and 1 mg of amine-PEG$_3$-Biotin (Thermo Scientific, Waltham, MA, USA) were dissolved in 200 µL water, and then 5 mg $NaCNBH_3$ was added. The mixture was incubated at 70 °C for 24 h, then another 5 mg $NaCNBH_3$ was added, and the reaction was incubated for another 24 h. After completing the reaction, the mixture was desalted with a spin column (3000 molecular weight cut-off). Biotinylated heparin was freeze-dried for chip preparation. A heparin SA chip for the SPR study was made using the following protocol: 20 µL solution of the biotinylated heparin (0.1 mg/mL) in HBS-EP$^+$ buffer was injected over flow cells 2 to 4 of the SA chip at a flow rate of 10 µL/min. Furthermore, flow cell 1 was immobilized using biotin as a reference channel using the same method.

3.3. Binding Kinetics and Affinity Studies of the Interaction between Heparin and the MPXV A35 Protein

The MPXV A35 protein was diluted with HBS-EP$^+$ buffer (pH 7.4). Different dilutions of A35 protein were injected at a flow rate of 30 µL/min. At the end of each injection, the same buffer was allowed to flow over the sensor surface to facilitate dissociation for 180 s. The SPR chip was regenerated by injecting it with 30 µL of 2 M NaCl. The response was monitored using a sensorgram at 25 °C.

3.4. Inhibition Activity of the Marine Sulfated Glycans on Heparin–MPXV Protein Interactions

To evaluate the inhibition of the MPXV protein–heparin interaction, 250 nM of MPXV protein was premixed with 100 µg/mL of different glycans in HBS-EP$^+$ buffer (pH 7.4) and injected over the heparin chip with a flow rate of 30 µL/min. The same buffer was allowed to flow over the sensor surface to facilitate dissociation after each injection. A 30 µL injection of 2 M NaCl was used for the regeneration of the sensor surface. Sensorgrams were monitored at 25 °C. MPXV proteins were used in the control experiments to make sure the surface was completely regenerated. When the binding sites of MPXV proteins were occupied by our glycan samples, the binding of premixed proteins with glycan samples to the surface-immobilized heparin was decreased with an RU attenuation of the SPR.

4. Conclusions

The current study demonstrated that MPXV A29 and A35 were strongly bound to heparin. Solution competition analysis between surface-immobilized heparin with eight defined marine sulfated glycans (IbSF, desIbSF, IbFucCS, desIbFucCS, PpFucCS, LvSF, HfSF, HfFucCS) from sea cucumber was performed by using an SPR competition assay. These results showed that the natural marine sulfated glycans (IbSF, IbFucCS, PpFucCS, LvSF, HfSF, HfFucCS) provided outstanding inhibitory activity of chip-surface heparin binding to the MPXV A29 and A35 proteins. However, the fully desulfated IbSF (desIbSF) and fully desulfated desIbFucCS showed only a weak inhibition activity. Our findings demonstrate that some sulfated glycans from cucumbers are promising natural MPXV inhibitors through binding with two critical MPXV proteins, namely, A29 and A35. The study of molecular interactions should facilitate the development of therapeutics for the prevention and treatment of MPXV. Additional studies will be needed in the future to uncover the potential in vitro and in vivo properties of marine sulfated glycans against monkeypox infection.

Author Contributions: Conceptualization, F.Z. and R.J.L.; methodology, P.H. and D.S.; analysis, P.H. and Y.L.; resource, S.B.K., R.D., V.H.P. and M.F.; original draft preparation, P.H., Y.L. and F.Z.; review and editing, K.X., V.H.P., J.S.D. and R.J.L.; revision, P.H., V.H.P., F.Z. and R.J.L., funding acquisition, J.S.D., V.H.P., F.Z. and R.J.L. All authors have read and agreed to the published version of the manuscript.

Funding: This work was supported by the NIH (S10OD028523, R21AI156573 (R.J.L, F.Z.); GlycoMIP, which is a National Science Foundation Materials Innovation Platform funded through Cooperative Agreement DMR-1933525 (R.J.L., J.S.D., F.Z.); and the New York State Biodefense Commercialization Fund (J.S.D., F.Z.). Pomin acknowledges the NIH grants 1P20GM130460-01A1-7936 and 1R03NS110996-01A1.

Data Availability Statement: Data presented in this study are available on request.

Conflicts of Interest: The authors declare no conflict of interest.

References

1. Magnus, P.V.; Andersen, E.K.; Petersen, K.B.; Birch-Andersen, A. A pox-like disease in cynomolgus monkeys. *Acta Pathol. Microbiolog. Scand.* **1959**, *46*, 156–176. [CrossRef]
2. Arita, I.; Henderson, D. Smallpox and monkeypox in non-human primates. *Bull. World Health Organ.* **1968**, *39*, 277. [PubMed]
3. Ladnyj, I.; Ziegler, P.; Kima, E. A human infection caused by monkeypox virus in Basankusu Territory, Democratic Republic of the Congo. *Bull. World Health Organ.* **1972**, *46*, 593.

4. Cunha, B.E. Monkeypox in the United States: An occupational health look at the first cases. *AAOHN J.* **2004**, *52*, 164–168. [CrossRef]
5. 2022 Monkeypox Outbreak Global Map. Available online: https://www.cdc.gov/poxvirus/monkeypox/response/2022/worldmap.html (accessed on 8 March 2023).
6. Kugelman, J.; Johnston, S.; Mulembakani, P.; Kisalu, N.; Lee, M.; Koroleva, G.; McCarthy, S.; Gestole, M.; Wolfe, N.; Fair, J.; et al. Genomic variability of monkeypox virus among humans, Democratic Republic of the Congo. *Emerg. Infect. Disease J.* **2014**, *20*, 232. [CrossRef] [PubMed]
7. Bauer, S.; Zhang, F.; Linhardt, R.J. Implications of glycosaminoglycans on viral zoonotic diseases. *Diseases* **2021**, *9*, 85. [CrossRef]
8. Isidro, J.; Borges, V.; Pinto, M.; Sobral, D.; Santos, J.D.; Nunes, A.; Mixão, V.; Ferreira, R.; Santos, D.; Duarte, S.; et al. Phylogenomic characterization and signs of microevolution in the **2022** multi-country outbreak of monkeypox virus. *Nat. Med.* **2022**, *28*, 1569–1572. [CrossRef]
9. Mahase, E. Monkeypox: Single dose of smallpox vaccine offers 78% protection, UKHSA reports. *BMJ* **2022**, *379*, o2829. [CrossRef]
10. Freyn, A.W.; Atyeo, C.; Earl, P.L.; Americo, J.L.; Chuang, G.-Y.; Natarajan, H.; Frey, T.; Gall, J.; Moliva, J.I.; Hunegnaw, R.; et al. A monkeypox mRNA-lipid nanoparticle vaccine targeting virus binding, entry, and transmission drives protection against lethal orthopoxviral challenge. *BioRxiv* **2022**, BioRxiv:2022.12.17.520886.
11. Shi, D.; He, P.; Song, Y.; Cheng, S.; Linhardt, R.J.; Dordick, J.S.; Chi, L.; Zhang, F. Kinetic and structural aspects of glycosaminoglycan-monkeypox virus protein A29 interactions using surface plasmon resonance. *Molecules* **2022**, *27*, 5898. [CrossRef] [PubMed]
12. Song, Y.; He, P.; Rodrigues, A.L.; Datta, P.; Tandon, R.; Bates, J.T.; Bierdeman, M.A.; Chen, C.; Dordick, J.; Zhang, F.; et al. Anti-SARS-CoV-2 Activity of Rhamnan Sulfate from Monostroma nitidum. *Mar. Drugs* **2021**, *19*, 685. [CrossRef]
13. Dwivedi, R.; Sharma, P.; Farrag, M.; Kim, S.B.; Fassero, L.A.; Tandon, R.; Pomin, V.H. Inhibition of SARS-CoV-2 wild-type (Wuhan-Hu-1) and Delta (B.1.617.2) strains by marine sulfated glycans. *Glycobiology* **2022**, *32*, 849–854. [CrossRef]
14. Kim, S.B.; Zoepfl, M.; Samanta, P.; Zhang, F.; Xia, K.; Thara, R.; Linhardt, R.J.; Doerksen, R.J.; McVoy, M.A.; Pomin, V.H. Fractionation of sulfated galactan from the red alga Botryocladia occidentalis separates its anticoagulant and anti-SARS-CoV-2 properties. *J Biol Chem.* **2022**, *298*, 101856. [CrossRef]
15. Dwivedi, R.; Samanta, P.; Sharma, P.; Zhang, F.; Mishra, S.K.; Kucheryavy, P.; Kim, S.B.; Aderibigbe, A.O.; Linhardt, R.J.; Tandon, R.; et al. Structural and kinetic analyses of holothurian sulfated glycans suggest potential treatment for SARS-CoV-2 infection. *J Biol Chem.* **2021**, *297*, 1012207. [CrossRef]
16. Chakraborty, S.; Mohapatra, R.K.; Chandran, D.; Alagawany, M.; Sv, P.; Islam, M.A.; Chakraborty, C.; Dhama, K. Monkeypox vaccines and vaccination strategies: Current knowledge and advances. An update—Correspondence. *Int. J. Surg.* **2022**, *105*, 106869. [CrossRef] [PubMed]
17. Ahmed, S.F.; Sohail, M.S.; Quadeer, A.A.; McKay, M.R. Vaccinia-virus-based vaccines are expected to elicit highly cross-reactive immunity to the 2022 monkeypox virus. *Viruses* **2022**, *14*, 1960. [CrossRef]
18. Kamhi, E.; Joo, E.J.; Dordick, J.S.; Linhardt, R.J. Glycosaminoglycans in infectious disease. *Biol. Rev.* **2013**, *88*, 928–943. [CrossRef]
19. Wang, P.; Chi, L.; Zhang, Z.; Zhao, H.; Zhang, F.; Linhardt, R.J. Heparin: An old drug for new clinical applications. *Carbohydr. Polym.* **2022**, *295*, 119818. [CrossRef]
20. Hoffmann, M.; Snyder, N.L.; Hartmann, L. Polymers inspired by heparin and heparan sulfate for viral targeting. *Macromolecules.* **2022**, *55*, 7957–7973. [CrossRef] [PubMed]
21. Chen, S.; Hu, Y.; Ye, X.; Li, G.; Yu, G.; Xue, C.; Chai, W. Sequence determination and anticoagulant and antithrombotic activities of a novel sulfated fucan isolated from the sea cucumber *Isostichopus badionotus*. *Biochim. Biophys. Acta (BBA) Gen. Subj.* **2012**, *1820*, 989–1000. [CrossRef] [PubMed]
22. Chen, S.; Xue, C.; Yin, L.a.; Tang, Q.; Yu, G.; Chai, W. Comparison of structures and anticoagulant activities of fucosylated chondroitin sulfates from different sea cucumbers. *Carbohydr. Polym.* **2011**, *83*, 688–696. [CrossRef]
23. Castro, M.O.; Pomin, V.H.; Santos, L.L.; Vilela-Silva, A.-C.E.S.; Hirohashi, N.; Pol-Fachin, L.; Verli, H.; Mourão, P.A.S. A Unique 2-Sulfated β-Galactan from the Egg Jelly of the Sea Urchin Glyptocidaris crenularis: Conformation Flexibility Versus Induction of the Sperm Acrosome Reaction*. *J Biol Chem.* **2009**, *284*, 18790–18800. [CrossRef] [PubMed]
24. Shi, D.; Qi, J.; Zhang, H.; Yang, H.; Yang, Y.; Zhao, X. Comparison of hydrothermal depolymerization and oligosaccharide profile of fucoidan and fucosylated chondroitin sulfate from *Holothuria floridana*. *Int. J. Biol. Macromol.* **2019**, *132*, 738–747. [CrossRef] [PubMed]

marine drugs

Article

Comparative Analyses of Fucoidans from South African Brown Seaweeds That Inhibit Adhesion, Migration, and Long-Term Survival of Colorectal Cancer Cells

Blessing Mabate [1], Chantal Désirée Daub [1], Brett Ivan Pletschke [1,*] and Adrienne Lesley Edkins [2,*]

1 Enzyme Science Programme (ESP), Department of Biochemistry and Microbiology, Faculty of Science, Rhodes University, Makhanda 6140, South Africa
2 Biomedical Biotechnology Research Unit (BioBRU), Department of Biochemistry and Microbiology, Rhodes University, Makhanda 6139, South Africa
* Correspondence: b.pletschke@ru.ac.za (B.I.P.); a.edkins@ru.ac.za (A.L.E.); Tel.: +27-466038081 (B.I.P.); +27-466038446 (A.L.E.)

Abstract: Human colorectal cancer (CRC) is a recurrent, deadly malignant tumour with a high incidence. The incidence of CRC is of increasing alarm in highly developed countries, as well as in middle to low-income countries, posing a significant global health challenge. Therefore, novel management and prevention strategies are vital in reducing the morbidity and mortality of CRC. Fucoidans from South African seaweeds were hot water extracted and structurally characterised using FTIR, NMR and TGA. The fucoidans were chemically characterised to analyse their composition. In addition, the anti-cancer properties of the fucoidans on human HCT116 colorectal cells were investigated. The effect of fucoidans on HCT116 cell viability was explored using the resazurin assay. Thereafter, the anti-colony formation potential of fucoidans was explored. The potency of fucoidans on the 2D and 3D migration of HCT116 cells was investigated by wound healing assay and spheroid migration assays, respectively. Lastly, the anti-cell adhesion potential of fucoidans on HCT116 cells was also investigated. Our study found that *Ecklonia* sp. Fucoidans had a higher carbohydrate content and lower sulphate content than *Sargassum elegans* and commercial *Fucus vesiculosus* fucoidans. The fucoidans prevented 2D and 3D migration of HCT116 colorectal cancer cells to 80% at a fucoidan concentration of 100 μg/mL. This concentration of fucoidans also significantly inhibited HCT116 cell adhesion by 40%. Moreover, some fucoidan extracts hindered long-term colony formation by HCT116 cancer cells. In summary, the characterised fucoidan extracts demonstrated promising anti-cancer activities in vitro, and this warrants their further analyses in pre-clinical and clinical studies.

Keywords: cancer; migration; adhesion; fucoidans; human colorectal cancer; *Ecklonia radiata*; *Ecklonia maxima*; *Sargassum elegans*

Citation: Mabate, B.; Daub, C.D.; Pletschke, B.I.; Edkins, A.L. Comparative Analyses of Fucoidans from South African Brown Seaweeds That Inhibit Adhesion, Migration, and Long-Term Survival of Colorectal Cancer Cells. *Mar. Drugs* **2023**, *21*, 203. https://doi.org/10.3390/md21040203

Academic Editors: Yuya Kumagai, Hideki Kishimura and Benwei Zhu

Received: 4 March 2023
Revised: 20 March 2023
Accepted: 22 March 2023
Published: 24 March 2023

1. Introduction

Cancer is a complex, multifactorial disease characterised by the uncontrollable growth of abnormal cancerous cells [1]. Cancers may progress to invade and spread to other tissues and organs using the circulatory and lymphatic systems through metastasis [2]. Cancer has one of the highest mortality rates and significantly contributes to lower global life expectancy [3]. The cancer burden globally is expected to increase from 2020 by approximately 47%, translating to about 28.4 million new cases per year by 2040. However, the increased number of cancer cases may be affected by the social-economic status of the global populace. Additionally, the rise may be linked to increased risk factors associated with globalisation and the growing economy [4]. These risk factors may include increased processed food consumption, lack of physical activity, and increasing obesity.

Colorectal cancer (CRC) is the third most diagnosed cancer (accounting for 10% of all cases) and the second most frequent cause of cancer-related deaths (accounting for

9.4% of oncological deaths). Thus, it constitutes a substantial portion of the global cancer burden [4,5]. Treatment strategies include chemotherapy, radiation therapy, surgery, or combination therapies [6]. Although surgical resection of the primary tumour in the early disease stages proves effective, patients may be diagnosed at more advanced stages [7,8]. The indiscriminate toxic effects of chemotherapeutic agents used for CRC treatment result in debilitating side effects and limit therapeutic outcomes [7,9].

With challenges of side effects, affordability, and access to current therapeutic remedies, the search for novel treatment and preventive strategies with minimal adverse effects must proceed urgently. Furthermore, marine bio-products have historically been deemed therapeutic advantages among other bio-compounds [10]. Natural compounds have gained attention over the past decades as these demonstrate targeted specific anti-cancer properties while demonstrating low toxicity [1]. The lower incidences of chronic diseases, such as heart disease, diabetes, and cancer in China and Japan have led researchers to investigate the contents of brown seaweeds, which have been used in their cuisines and medicinal applications [11]. Among the more than 3000 natural products derived from seaweeds, fucoidans have received significant attention for their most promising anti-cancer properties [1,11].

Fucoidan is a heparin-like structured, naturally derived polysaccharide compound present in the cell wall matrix of brown seaweeds [12]. This heterogeneous polysaccharide is predominantly comprised of L-fucose with smaller quantities of varying monosaccharides and sulphate, which contribute to its complex structural characteristics and have an unquestionable effect on its broad range of biological activities [1]. These biological activities include anti-oxidant [13], anti-coagulant [14], anti-thrombotic, anti-inflammatory, anti-viral, anti-lipidemic [15], anti-diabetic [16], anti-metastatic and anti-cancer activities [17].

Fucoidans have anti-cancer effects against various cancer cell lines by causing cell cycle arrest [18], inducing apoptosis [9], preventing angiogenesis [9,19], and inhibiting migration and metastasis [1]. As tumour migration is a hallmark of cancers, it is plausible to target this process to alleviate tumour progression. Moreover, fucoidans inhibit metastasis by blocking cell migration and colony formation. Fucoidan isolated from *F. vesiculosus* significantly inhibited the migration of the human colon cancer cell line HT-29 by suppressing PI3k/Akt/mTOR/p70S6K1 [19]. Whereas the treatment of colorectal carcinoma cells, DLD-1 and HCT116, with fucoidan from *Padina boryana*, proved successful in inhibiting colony formation [20].

The anti-cancer effect of fucoidan on colon cancer cell lines has been reported primarily using the commercially available *F. vesiculosus* fucoidan. However, the diversity of brown seaweeds is broad, and their bioactivities have been linked to the source of seaweed and its structural and chemical characteristics. Additionally, in addition to the limited literature on fucoidan effects on colon cancers, there is also limited literature available on the biological activities, including the anti-cancer properties of South African seaweed-derived fucoidans. However, the country harbours one of the most extensive coastlines globally, with a rich seaweed biodiversity [21]. The present study characterised fucoidan extracts from native South African brown seaweeds and linked their structural differences to their anti-cancer properties against the HCT116 cell line.

2. Results and Discussion

2.1. Fucoidan Yield

The fucoidans in this study were hot water extracted, except for the *F. vesiculosus* fucoidan, which was purchased commercially. Considerable amounts of fucoidans were successfully extracted with an average fucoidan/defatted seaweed dry weight ratio of 5.4, 5.9 and 2.2% for *E. maxima*, *E. radiata* and *S. elegans*, respectively. The resulting yields of the extracted fucoidans were within the expected range (1.1–4.8%) for water extracted fucoidans [22].

2.2. Structural Analysis of Fucoidans

2.2.1. FTIR Analysis

Fucoidan extracts were structurally analysed by Fourier-transform infrared spectroscopy (FTIR) (Figure 1) and displayed similar spectra to previously characterised fucoidans [22,23]. All the profiled fucoidans displayed a spectral band between 3500 cm^{-1} and 3200 cm^{-1}, characteristic of polysaccharides. This peak is associated with the stretching vibrations of the O-H groups within carbohydrates. The bands in the region 2900 to 3000 cm^{-1} observed in all the fucoidans are assigned to the C-H stretching in the pyranose ring and methyl groups associated with the fucose [24].

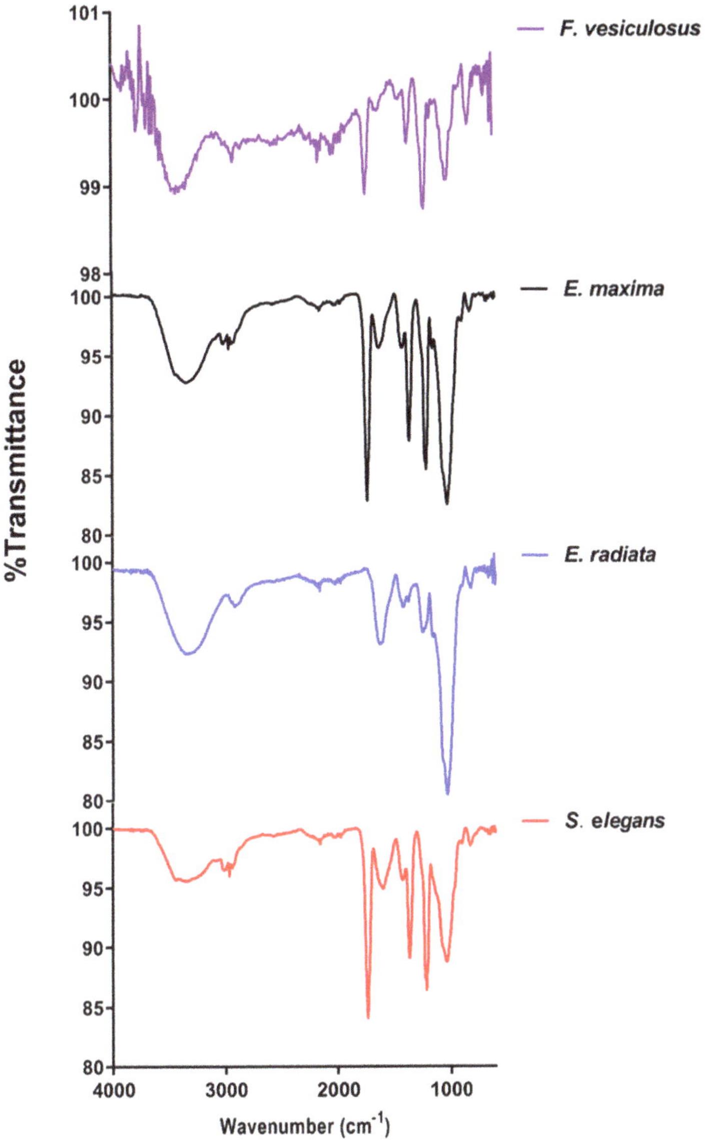

Figure 1. FTIR spectra of the fucoidans under study. The overlaid spectra were obtained from water-extracted fucoidans and the commercial *F. vesiculosus* fucoidan.

Typically, the carbonyl groups and stretching of O-acetyl groups are depicted by the peaks around 1650 cm^{-1} [25]. Additionally, the stretching of the S=O bond linked with sulphate groups is characterised by peaks between 1210 and 1270 cm^{-1} [22]. Stretching vibrations of the glycosidic C–O bonds within the fucoidans structures are represented by peaks close to the wavenumber 1100 cm^{-1} [26]. Furthermore, the peaks at wavenumber 854 cm^{-1} depict sulphate groups on fucoidans linked to carbonyl side chains [13]. This peak at around 854 cm^{-1} was more pronounced for the *F. vesiculosus* commercial fucoidan. This suggested that *F. vesiculosus* fucoidan had a relatively higher sulphate content than the extracted fucoidans (Figure 1).

2.2.2. Proton NMR Analysis of Extracted Fucoidans

The structural composition of the extracted fucoidans was also elucidated by proton NMR. The fucoidans generally exhibited chemical shifts (Figure 2) similar to several characterised fucoidans [14,27,28]. The chemical shifts in all fucoidans showed peaks at 1.28 ppm and 1.45 ppm suggesting the presence of alternating α (1–3) and α (1–4) linkages of fucose residues linked with sulphates (α-L-Fuc, α-L-Fuc (2-SO_3^-) and α-L-Fuc (2,3-diSO_3^-) [28]. The *F. vesiculosus* fucoidan displayed relatively more prominent peaks in the 1.28 ppm and 1.45 ppm range, suggesting a higher sulphate content than the extracted fucoidans (Figure 2). A higher sulphate content in the fucoidans may improve their biological activities.

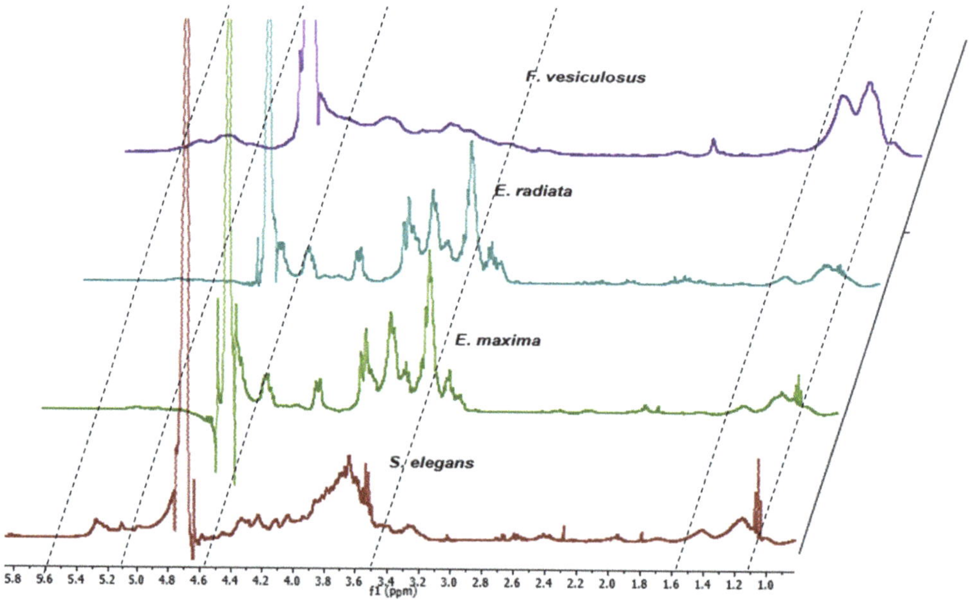

Figure 2. ^{1}H NMR for the different seaweed fucoidans. Overlaid proton NMR spectra of extracted fucoidans and commercial *F. vesiculosus* fucoidan.

Vibration bands at 1.45 ppm are assigned to symmetric CH_3 deformations emanating from methyl proton on C6 of fucose [14]. The peaks at 2.1 ppm are assigned to the H-6 methylated protons of *L*-fucopyranosides [27]. The peaks in the range of 3.5–4.5 ppm are characteristic of the (H2 to H5) ring protons of *L*-fucopyranosides. The exhibited peaks in the ring proton region also suggest variable fucosyl sulphates located at variable glycosidic linkages with varying monosaccharide patterns. The definitive peaks in Figure 2 at 3.3 ppm and 3.7 ppm in the fucoidans suggest the presence of hexoses, including glucose, galactose, and mannose [27]. Our results show that the spectra of *E. maxima* and *E. radiata* fucoidans displayed more pronounced peaks at the 3.3 ppm to 3.7 ppm region than the *F. vesiculosus* and *S. elegans* fucoidans (Figure 2). This could suggest that *Ecklonia* sp. fucoidans have higher sugar content. Furthermore, the extracted fucoidans had limited to negligible uronic acid contamination as there were no chemical shifts in the region around 5.8 ppm (Figure 2) [29].

2.2.3. Thermogravimetric Analysis of Fucoidans

The TGA decomposition profiles of the fucoidans validated the compounds as polysaccharides, as their decomposition started just above 200 °C (Figure 3), characteristic of the organic polymers [30].

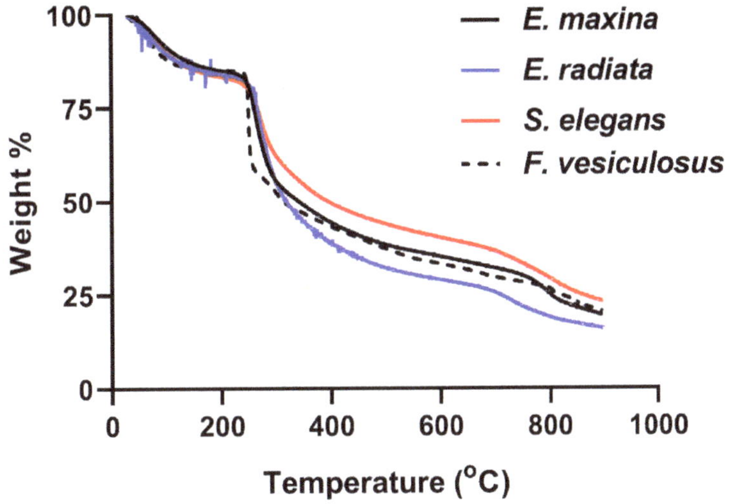

Figure 3. Thermal gravimetric analysis (TGA) analysis of the fucoidan extracts. Superimposed thermograms for the water-extracted fucoidans from seaweeds and commercial *F. vesiculosus* fucoidan.

The TGA plots of the fucoidans showed about 20% loss in mass at a temperature of 240 °C, associated with the loss in moisture content through evaporation [31] and some volatile matter [32]. The most significant loss of mass (~45%) occurred between 240 °C and 420 °C, which accounted for the arbitrary depolymerisation and decomposition of organic constituents, such as carbohydrates. Notably, *F. vesiculosus* fucoidan depolymerisation and decomposition of organic matter occurred relatively more rapidly than the other fucoidans, as shown by the steeper slope in Figure 3. Its relatively low carbohydrate content may be the reason for this observation (Table 1). Above 420 °C, combustion of carbon black occurred. The remaining residual mass at 600 °C accounted for the ash content, usually containing sulphates, phosphates, and carbonates [33]. The profiles of the extracts were characteristic of previously profiled fucoidan extracts in the literature [34,35].

The structural analysis of fucoidans through FTIR, proton NMR and TGA confirmed the integrity of our extracts, as they showed comparable patterns to the commercial *F. vesiculosus* fucoidan. It was also evident that *Ecklonia* sp. fucoidans displayed similar yet unique profiles to the *S. elegans* and *F. vesiculosus* fucoidans. Our observations support the findings of Ermakova and colleagues that diverse seaweed species yield diverse fucoidan structures [36]. These differences may be caused by the survival needs of the seaweeds, influenced by their habitat. Considering the unique profiles observed within the structural analyses of the fucoidans, these were further characterised chemically to assess their composition.

Table 1. Composition of fucoidan structures.

	w/w % ± SD			
Component	*E. maxima*	*E. radiata*	*S. elegans*	*F. vesiculosus*
Total carbohydrates [a]	72.8 ± 5.2	88 ± 7.4	44.4 ± 6.2	41.3 ± 9.5
L-fucose [b]	4.56 ± 0.8	3.7 ± 0.1	4.9 ± 0.9	8.2 ± 0.4
D-glucose [b]	8.1 ± 3.4	7.1 ± 2.3	5.7 ± 1.7	5.1 ± 2.1
D-galactose [b]	4.8 ± 0.1	4.9 ± 1.2	5.7 ± 0.5	7.1 ± 1.83
D-mannose [b]	3.0 ± 0.5	4.2 ± 0.2	7.1 ± 1.8	4.5 ± 0.8
Total sulphates [c]	7.2 ± 1.2	8.8 ± 1.4	9.7 ± 1.8	14.7 ± 2.3
Total phenolics [d]	1.9 ± 0.6	1.9 ± 0.4	2.8 ± 0.8	0 ± 0.04
Uronic acids [e]	2.6 ± 1.2	2.2 ± 0.7	4.8 ± 0.6	2.2 ± 0.8
Total protein [f]	2.1 ± 0.6	2.4 ± 0.9	4.6 ± 2.4	1.9 ± 0.6
Total ash [g]	19.7 ± 0.6	16.0 ± 2.1	23.1 ± 3.5	20.4 ± 2.8
MW [h]	27.4 kDa	8.5 kDa	74.9 kDa	84.4 kDa

Determined by [a] Phenol sulphuric acid method; [b] HPLC (RID); [c] Barium chloride gelatin method; [d] Folin-Ciocalteu method; [e] MegazymeTM uronic acid kit; [f] Bradford's assay; [g] TGA; [h] size exclusion HPLC.

2.3. Composition of Fucoidans

The fucoidans were partially characterised chemically by determining their total sugar contents, monosaccharides distributions and impurities (including protein, phenolics and uronic acids). *E. maxima* and *E. radiata* fucoidans contained high amounts of total carbohydrates, with 72.8% and 88% (*w*/*w*), respectively (Table 1). The *S. elegans* and *F. vesiculosus* fucoidans had approximately 40% (*w*/*w*) total carbohydrate content (Table 1) and were, therefore, comparatively lower than that of the *Ecklonia* sp. extracted fucoidans.

After hydrolysing the fucoidans using 2 M TFA, monosaccharides were quantified using HPLC and Megazyme kits (Table 1). The predominant monosaccharides detected in all fucoidans were fucose, glucose, galactose, and mannose. Generally, *Ecklonia* sp. fucoidans had a relatively high monosaccharide content, with glucose, fucose, galactose and mannose being the most prominent sugars (Table 1). These findings are consistent with the findings of January and colleagues, who detected considerable amounts of glucose, galactose, and mannose in their *E. maxima* fucoidan extract [37]. The commercial *F. vesiculosus* fucoidan contained relatively higher levels of fucose than that of the extracted fucoidans (Table 1). Furthermore, *S. elegans* fucoidan had notably higher mannose content than the other fucoidans (Table 1). The monosaccharide distribution of the extracts is representative of the characteristic fucoidans.

Commercial *F. vesiculosus* had the highest sulphate content (about 15%), followed by *S. elegans* fucoidan, which had 9.7% (Table 1). *S. elegans* and *F. vesiculosus* fucoidans had higher sulphate contents than the *Ecklonia* sp.-derived fucoidans (between 7–8%). The higher sulphates within *F. vesiculosus* and *S. elegans* fucoidan determined by colourimetry agreed with the structural characterisation data (Figures 1 and 2). FTIR spectra at wavenumber around 845 cm^{-1} showed a more pronounced peak for the *F. vesiculosus* fucoidan than all extracts (Figure 1). The pronounced NMR peaks indicative of sulphates between ppm 1.2 and 1.6 were evident for the *F. vesiculosus* and *S. elegans* than for *Ecklonia* sp. fucoidans (Figure 2). Additionally, the ash content was higher within the *S. elegans* and *F. vesiculosus* fucoidans (Table 1), suggesting more sulphates among these fucoidans than the *Ecklonia* sp. fucoidans. The ash content detected from the fucoidans was between 19 and 24%, consistent with the ash contents in some characterised fucoidans [15,38]. Furthermore, the fucoidans had minimal protein and uronic acid contamination, with *S. elegans* having the highest at ~4% of each. Insignificant amounts (<2%) of phenolics were detected within the fucoidans (Table 1). The molecular weights of the fucoidans were determined by size exclusion HPLC.

The molecular size of *E. maxima* fucoidan was 27.4 kDa, *E. radiata* fucoidan was 8.5 kDa, *S. elegans* fucoidan was 74.9 kDa, and *F. vesiculosus* fucoidan was 84.4 kDa. Structural and chemical characterisation data suggest that the extracted crude fucoidans were relatively pure as they showed similar profiles to the commercial *F. vesiculosus* fucoidan and other previously characterised fucoidans in literature.

2.4. Fucoidans' Cytotoxicity to HCT116 Cancer Cells

The potential cytotoxicity of all the fucoidan extracts towards the HCT116 colon cancer cell line was examined and compared to the chemotherapeutic drug 5-fluorouracil (5FU). The colon cancer cell line HCT116 was selected with the probable oral route of administration of fucoidans. For decades 5FU has played a pivotal role in the treatment of colorectal cancer [39]. Thus, it was chosen as a positive control for our experiments. The 5-FU treatments showed robust anti-cancer activity with an IC_{50} value of 9.9 µM. The reduction in cell viability due to treatment with fucoidan extracts was expressed as the percentage of viable cells remaining after treatment compared to the vehicle-treated control cells. Even at 2.5 mg/mL loading, none of the fucoidans displayed any significant cytotoxic effect on the HCT116 cells (Figure 4). About 4 g/day of fucoidan has been used in combination with other chemotherapeutics, including 5-FU, in colorectal cancer patients. Although patient survival was improved when fucoidan was included in the treatment, a significant observation was reduced side effects [40].

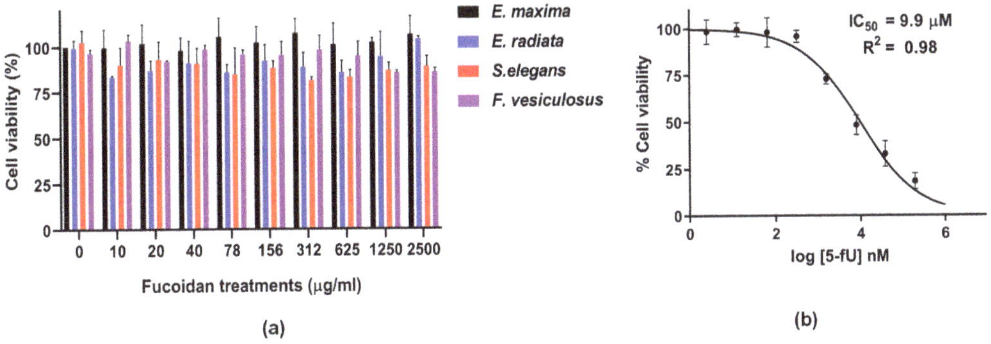

Figure 4. Fucoidans' cytotoxicity on HCT116 cells assessed by the resazurin assay. (**a**) Cell viability after treatment with fucoidans, (**b**) IC_{50} curve of 5-FU (positive control) demonstrates the compound's cytotoxic effect on HCT116 cells. The data represent values obtained from 3 biological replicates expressed as means ± SD (n = 3).

The lack of cytotoxicity of the fucoidans could be attributed to the large molecular sizes (Table 1), making penetration into the cells difficult. Large molecular sizes of fucoidans have been reported to limit the bio-accessibility of these compounds, posing a challenge for their applications [41]. Native *Undaria pinnatifida* fucoidan had minimal anti-tumour activity compared to its depolymerised counterpart against the human lung cancer cell line A549 [42]. This observation suggests a need for depolymerising fucoidans to increase toxicity while at the same time maintaining their bioactivities. We acknowledge that size cannot be the only determining factor, but other fucoidans' characteristic factors, including sulphation, and monosaccharide distribution, will contribute to their bioactivities.

2.4.1. The Effect of Fucoidans on HCT116 Colony Formation

Having established that fucoidans did not show substantial cytotoxicity, these compounds were further tested for their ability to inhibit colony formation. This assay has been the method of choice to determine replicative cell death after ionising radiation, although it is also used to determine the effectiveness of other cytotoxic agents [43]. *S. elegans* and *F.*

vesiculosus fucoidans were significant inhibitors of HCT116 colony formation ($p < 0.05$) (Figure 5). The positive control 4-NQO was used in this assay and showed the dose-dependent inhibition of HCT116 cell colony formation.

(a)

(b)

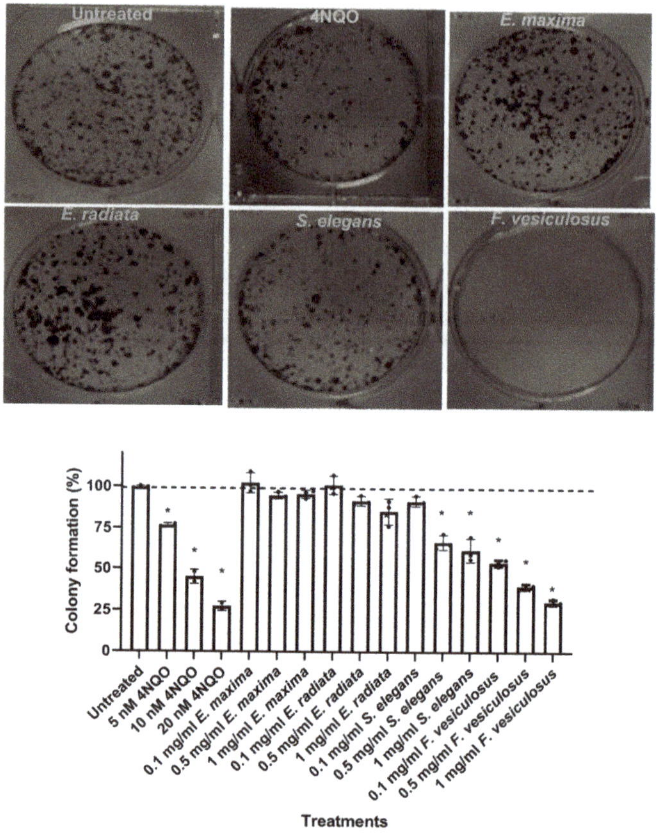

Figure 5. The dose-dependent clonogenic effect of fucoidan on HCT116 cancer cells. (**a**) Visual representation of the effect of fucoidan extracts (1 mg/mL) on HCT116 colony formation; (**b**) Dose-dependent effect of compounds on HCT116 cells' colony formation. The HCT116 colony cells were calculated and expressed as the means ± SD percentages ($n = 3$). The * shows a significant treatment difference versus the untreated control ($p < 0.05$) analysed by One-way ANOVA.

The *S. elegans* fucoidan exhibited about 40% colony formation inhibition at 0.5 mg/mL. The *F. vesiculosus* fucoidan inhibited HCT116 cell colony formation by over 50% at 0.1 mg/mL concentration (Figure 5). The inhibition by *F. vesiculosus* and *S. elegans* fucoidans may be attributed to the superior sulphate content compared to that of the *Ecklonia* sp. derived fucoidans (Table 1). A limited number of studies have reported the ability of fucoidans to decrease tumour cell survival using this assay. Nevertheless, our findings agree with those of Shin and colleagues, who reported that manganese dioxide nanoparticles coated with fucoidan decreased colony formation by a pancreatic cancer cell line [44]. Another independent study reported fucoidan inhibited colony formation of HepG2 liver cancer cells [20].

2.4.2. Fucoidans Inhibit the 2D Migration of HCT116 Cancer Cells

Fucoidans were next tested for effects on the 2-dimensional (2D) migration of human HCT116 colorectal cancer cells using the wound healing assay. The *F. vesiculosus* and *S.*

elegans fucoidans significantly inhibited cell migration compared to the untreated control (Figure 6). *S. elegans* fucoidan showed a dose-dependent inhibition of HCT116 cell migration at all concentrations tested, with inhibition reaching up to 30% at about 0.25 mg/mL (Figure 6), while cell migration inhibition by fucoidan from *F. vesiculosus* was only significant at 0.5 mg/mL.

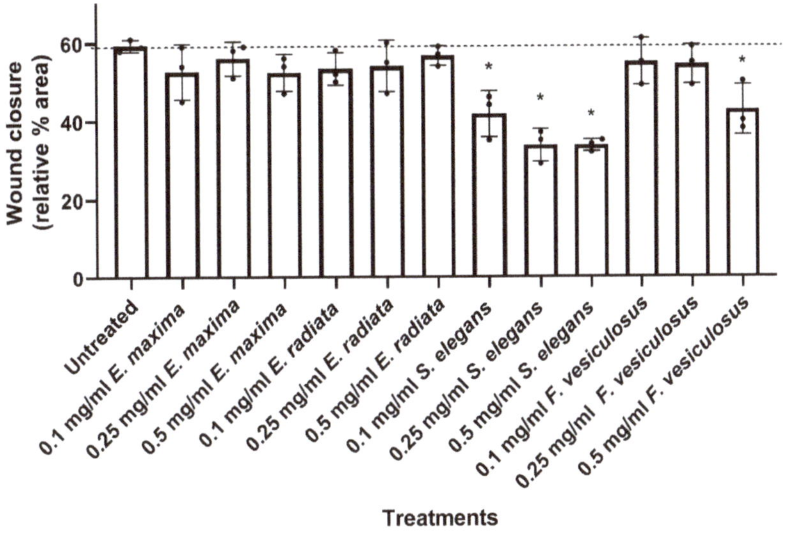

Figure 6. The effect of fucoidan extracts on 2D HCT116 cell migration. Quantified migration profiles of HCT116 cells treated with *E. maxima, E. radiata, S. elegans* and *F. vesiculosus* fucoidan extracts relative to the untreated control. The data are represented as means ± SD of biological replicates ($n = 3$). The asterisk * represents treatment concentrations that had a statistically significant effect on the migration of the cells at $p < 0.05$ tested by One-way ANOVA.

The *Ecklonia* sp. fucoidans did not significantly inhibit HCT116 cancer cell migration, even at high concentrations (Figure 6). This observation may be linked to the high amount of sugars within their structure (Table 1). Literature has suggested that fucoidans consisting of sugars, including galactose, may provide the nutrition required for wound healing [45]. However, fucoidans with a higher sulphate concentration were associated with a better bioactivity [36,46]. Thus, we can infer that *S. elegans* fucoidan showed better inhibitory action to wound healing of the HCT116 cells due to its unique structural properties, including high sulphation (Figures 1 and 2).

2.4.3. Fucoidans Inhibit HCT116 3D Spheroid Migration

Next, we tested the ability of fucoidans to prevent the migration of cells from a three-dimensional sphere onto tissue culture plastics. In this assay, the fucoidans inhibited the migration of the HCT116 cells from spheres in a time-dependent manner (Figure 7a). The commercial *F. vesiculosus, S. elegans* and *E. radiata* fucoidans displayed comparable efficacies, showing more than 80% inhibition at 0.1 mg/mL concentration. Furthermore, inhibition of HCT116 spheroid migration by the fucoidans was dose-dependent (Figure 7b). Although *E. maxima* fucoidan showed a slightly lower inhibition potential than the other fucoidans, it still significantly ($p < 0.05$) inhibited migration from HCT116 spheres (Figure 7b).

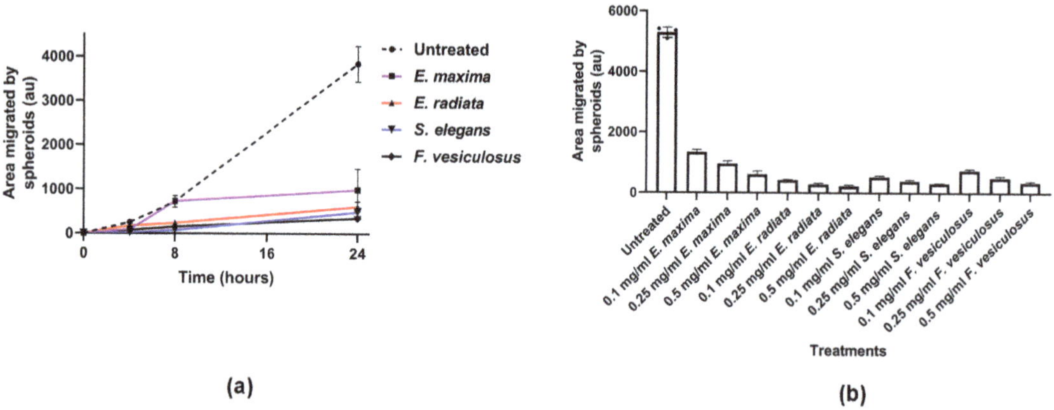

Figure 7. The effect of fucoidans on the 3D HCT116 spheroid migration. (**a**) Time-dependent effect of fucoidans at a fixed concentration (0.1 mg/mL) on spheroid migration; (**b**) Quantification of the dose-dependent effect of fucoidans on 3D spheroid HCT116 migration. The data are represented as means ± SD of biological replicates of spheroids ($n = 3$). One-way ANOVA was used to compare treatments to the untreated experiments, where significance was considered at $p < 0.05$. No asterisks * are shown since all treatments differed significantly from the untreated experiments.

Notably, the fucoidan extracts showed potency in inhibiting HCT116 cell migration during time- and dose-dependent experiments. The anionic nature, which is the common characteristic of fucoidans, could be critical in disrupting the migration of HCT116 cells. Limited reports in the literature have investigated the effects of fucoidans on spheroid-based migration. However, a study by Han and colleagues showed that tumour migration of a human colon cancer cell line (HT-29) was inhibited by fucoidan [17]. Indeed, very few investigations on the potency of chemotherapeutics on spheroid migration have been reported [47]. In addition, spheroid culture systems provide similar physicochemical environments to in vivo models, making them ideal for studying tumour migration—however, their use in fucoidan studies is seldom reported. The fucoidans in the current study demonstrated their high potency in inhibiting 3D HCT116 migration from spheroids, which may be important in controlling the proliferation of colorectal cancers. Another merit of employing spheroid culture systems is that they involve cell-to-cell and cell-to-matrix interactions, which overcomes the limitations of traditional monolayer cell cultures, which are two-dimensional (2D) [47,48]. Fucoidans maybe be interfering with cell-to-matrix adhesion or even with cell-to-cell interactions.

2.4.4. Fucoidans Disrupt Cancer Cell Sphere Formation

Next, the HCT116 cells were pretreated with 0.1 mg/mL and 0.5 mg/mL of fucoidans to determine whether fucoidans inhibit sphere formation. Representative morphological data of the HCT116 cell spheres pretreated with 0.5 mg/mL of *F. vesiculosus* illustrated a common observation for all fucoidans tested (Figure 8). Fucoidan treatment disrupted the formation of spheres compared to those from untreated samples (Figure 8).

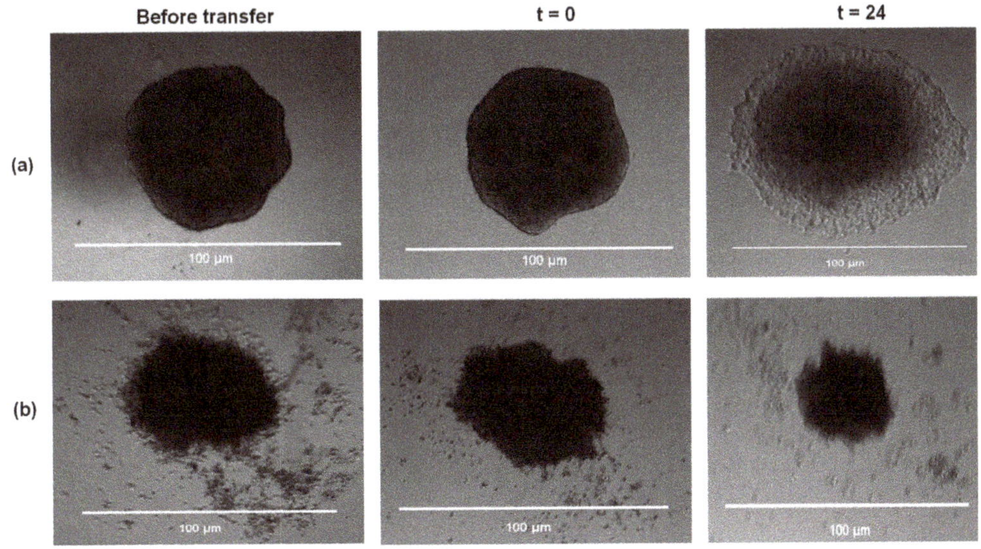

Figure 8. A representative visual illustration of HCT116 spheroid pretreated with fucoidan. The images show spheroids before transfer to fresh medium, at t = 0, and after 24 h (t = 24). (**a**) representative sphere formed from an untreated HCT116 culture; (**b**) sphere formed from HCT116 cells pretreated with *F. vesiculosus* fucoidan at 0.5 mg/mL final concentration.

The HCT116 sphere sizes formed after pre-treatment with fucoidans were quantified (Figure 9a). All the fucoidans significantly reduced the size of spheroids formed compared to the untreated sample (Figure 9a; $p < 0.05$).

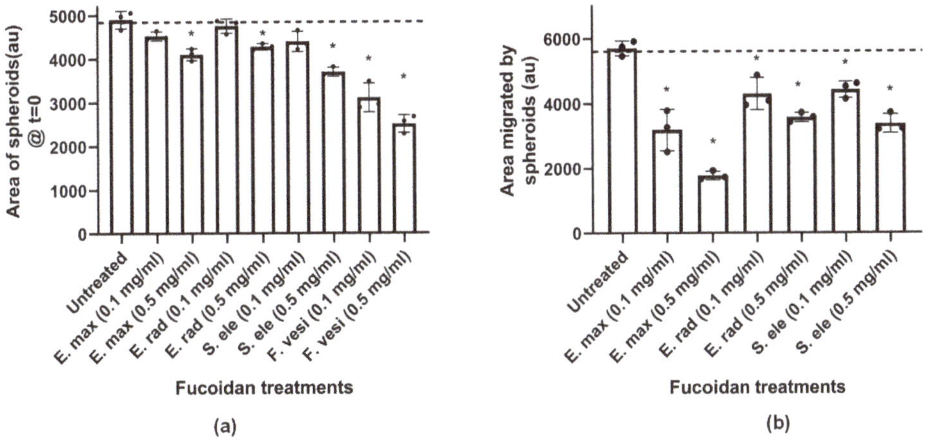

Figure 9. Fucoidans hinder HCT116 spheroid formation and reduce migration from spheres. (**a**) Size of HCT116 spheroids; (**b**) Distance migrated on tissue culture plastic from pretreated spheroids. The data are represented as means ± SD of biological replicates of spheroids sizes and migration ($n = 3$). The asterisk * represents treatment concentrations that were statistically significant from the untreated cells at $p < 0.05$ tested using One-way ANOVA.

The pretreated spheroids were subsequently transferred to an untreated medium to investigate the migration of cells from the spheres back onto tissue culture plastic (Figure 9b). Interestingly, all the spheres pretreated with fucoidan showed reduced migration compared to untreated spheroids (Figure 9b; $p < 0.05$). Therefore, pretreatment of the HCT116 cell culture indicated that fucoidans hindered spheroid formation and subsequent migration onto the tissue culture plastic matrix. In addition, the spheres which were pretreated with *F. vesiculosus* fucoidan were distorted and failed to migrate. Although investigations on spheroid formation are largely unexplored as far as the use of fucoidans is concerned, Han and colleagues reported that *F. vesiculosus* fucoidan disrupted HT-29 spheroid formation [19]. Their findings concur with our sphere formation results (Figure 8). Although this technique is a useful tool, it is limited to very few in vitro studies. However, our findings can be used as a motivation to further pursue the potential of fucoidans in in vivo and clinical settings.

2.4.5. Fucoidans Inhibit HCT116 Cell Adhesion

The effect of fucoidan extracts on HCT116 cell adhesion was also investigated. The fucoidans significantly prevented the adhesion of HCT116 cells to tissue culture plastic (Figure 10).

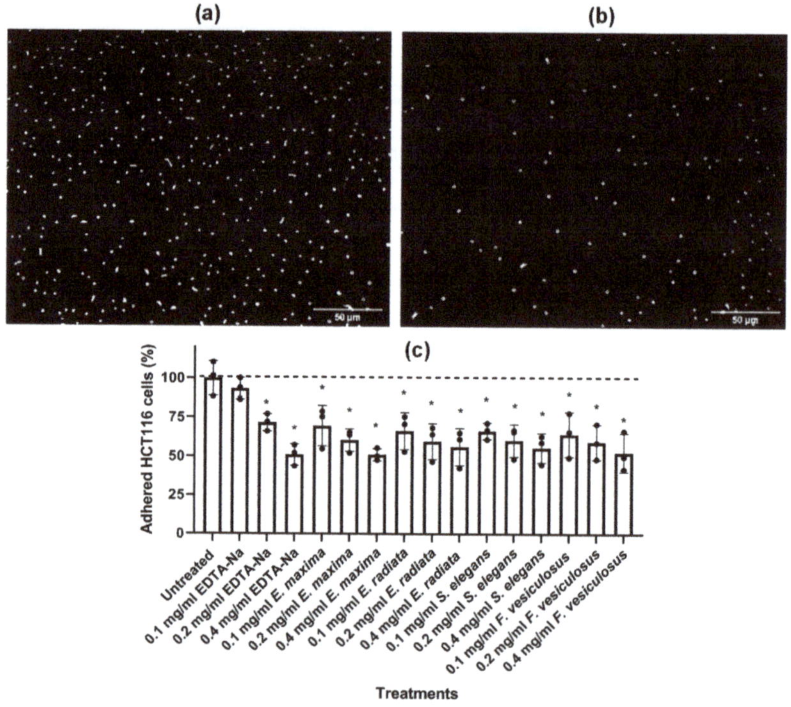

Figure 10. Fucoidan inhibits the adhesion of HCT116 cancer cells. (**a**) untreated cells; (**b**) cells treated with fucoidan under light microscopy; (**c**) Quantification of HCT116 cancer cells adhesion by crystal violet. The data are represented as means ± SD of three biological replicates (n = 3). The asterisk * represents treatment concentrations that were statistically significant from the untreated cells at $p < 0.05$ tested using One-way ANOVA.

The dose-dependent inhibition of HCT116 cancer cell adhesion by fucoidan was quantified by crystal violet (Figure 10c). EDTA-Na, a known chelator of metal ions required for cell adhesion, was used as a positive control. All fucoidans were efficient inhibitors of cell adhesion. Cell adhesion within cancer cells is vital for various biological processes, including cellular organisation, communication, differentiation, migration, and metastasis [49]. The cancer cell adhesion is dependent on several adhesion molecules and receptors, including integrins, selectins, glycoproteins, and proteoglycans [49]. The fucoidans may have hindered the proper functioning of these molecules, thereby impacting the adhesion of cancerous cells. Some fucoidans prevent the adhesion of cancer cells onto the extracellular matrix (ECM). Fucoidan from *A. nodosum* inhibited the MDA-MB-231 cancerous cells adhering to fibronectin ECM [50], consistent with our findings on tissue culture plastic. Fucoidans are negatively charged polysaccharides due to their sulphated nature, which may interfere with integrins that require Mg^{2+} as a cofactor for adhesion [49]. Thus, it is possible to suggest our fucoidans inhibited the HCT116 cancer cells' adhesion in a similar mechanism. This observed effect of fucoidans on cell adhesion might also explain the effect of these compounds in inhibiting the formation and migration from spheres (Figures 8 and 9). However, HCT116 cells' adhesion cannot be the only process affected by fucoidans, as *E. maxima* and *S. elegans* extracts show similar anti-adhesion properties but show radically different effects in the colony formation assay (Figure 5). A complex combination of structural characteristics, including the degree of sulphation, molecular size, and carbohydrate content, should be essential to fucoidans' biological activities. The observed anticancer activities of fucoidans may be useful as a preventive/treatment strategy for CRC since they are likely to be administered orally.

3. Materials and Methods

Fucus vesiculosus fucoidan (Cat. No. F5631) was purchased from Sigma-Aldrich (St. Louis, MO, USA). The analytical kits used in this study were purchased from Megazyme™ (Bray, WC, Ireland). The other reagents were purchased from Sigma-Aldrich, MERCK, Flucka Saarchem (Darmstadt, HE, Germany), and Celtic Diagnostic and Life Technologies (Cape Town, South Africa).

3.1. Sampling and Seaweed Processing

The brown seaweeds, *Ecklonia radiata* and *Sargassum elegans,* were harvested between February and March 2019 from Kelly's beach in Port Alfred (coordinates 33°36′36.8424″ S; 26°53′23.4996″ E) in the Eastern Cape province, South Africa. *Ecklonia maxima* seaweed was kindly donated by the HIK-Abalone farm located in Hermanus, Western Cape province, South Africa. Most of the *E. radiata* seaweed was collected as beach cast. However, some were harvested together with the *S. elegans* from rock pools. The beach cast and rockpool collected *E. radiata* were mixed and processed as a single batch. The harvested seaweeds were stored on ice during transportation to the laboratory. Upon arrival at the laboratory, the seaweed was washed 3× with distilled water, cut into smaller pieces and oven-dried at 40 °C for 72 h. The dried seaweed was pulverised using a coffee grinder, and the resulting powder was stored at room temperature until use.

3.2. Hot Water Extraction

The seaweeds were defatted, and pigments were extracted using a high methanol percentage mixture, with a solvent ratio of 4:2:1 for MeOH: $CHCl_3$: H_2O [51,52]. The fucoidans were hot water extracted as described by Lee and co-workers with minor modifications [53]. A mass of 15 g dry defatted seaweed powder was suspended in 450 mL of distilled water in a ratio of 1:30 (*w*/*v*). The mixture was heated to 70 °C with agitation overnight. The extracted fucoidan yield was expressed as a percentage of the dry defatted seaweed weight (% dry wt).

3.3. Structural Validation of Extracted Fucoidans

3.3.1. Fourier Transform Infrared Spectrometry (FTIR) Analysis

A hundred milligrams of ground fucoidan was scanned using Fourier-transform infrared spectroscopy (FTIR) on a 100 FT-IR spectrometer system (Perkin Elmer, Wellesley, MA, USA). The signals were automatically recorded by averaging four scans over 4000–650 cm^{-1}. The baseline and ATR corrections for penetration depth and frequency variations were performed using Spectrum One software (version 1.2.1) (Perkin Elmer, Wellesley, MA, USA).

3.3.2. NMR Spectroscopy Analysis

Fucoidan samples (10 mg) were dissolved in 1 mL D_2O. After centrifugation at 13,000× *g* for 2 min, any insoluble matter was removed by filtering the supernatant through a 0.45-μm filter. The deuterium-exchanged samples were subjected to ^{1}H-NMR analysis, and spectra were recorded at 23 °C using a 400 MHz spectrometer (Bruker, Fällanden, Switzerland) with Topspin 3.5 software (Bruker, Billerica, MA, USA).

3.3.3. Thermogravimetric Analysis

Fucoidans were subjected to thermogravimetric analysis using a Pyris Diamond model thermogravimetric analyser (PerkinElmer®, Shelton, CT, USA). Samples of 4 mg fucoidan were analysed in an aluminium crucible. Pure nitrogen (purity of 99.99%) was used as the carrier gas during all the experiments to reduce the mass transfer effect. The gas flow rate was at 20 mL/min. The fucoidans were heated from 30 °C to 900 °C at a heating rate of 30 °C/min. A separate blank using an empty tray was run for baseline correction. Lastly, the mass loss relative to the temperature increment was automatically recorded, and the derivative thermogram (DTG) was plotted using GraphPad Prism version 6.

3.4. Chemical Characterisation of Fucoidans

Using *L*-fucose as a standard, the phenol-sulphuric acid method estimated the total sugar content within the fucoidans [54]. The total reducing sugar content in 2 M TFA partially hydrolysed fucoidans was quantified using the dinitrosalicylic acid (DNS) assay [55]. Furthermore, the protein contamination was measured using Bradford's method, utilising bovine serum albumin (BSA) as a standard [56]. The sulphate content in formic acid (60% *v*/*v*) desulphurised fucoidan was measured using a barium chloride–gelatin method as described previously [57], which was scaled down to microtitre volumes.

Polyphenols within the fucoidans were quantified using a modified Folin–Ciocalteu method with gallic acid as a standard [58]. Moreover, quantitative analyses of *L*-fucose, D-fructose, D-galactose, D-xylose, L-arabinose, and D-mannose in the fucoidans were performed using high-performance liquid chromatography (HPLC) method [16]. A Shimadzu HPLC (RID) instrument (Kyoto, Japan) and a Fortis Amino column (Fortis Technologies Ltd., Cheshire, UK) was utilised in the HPLC method. The ash contents in fucoidans were derived from derivative thermogravimetry (DTG) data.

3.5. Determination of Fucoidans Molecular Weights by HPLC

The molecular weights of fucoidans were determined using size exclusion high-performance liquid chromatography with a refractive index detector (HPLC-RID). The fucoidan extracts were separated using a Shodex OHpak SB-806M HQ (8.0 mm I.D. × 300 mm) column (Showa Denko, Tokyo, Japan) according to the manufacturer's recommendations. The mobile phase (0.1 M $NaNO_3$ aq) used was filtered through 0.22 μm nylon membranes (Membrane solutions, Auburn, USA). The flow rate was adjusted to 0.6 mL/min, the column temperature was at 30 °C, and the sample injection volume was 20 μL. Pullulan standards (Shodex, Tokyo, Japan) were used to construct the standard curve for interpolating fucoidan molecular weights.

3.6. Cell Culture

The HCT116 human colon cancer cell line was from the American Type Culture Collection (ATCC CCL-247). The cell line was cultured in Dulbecco's Modified Eagle's Medium (DMEM) with GlutaMAX™-I, supplemented with 10% (*v*/*v*) fetal bovine serum (FBS) and 1% (*v*/*v*) sodium pyruvate. The cell culture was maintained at 9% CO_2 in a humidified incubator at 37 °C.

3.7. Cytotoxicity Screening

The susceptibility of the HCT116 cell line to the fucoidan extracts was determined using an optimised resazurin assay [16]. Briefly, cells were seeded at a density of

1×10^5 cells/well in DMEM growth medium in a 96-well plate. After the cells adhered to the plate matrix overnight, they were treated with varying doses of fucoidan (0.1 mg/mL to 2.5 mg/mL). The anti-cancer agent 5-fluorouracil (5-FU) in a concentration range of 0.0064 µM to 2500 µM was included as a positive control for cytotoxicity. The experiments were incubated for 72 h before treatment with resazurin. Cell viability was measured by fluorescence (excitation = 560 nm and emission = 590 nm).

3.8. Clonogenic Assay

HCT116 cells were seeded at a density of 1.5×10^3 cells/mL in a six-well plate and allowed to adhere overnight. The cells were treated with fucoidan extracts or 4-nitroquinoline 1-oxide (4NQO), which was used as a positive control. The cultures were incubated at 37 °C for 48 h, upon which half the volume of spent medium was removed and replaced with fresh medium lacking treatment. The cultures were incubated, and the medium changed every two days until individual colonies of at least 50 cells/colony were visible. The medium was removed, and the cells were washed once with PBS. The cells were fixed for 10 min by a 3:1 methanol to the acetic acid mixture. The fixative was removed, and the plate was allowed to air dry for 2 min. The HCT116 cell colonies were stained with 5% (*w*/*v*) crystal violet in methanol for 4–6 h, washed three times in PBS and rinsed in water. The plates were air-dried, and the images were captured using a ChemiDoc™-XRS (BioRad, Hercules, CA, USA). The cells were solubilised completely using 1 M acetic acid, and the absorbance was read at a wavelength of 590 nm. The % colony formation was expressed as percentiles relative to the untreated experiments.

3.9. Wound Healing Assay

A volume of 500 µL/well of HCT116 cells were seeded at 7×10^5 cells/mL into 24 well plates. The cells were allowed to adhere and grow to 100% confluence overnight at 37 °C. A wound was made down the centre of the well with a pipette tip. After wounding, the floating cells were removed, and fresh medium without or with varying doses of fucoidan (0.1–0.5 mg/mL) treatments was added. Pre-migration images of the wounds were taken at 4× magnification. The plates were further incubated at 37 °C for 12 h, whereafter, images were taken at the same position as the premigration images. The images were analysed on ImageJ using a wound healing plugin [59], and wound closure was calculated using the formula below where the percentage wound area was calculated relative to the wound size at t = 0:

$$\text{Wound closure} = \%\text{wound area}(t = 0) - \%\text{wound area}\ (t = 12)$$

3.10. Sphere-Based Tumour Migration Assays

HCT116 cells were resuspended in an appropriate volume of Dulbecco's Modified Eagle's Medium (DMEM) (final concentration of 1×10^4 cells/10 µL) for the formation of spheres in an optimised hanging drop method [60]. About 5 mL of sterile PBS was pipetted into the bottom portion of the tissue culture plate (100 mm diameter) to create a humidified environment., Multiple 10 µL culture drops were deposited inside the lid of the culture dish. The lid with the hanging drops was placed back on top of the PBS-containing dish, taking care to avoid disturbing the droplets. The plate was incubated for 48 h at 37 °C to allow the spheres to grow. The spheres were then transferred to a 24-well plate prefilled with 300 µL medium and respective treatments with compounds ranging from 0.1 mg/mL to 0.5 mg/mL. In some experiments, the HCT116 culture (at a density of 10,000 cells/10 µL) was pretreated with 0.5 mg/mL and 0.1 mg/mL of the compounds during sphere formation. Untreated or pretreated spheres transferred to the adherent plate were allowed to adhere by incubation at 37 °C for 4 h. Images were taken at 4× magnification and this time was taken as t = 0 (4 h post-seeding of spheres into adherent plates). The spheroids were monitored over time for t = 24 h. The areas of migration were quantified using Fiji/ImageJ (Version 1.53f51). The results presented were represented by three experimental biological replicates. The data were normalised to the initial size of each spheroid at time 0 to determine cell migration from the spheroid. The migration of cells from spheres was calculated as follows:

$$\text{Distance migrated} = \text{area measured at t} = 24 \text{ hrs} - \text{area at t} = 0 \text{ h}$$

3.11. Cell Adhesion Assays

HCT116 cells were seeded at a density of 6×10^4 cells/well in a 96-well plate and treated with varying concentrations of fucoidan (0.1–0.4 mg/mL) or left untreated as the control. The culture was incubated at 37 °C with 9% CO_2 for 8 h. The spent medium was decanted from the plate, and the adhered cells were washed thrice with 1 × sterile PBS (137 mM NaCl, 2.7 mM KCl, 10 mM Na_2HPO_4 and 2 mM KH_2PO_4, pH = 7). The cells were fixed by adding 100 µL/well of a 3:1 methanol: acetic acid solution and incubated at room temperature for 15 min. The methanol-acetic acid mixture was washed off using sterile distilled H_2O and blotted dry on a paper towel. The cells were stained with 0.1% (*w*/*v*) crystal violet dye (40 µL/well) and incubated at room temperature for 20 min with gentle agitation at 30 rpm. The crystal violet dye was discarded, and the plate was washed four times with distilled water. A volume of 100 µL/well of 1% (*w*/*v*) SDS was added, the plate incubated overnight, and the optical density was then measured at a wavelength of 590 nm.

4. Conclusions

The extracted compounds were unique in composition, with *Ecklonia* sp. fucoidans having a relatively high carbohydrate content compared to *S. elegans* and commercially purchased *F. vesiculosus*. Furthermore, the *Ecklonia* sp. fucoidans had a comparatively low degree of sulphation compared to the other fucoidans, despite having comparatively lower molecular weights. Their low molecular weight could have had an impact on the anti-adhesion and anti-spheroid migration of the HCT116 cancer cells. Although slightly larger, the *S. elegans* and *F. vesiculosus* fucoidans had a relatively higher sulphate content than the *Ecklonia* sp. fucoidans, which may have enhanced the anti-cancer activities of these fucoidans observed by the anti-colony formation, anti-adhesion and anti-spheroid migration of the HCT116 cells. Our study reaffirms that molecular weight and sulphation of fucoidan, along with other properties, may be important for biological activity. This study also showed that fucoidans differ in structure and activity depending on the type (genus and species) of seaweed. Although there are structural differences between the fucoidans studied, their anti-cancer effects suggest some potential health benefits of seaweed fucoidans that warrant further analysis.

Author Contributions: Conceptualisation, B.M., C.D.D., A.L.E. and B.I.P.; Investigation, B.M. and C.D.D.; writing—original draft preparation, B.M. and C.D.D.; writing—review and editing, B.M., C.D.D., A.L.E. and B.I.P.; supervision, A.L.E. and B.I.P.; project administration, A.L.E. and B.I.P.; funding acquisition, B.I.P. and A.L.E. All authors have read and agreed to the published version of the manuscript.

Funding: B.M. was funded by the German Academic Exchange Service (DAAD) In-Region Scholarship (grant no. 57408782). C.D.D. received financial support for this study from the Pearson Young Memorial scholarship. A.L.E is supported by the National Research Foundation of South Africa (Grant Numbers 98566 and 105829), and both A.L.E. and B.I.P. are supported by Rhodes University (RRG). This research was supported in part by KelpX.

Institutional Review Board Statement: Not applicable.

Data Availability Statement: Data are available upon request.

Conflicts of Interest: The authors declare no conflict of interest.

References

1. Lin, Y.; Qi, X.; Liu, H.; Xue, K.; Xu, S.; Tian, Z. The anti-cancer effects of fucoidan: A review of both in vivo and in vitro investigations. *Cancer Cell Int.* **2020**, *20*, 154. [CrossRef] [PubMed]
2. Marudhupandi, T.; Kumar, T.T.A.; Lakshmanasenthil, S.; Suja, G.; Vinothkumar, T. In vitro anti-cancer activity of fucoidan from Turbinaria conoides against A549 cell lines. *Int. J. Biol. Macromol.* **2015**, *72*, 919–923. [CrossRef] [PubMed]

3. WHO. Cancer. 2021. Available online: https://www.who.int/news-room/fact-sheets/detail/cancer (accessed on 5 January 2022).
4. Sung, H.; Ferlay, J.; Siegel, R.L.; Laversanne, M.; Soerjomataram, I.; Jemal, A.; Bray, F. Global Cancer Statistics 2020: GLOBOCAN Estimates of Incidence and Mortality Worldwide for 36 Cancers in 185 Countries. *CA Cancer J. Clin.* **2021**, *71*, 209–249. [CrossRef] [PubMed]
5. Motsuku, L.; Chen, W.C.; Muchengeti, M.M.; Naidoo, M.; Quene, T.M.; Kellett, P.; Mohlala, M.I.; Chu, K.M.; Singh, E. Colorectal cancer incidence and mortality trends by sex and population group in South Africa: 2002–2014. *BMC Cancer* **2021**, *21*, 129. [CrossRef]
6. Senthilkumar, K.; Manivasagan, R.; Venkatesan, J.; Kim, S.K. Brown seaweed fucoidan: Biological activity and apoptosis, growth signalling mechanism in cancer. *Int. J. Biol. Macromol.* **2013**, *60*, 366–374. [CrossRef]
7. Kim, E.J.; Park, S.Y.; Lee, J.Y.; Park, J.H.Y. Fucoidan present in brown algae induces apoptosis of human colon cancer cells. *BMC Gastroenterol.* **2010**, *10*, 96. [CrossRef]
8. Siegel, R.L.; Jakubowski, C.D.; Fedewa, S.A.; Davis, A.; Azad, N.S. Colorectal Cancer in the Young: Epidemiology, Prevention, Management. *Am. Soc. Clin. Oncol Educ. Book* **2020**, *40*, e75–e88. [CrossRef]
9. Jin, J.O.; Chauhan, P.S.; Arukha, A.P.; Chavda, V.; Dubey, A.; Yadav, D. The Therapeutic Potential of the Anti-cancer Activity of Fucoidan: Current Advances and Hurdles. *Mar. Drugs* **2021**, *19*, 265. [CrossRef]
10. Yuan, H.; Ma, Q.; Ye, L.; Piao, G. The Traditional Medicine and Modern Medicine from Natural Product. *Molecules* **2016**, *21*, 559. [CrossRef]
11. Van Weelden, G.; Bobiński, M.; Okła, K.; Van Weelden, W.J.; Romano, A.; Pijnenborg, J.M.A. Fucoidan Structure and Activity in Relation to Anti-Cancer Mechanisms. *Mar. Drugs* **2019**, *17*, 32. [CrossRef]
12. Gupta, S.; Abu-Ghannam, N. Bioactive and possible health effects of edible brown seaweeds. *Trends Food Sci. Technol.* **2011**, *22*, 315–326. [CrossRef]
13. Fernando, S.; Sanjeewa, K.K.A.; Samarakoon, K.W.; Lee, W.W.; Kim, H.S.; Kim, E.A.; Gunasekara, U.K.D.S.S.; Abeytunga, D.T.U.; Nanayakkara, C.; de Silva, E.D.; et al. FTIR characterisation and antioxidant activity of water soluble crude polysaccharides of Sri Lankan marine algae. *ALGAE* **2017**, *32*, 75–86. [CrossRef]
14. Kopplin, G.; Rokstad, A.M.; Mélida, H.; Bulone, V.; Skjåk-Bræk, G.; Aachmann, F.L. Structural Characterisation of Fucoidan from Laminaria hyperborea: Assessment of Coagulation and Inflammatory Properties and Their Structure−Function Relationship. *ACS Appl. Bio Mater.* **2018**, *1*, 1880–1892. [CrossRef]
15. Li, B.; Lu, F.; Wei, X.; Zhao, R. Fucoidan: Structure and bioactivity. *Molecules* **2008**, *13*, 1671–1695. [CrossRef] [PubMed]
16. Mabate, B.; Daub, C.D.; Malgas, S.; Edkins, A.L.; Pletschke, B.I. A Combination Approach in Inhibiting Type 2 Diabetes-Related Enzymes Using Ecklonia radiata Fucoidan. *Pharmaceutics* **2021**, *13*, 1979. [CrossRef]
17. Han, Y.S.; Lee, J.H.; Lee, S.H. Fucoidan inhibits the migration and proliferation of HT-29 human colon cancer cells via the phosphoinositide-3 kinase/Akt/mechanistic target of rapamycin pathways. *Mol. Med. Rep.* **2015**, *2*, 3446–3452. [CrossRef]
18. Park, H.Y.; Park, S.H.; Jeong, J.W.; Yoon, D.; Han, M.H.; Lee, D.S.; Choi, G.; Yim, M.-J.; Lee, J.M.; Kim, D.-H.; et al. Induction of p53-Independent Apoptosis and G1 Cell Cycle Arrest by FuFucoidan in HCT116 Human Colorectal Carcinoma Cells. *Mar. Drugs* **2017**, *15*, 154. [CrossRef]
19. Han, Y.S.; Lee, J.H.; Lee, S.H. Antitumor Effects of Fucoidan on Human Colon Cancer Cells via Activation of Akt Signaling. *Biomol. Ther.* **2015**, *23*, 225–232. [CrossRef]
20. Arumugam, P.; Arunkumar, K.; Sivakumar, L.; Murugan, M.; Murugan, K. Anti-cancer effect of fucoidan on cell proliferation, cell cycle progression, genetic damage and apoptotic cell death in HepG2 cancer cells. *Toxicol. Rep.* **2019**, *6*, 556–563. [CrossRef]
21. Bolton, J.J.; Stegenga, H. Seaweed species diversity in South Africa. *S. Afr. J. Mar. Sci.* **2002**, *24*, 9–18. [CrossRef]
22. Kumar, T.V.; Lakshmanasenthil, S.; Geetharamani, D.; Marudhupandi, T.; Suja, G.; Suganya, P. Fucoidan—A inhibitor from Sargassum wightii with relevance to type 2 diabetes mellitus therapy. *Int. J. Biol. Macromol.* **2015**, *72*, 1044–1047. [CrossRef] [PubMed]
23. Zhao, D.; Ding, X.; Hou, Y.; Hou, W.; Liu, Y.; Xu, T.; Yang, D. Structural characterisation, immune regulation and antioxidant activity of a new heteropolysaccharide from Cantharellus cibarius Fr. *Int. J. Mol. Med.* **2018**, *41*, 2744–2754. [CrossRef] [PubMed]
24. Zhao, D.; Xu, J.; Xu, X. Bioactivity of fucoidan extracted from Laminaria japonica using a novel procedure with high yield. *Food Chem.* **2018**, *245*, 911–918. [CrossRef] [PubMed]
25. Pereira, L.; Gheda, S.F.; Ribeiro-Claro, P.J.A. Analysis by Vibrational Spectroscopy of Seaweed Polysaccharides with Potential Use in Food, Pharmaceutical, and Cosmetic Industrie. *Int. J. Carbohydr. Chem.* **2013**, *7*, 537202. [CrossRef]
26. Alwarsamy, M.; Gooneratne, R.; Ravichandran, R. Effect of fucoidan from Turbinaria conoides on human lung adenocarcinoma epithelial (A549) cells. *Carbohydr. Polym.* **2016**, *152*, 207–213. [CrossRef]
27. Shan, X.; Liu, X.; Hao, J.; Cai, C.; Fan, F.; Dun, Y.; Zhao, X.L.; Liu, X.X.; Li, C.X.; Yu, G.L. In vitro and in vivo hypoglycemic effects of brown algal fucoidans. *Int. J. Biol. Macromol.* **2016**, *82*, 249–255. [CrossRef]
28. Nguyen, T.T.; Mikkelsen, M.D.; Tran, V.H.N.; Trang, V.T.D.; Rhein-Knudsen, N.; Cao, H.T.T. Enzyme-Assisted Fucoidan Extraction from Brown Macroalgae Fucus distichus subsp. evanescens and Saccharina latissima. *Mar. Drugs* **2020**, *18*, 296. [CrossRef]
29. Liu, X.; Yu, W. Evaluating the Thermal Stability of High Performance Fibers by TGA. *J. Appl. Polym. Sci.* **2006**, *99*, 937–944. [CrossRef]

30. White, J.E.; Catallo, W.J.; Legendre, B.L. Biomass pyrolysis kinetics: A comparative critical review with relevant agricultural residue case studies. *J. Anal. Appl. Pyrolysis* **2011**, *91*, 1–33. [CrossRef]
31. Chen, Z.; Hu, M.; Zhu, X.; Guo, D.; Liu, S.; Hu, Z.; Xiao, B.; Wang, J.; Laghari, M. Characteristics and kinetic study on pyrolysis of five lignocellulosic biomass via thermogravimetric analysis. *Bioresour. Technol.* **2015**, *192*, 441–450. [CrossRef]
32. Carpio, R.B.; Zhang, Y.; Kuo, C.T.; Chen, W.T.; Schideman, L.C.; Leon, R.L. Characterisation and thermal decomposition of demineralised wastewater algae biomass. *Algal Res.* **2019**, *38*, 101399. [CrossRef]
33. Morimoto, M.; Takatori, M.; Hayashi, T.; Mori, D.; Takashima, O.; Yoshida, S.; Sato, K.; Kawamoto, H.; Tamura, J.-I.; Izawa, H.; et al. Depolymerisation of sulfated polysaccharides under hydrothermal conditions. *Carbohydr. Res.* **2014**, *384*, 56–60. [CrossRef]
34. Saravanaa, P.S.; Choa, Y.N.; Patilb, M.P.; Choa, Y.J.; Kimb, G.D.; Park, Y.B.; Woo, H.-C.; Chun, B.-S. Hydrothermal degradation of seaweed polysaccharide: Characterisation and biological activities. *Food Chem.* **2018**, *268*, 179–187. [CrossRef]
35. Ermakova, S.; Sokolova, R.; Kim, S.M.; Um, B.H.; Isakov, V.; Zvyagintseva, T. Fucoidans from brown seaweeds Sargassum hornery, Eclonia cava, Costaria costata: Structural characteristics and anti-cancer activity. *Appl. Biochem. Biotechnol.* **2011**, *164*, 841–885. [CrossRef]
36. January, G.G.; Naidoo, R.K.; Kirby-McCullough, B.; Bauerd, R. Assessing methodologies for fucoidan extraction from South African brown algae. *Algal Res.* **2019**, *40*, 101517. [CrossRef]
37. Catarino, M.D.; Silva, A.M.S.; Cardoso, S.M. Phytochemical Constituents and Biological Activities of *Fucus* spp. *Mar. Drugs* **2018**, *16*, 249. [CrossRef]
38. Lee, J.J.; Beumer, J.H.; Chu, E. Therapeutic Drug Monitoring of 5-Fluorouracil. Cancer chemotherapy and pharmacology. *Cancer Chemother Pharmacol.* **2016**, *78*, 447. [CrossRef]
39. Ikeguchi, M.; Yamamoto, M.; Arai, Y.; Maeta, Y.; Ashida, K.; Katano, K.; Miki, Y.; Kimura, T. Fucoidan reduces the toxicities of chemotherapy for patients with unresectable advanced or recurrent colorectal cancer. *Oncol. Lett.* **2011**, *2*, 319–322. [CrossRef]
40. Wang, Y.; Xing, M.; Cao, Q.; Ji, A.; Liang, H.; Song, S. Biological Activities of Fucoidan and the Factors Mediating Its Therapeutic Effects: A Review of Recent Studies. *Mar. Drugs* **2019**, *17*, 183. [CrossRef]
41. Yang, C.; Chung, D.; Shina, I.S.; Lee, H.; Kim, J.; Lee, Y. Effects of molecular weight and hydrolysis conditions on anti-cancer activity of fucoidans from sporophyll of Undaria pinnatifida. *Int. J. Biol. Macromol.* **2008**, *43*, 433–437. [CrossRef]
42. Franken, N.A.P.; Rodermond, H.M.; Stap, J.; Haveman, J.; Bree, C.V. Clonogenic assay of cells in vitro. *Nat. Protoc.* **2006**, *1*, 2315–2319. [CrossRef] [PubMed]
43. Shin, S.W.; Jung, W.; Choi, C.; Kim, S.Y.; Son, A.; Kim, H.; Lee, N.; Park, H.C. Fucoidan-Manganese Dioxide Nanoparticles Potentiate Radiation Therapy by Co-Targeting Tumor Hypoxia and Angiogenesis. *Mar. Drugs* **2018**, *16*, 510. [CrossRef] [PubMed]
44. Wild, T.; Rahbarnia, A.; Kellner, M.; Sobotka, L.; Eberlein, T. Basics in nutrition and wound healing. *Nutrition* **2010**, *26*, 862–866. [CrossRef]
45. Ale, M.T.; Mikkelsen, J.D.; Meyer, A.S. Important Determinants for Fucoidan Bioactivity: A Critical Review of Structure-Function Relations and Extraction Methods for Fucose-Containing Sulfated Polysaccharides from Brown Seaweeds. *Mar. Drugs* **2011**, *9*, 2106–2130. [CrossRef] [PubMed]
46. Vinci, M.; Box, C.; Zimmermann, M.; Eccles, S.A. Tumor Spheroid-Based Migration Assays for Evaluation of Therapeutic Agents. In *Target Identification and Validation in Drug Discovery: Methods and Protocols, Methods in Molecular Biology*; Moll, J., Colombo, R., Eds.; Springer Science & Business Media: New York, NY, USA, 2013; pp. 253–266.
47. Ryu, N.E.; Lee, S.H.; Park, H. Spheroid Culture System Methods and Applications for Mesenchymal Stem Cells. *Cells* **2019**, *8*, 1620. [CrossRef]
48. Lazarovici, P.; Marcinkiewicz, C.; Lelkes, P.I. Cell-Based Adhesion Assays for Isolation of Snake Venom's Integrin Antagonists. In *Snake and Spider Toxins: Methods and Protocols, Methods in Molecular Biology*; Priel, A., Ed.; Springer Science+Business Media: New York, NY, USA, 2020; pp. 205–220.
49. Liu, J.M.; Bignon, J.; Haroun-Bouhedja, F.; Bittoun, P.; Vassy, J. Inhibitory Effect of Fucoidan on the Adhesion of Adenocarcinoma Cells to Fibronectin. *Anti-Cancer Res.* **2005**, *25*, 2129–2134.
50. Suresh, V.; Senthilkumar, N.; Thangam, R.; Rajkumar, M.; Anbazhagan, C.; Rengasamy, R. Separation, purification and preliminary characterisation of sulfated polysaccharides from Sargassum plagiophyllum and its in vitro anti-cancer and antioxidant activity. *Process Biochem.* **2013**, *48*, 364–373. [CrossRef]
51. Yuan, Y.; Macquarrie, D. Microwave assisted extraction of sulfated polysaccharides (fucoidan) from Ascophyllum nodosum and its antioxidant activity. *Carbohydr. Polym.* **2015**, *129*, 101–107. [CrossRef]
52. Lee, S.H.; Ko, C.I.; Ahn, G.; You, S.; Kim, J.S.; Heu, M.S.; Kim, J.; Jee, Y.; Jeon, Y.-J. Molecular characteristics and anti-inflammatory activity of the fucoidan extracted from Ecklonia cava. *Carbohydr. Polym.* **2012**, *89*, 599–606. [CrossRef]
53. Dubois, M.; Gilles, K.A.; Hamilton, J.K.; Rebers, P.A.; Smith, F. Colorimetric method for determination of sugars and related substances. *Anal. Chem.* **1956**, *28*, 350–356. [CrossRef]
54. Miller, G.L. Use of Dinitrosalicylic Acid Reagent for Determination of Reducing Sugar. *Anal. Chem.* **1959**, *31*, 426–428. [CrossRef]
55. Bradford, M.M. A rapid and sensitive for the quantitation of microgram quantities of protein utilising the principle of protein–dye binding. *Anal. Biochem.* **1976**, *72*, 248–252. [CrossRef]
56. Dodgson, K.S.; Price, R.G. A note on determination of ester sulphate content of sulphated polysaccharides. *Biochem. J.* **1962**, *84*, 106–110. [CrossRef]

57. Huang, D.; Ou, B.; Prior, R.L. The chemistry behind antioxidant capacity assay. *J. Agric. Food Chem.* **2005**, *53*, 1841–1856. [CrossRef] [PubMed]
58. Suarez-Arnedo, A.; Figueroa, F.T.; Clavijo, C.; Arbeláez, P.; Cruz, J.C.; Muñoz-Camargo, C. An image J plugin for the high throughput image analysis of in vitro scratch wound healing assays. *PLoS ONE* **2020**, *15*, e0232565. [CrossRef]
59. Keller, G.M. In vitro differentiation of embryonic stem cells. *Curr. Opin. Cell Biol.* **1995**, *7*, 862–869. [CrossRef]
60. Daub, C.D.; Mabate, B.; Malgas, S.; Pletschke, B.I. Fucoidan from Ecklonia maxima is a powerful inhibitor of the diabetes-related enzyme, α-glucosidase. *Int. J. Biol.* **2020**, *151*, 412–420. [CrossRef]

marine drugs

MDPI

Article

Chitooligosaccharides Derivatives Protect ARPE-19 Cells against Acrolein-Induced Oxidative Injury

Cheng Yang [1], Rongrong Yang [1], Ming Gu [1], Jiejie Hao [1,2], Shixin Wang [1,3,*] and Chunxia Li [1,2,3,*]

1 Shandong Key Laboratory of Glycoscience and Glycotechnology, Key Laboratory of Marine Drugs of Ministry of Education, School of Medicine and Pharmacy, Ocean University of China, Qingdao 266003, China
2 Laboratory for Marine Drugs and Bioproducts, Pilot National Laboratory for Marine Science and Technology (Qingdao), Qingdao 266237, China
3 Laboratory of Marine Glycodrug Research and Development, Marine Biomedical Research Institute of Qingdao, Qingdao 266071, China
* Correspondence: shixin113@126.com (S.W.); lchunxia@ouc.edu.cn (C.L.); Tel.: +86-532-8203-1631 (C.L.); Fax: +86-532-8203-3054 (C.L.)

Abstract: Age-related macular degeneration (AMD) is the leading cause of vision loss among the elderly. The progression of AMD is closely related to oxidative stress in the retinal pigment epithelium (RPE). Here, a series of chitosan oligosaccharides (COSs) and *N*-acetylated derivatives (NACOSs) were prepared, and their protective effects on an acrolein-induced oxidative stress model of ARPE-19 were explored using the MTT assay. The results showed that COSs and NACOs alleviated APRE-19 cell damage induced by acrolein in a concentration-dependent manner. Among these, chitopentaose (COS–5) and its *N*-acetylated derivative (N–5) showed the best protective activity. Pretreatment with COS–5 or N–5 could reduce intracellular and mitochondrial reactive oxygen species (ROS) production induced by acrolein, increase mitochondrial membrane potential, GSH level, and the enzymatic activity of SOD and GSH-Px. Further study indicated that N–5 increased the level of nuclear Nrf2 and the expression of downstream antioxidant enzymes. This study revealed that COSs and NACOSs reduced the degeneration and apoptosis of retinal pigment epithelial cells by enhancing antioxidant capacity, suggesting that they have the potential to be developed into novel protective agents for AMD treatment and prevention.

Keywords: chitosan oligosaccharide; *N*-acetylated chitosan oligosaccharide; ARPE-19; oxidative stress; Nrf2

Citation: Yang, C.; Yang, R.; Gu, M.; Hao, J.; Wang, S.; Li, C. Chitooligosaccharides Derivatives Protect ARPE-19 Cells against Acrolein-Induced Oxidative Injury. *Mar. Drugs* **2023**, *21*, 137. https://doi.org/10.3390/md21030137

Academic Editors: Yuya Kumagai, Hideki Kishimura and Benwei Zhu

Received: 30 January 2023
Revised: 13 February 2023
Accepted: 20 February 2023
Published: 22 February 2023

1. Introduction

Age-related macular degeneration (AMD) is one of the main causes of irreversible central visual loss in the elderly worldwide [1,2]. In 2020, the number of AMD patients worldwide was 19.6 million, and this number was predicted to be 288 million in 2040 [1,3,4]. According to the symptoms, AMD can be divided into dry and wet forms with 80% and 20% prevalence, respectively [5]. Current treatments for wet AMD include laser therapy and VEGF antibody injection (such as Eylea) [6], while there is no preventive therapy for dry AMD [7]. Therefore, it is necessary to develop effective agents to prevent or cure dry AMD.

Numerous studies have indicated that AMD pathogenesis was related with chronic oxidative stress and the inflammation of retinal pigment epithelial (RPE) cells, which could lead to the eventual degeneration of the RPE [8–11]. Jin et al. [12] suggested that retinal pigment epithelium cell apoptosis was induced by ultraviolet and hydrogen peroxide via AMPK signaling. *Melissa officinalis* L. extracts and resveratrol were reported to improve cell viability and decrease reactive oxygen species (ROS) generation in RPE cells to prevent AMD [10,13]. These results demonstrated that the inhibition of RPE cell damage induced by

ROS could prevent the process of AMD [14]. Therefore, antioxidation could be an effective strategy to protect RPE cells for the amelioration of early AMD.

Chitin is extracted mainly from the shells of crabs, shrimps and insects and is one of the most abundant natural biopolymers [15–17]. Chitosan oligosaccharides (COSs) are the degraded product of chitin or chitosan and consist of glucosamine linked by β-1,4-glycosidic bonds, possess various biological effects, including anti-inflammatory, antimicrobial, immunomodulatory, antioxidant, and anticancer activities [18–21]. Fang demonstrated that COS attenuated oxidative-stress related retinal degeneration in a dose-dependent manner in a rat model [22]. Xu found that COSs protected against Cu(II)-induced neurotoxicity in primary cortical neurons by interfering with an increase in intracellular reactive oxygen species (ROS) [23]. Our previous study indicated that peracetylated chitosan oligosaccharide (PACOs) pretreatment significantly reduced lactate dehydrogenase release and reactive oxygen species production in PC12 cells [24]. In addition, Guo's group indicated that the antioxidant properties of chitosan were inversely related to its molecular weight (Mw) [25]. We performed a preliminary screening of structurally related compounds, and COSs and NACOs showed excellent antioxidant activity with the potential to prevent AMD. In the present study, we investigated the effect of a series of chitosan oligosaccharides and their *N*-acetylated derivatives on RPE cell damage and explored the possible mechanisms of action. The results showed that chitosan oligosaccharides had an excellent capacity for protecting RPE cells from acrolein-induced oxidative stress.

2. Results and Discussion

2.1. Characterization of Chitooligosaccharides and N-Acetylated Chitooligosaccharides

According to the previous method, chitooligosaccharides (COSs) and *N*-acetylated chitooligosaccharides (NACOs) were prepared via enzymatic hydrolysis [24] and acetylated modification [26].

The crude products were isolated and purified to provide monomers with different degree of polymerization (Figure 1A). NACOs were purified by column chromatography using graphitized carbon black as the stationary phase and ethanol–water as the mobile phases. This purification method was simple and efficient with the elimination of the tedious operation process of desalting, compared with gel exclusion and ion exchange purification methods [27]. The purity of these compounds was analyzed via HPLC (LC-10AD, Shimadzu, Kyoto, Japan) [28,29]. As shown in Figure 1B, the purity of COS (COS–2~6) and NACO (N–2~6) monomers was above 95%.

The structures of COSs and NACOSs were characterized using a quadrupole time of flight (Q-TOF) mass spectrometer, and nuclear magnetic resonance (NMR) and Fourier-transform infrared spectroscopy (FT-IR) analysis (Figure 1C–E). The Q-TOF MS analysis (positive ion mode) of COSs and NACOs samples are shown in Figure 1C and Table 1.

For the FT-IR spectra (Figure 1D), the bands at 3370 cm^{-1}, 2876 cm^{-1}, and 1073 cm^{-1} were corresponded to stretching vibrations of O-H, C-H and C-O, respectively. The spectra of *N*-acetyl chitosan oligosaccharides showed the characteristic absorptions of 1649 cm^{-1}, 1549 cm^{-1} and 1314 cm^{-1}, which were attributed to amide I, II and III bands of amide, respectively [30]. Moreover, there was no 1735 cm^{-1} band (-C(=O)O-) in the *N*-acetylated chitosan oligosaccharide, indicating no acetylation on the OH groups of COSs.

The structures of COSs and NACOSs were also characterized via NMR. Taking COS–3 and N–3 as examples, the 13C NMR signals in spectra (Figure 1E) were assigned in Table 2. Compared to COS–3, acetyl signal peaks appeared in the 13C NMR spectrum of N–3, with 174.8 ppm attributed to C=O, and peaks at 22.6~22.3 ppm attributed to CH_3 of acetyls.

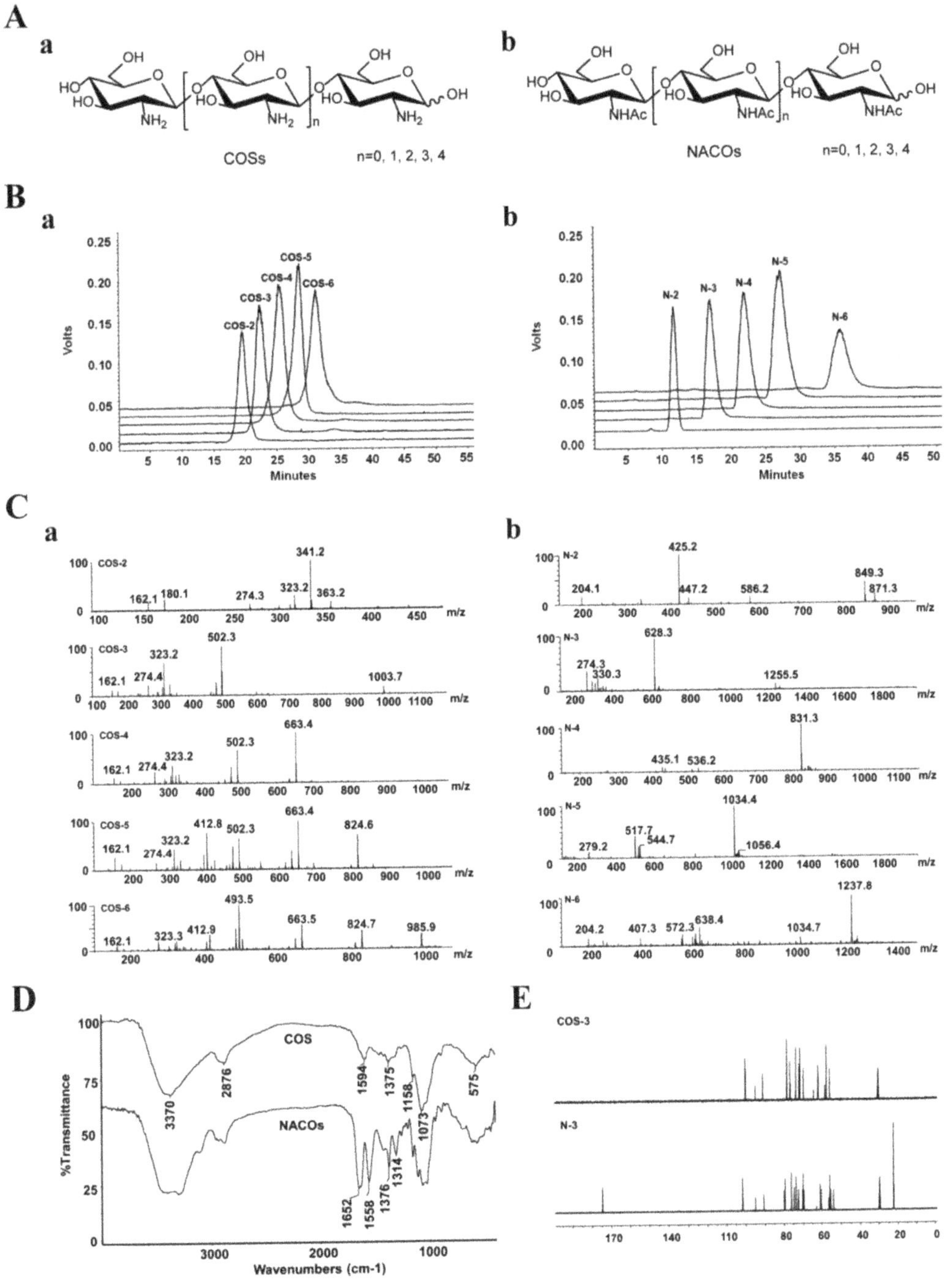

Figure 1. Characterization of COSs and NACOs. (**A**) Schematic structures of COSs (**a**) and NACOs (**b**). (**B**) HPLC chromatograms of COSs (**a**) and NACOs (**b**). (**C**) MS spectra of COSs (**a**) and NACOs (**b**). (**D**) IR spectra of COSs and NACOs. (**E**) ^{13}C NMR (125 MHz, D_2O) of COS–3 and N–3.

Table 1. The MS data of COS and NACO samples.

	Molecular Formula	Mw	*m*/*z*
COS–2	$C_{12}H_{24}N_2O_9$	340.1	$[M + H]^+ = 341.2$ $[M + Na]^+ = 363.2$
COS–3	$C_{18}H_{35}N_3O_{13}$	501.2	$[M + H]^+ = 502.3$ $[2M + H]^+ = 1003.7$
COS–4	$C_{24}H_{46}N_4O_{17}$	662.3	$[M + H]^+ = 663.4$
COS–5	$C_{30}H_{57}N_5O_{21}$	823.4	$[M + H]^+ = 824.6$ $[M + 2H]^+ = 412.8$
COS–6	$C_{36}H_{68}N_6O_{25}$	984.5	$[M + H]^+ = 985.9$ $[M + 2H]^+ = 493.5$
N–2	$C_{16}H_{28}N_2O_{11}$	424.4	$[M + H]^+ = 425.2$ $[M + Na]^+ = 447.2$
N–3	$C_{24}H_{41}N_3O_{16}$	627.6	$[M + H]^+ = 628.3$ $[2M + H]^+ = 1255.5$
N–4	$C_{32}H_{54}N_4O_{21}$	830.8	$[M + H]^+ = 831.3$
N–5	$C_{40}H_{67}N_5O_{26}$	1033.9	$[M + H]^+ = 1034.4$
N–6	$C_{48}H_{80}N_6O_{31}$	1237.1	$[M + H]^+ = 1237.8$

Table 2. The ^{13}C NMR date of COS–3 and N–3.

Sample		NMR Data (ppm)							
		C=O	CH3	C1	C2	C3	C4	C5	C6
COS–3	GlcN″			100.4	58.5	74.4	72.3	79.1	62.9
	GlcN′			100.2	58.5	79.1	77.4	72.8	62.7
	GlcNβ			95.3	59.3	70.6	79.1	72.6	62.7
	GlcNα			91.6	56.9	70.6	79.1	72.6	62.7
N–3	GlcNAc″	174.8	22.6 22.5 22.3	101.8	56.0	73.9	70.1	76.3	61.0
	GlcNAc′			101.6	55.4	72.6	79.6	74.9	60.4
	GlcNAcβ			95.2	56.5	72.9	79.6	75.0	60.5
	GlcNAcα			90.8	54.1	69.6	80.1	70.4	60.4

2.2. Protective Effect of COSs and NACOs against Acrolein-Induced Cell Death

The cytotoxicity of COS and NACO monomers (DP 2, 3, 4, 5, 6) was tested via MTT assay in ARPE-19 cells. After 24 h of incubation with 1 mM COSs or NACOs, the MTT test showed that both COSs and NACOs exhibited no significant cytotoxicity (Figure S1A). In addition, the effect of COSs and NACOs on the viability of ARPE-19 cells was tested with different concentrations (200, 400, 800 μM). It showed that COSs and NACOs did not affect cell proliferation. (Figure S2).

Acrolein, a major component of the gas phase of cigarette smoke and also a product of lipid peroxidation in vivo, has been shown to be a mitochondrial toxicant related to mitochondrial dysfunction [31]. Therefore, acrolein-induced cellular oxidative mitochondrial dysfunction in retinal pigment epithelial (RPE) cells had been used as a cellular model to evaluate antioxidants and mitochondrial protecting agents [32–34]. Here, AREP-19 cells were pretreated with different concentrations of COSs or NACOs (200, 400 and 800 μM) for 48 h, and then treated with 75 μM acrolein for 24 h, and cell viability was measured using the MTT test.

As shown in Figure 2, the cells exposed to 75 μM acrolein showed a significant decrease in cell viability (about 50%) compared to the untreated control group. However, after pretreatment with COSs or NACOs at 200, 400, and 800 μM for 48 h before acrolein exposure, the cell viability increased significantly. Furthermore, COSs and NACOs exhibited similar protective activity which was dose-dependent. In addition, we also prepared peracetylated chitosan oligosaccharides (PACOs) [24], but PACOs had a certain cytotoxicity to ARPE-19 (Figure S1B). Glucosamine pentamer (COS–5) and *N*-acetylated chitopentaose (N–5) showed the highest protective activity, which indicated that the pentaose skeleton may be the suitable structure for binding to the receptors or targets, such as heparin core pentasaccharide, for anticoagulant activity [35].

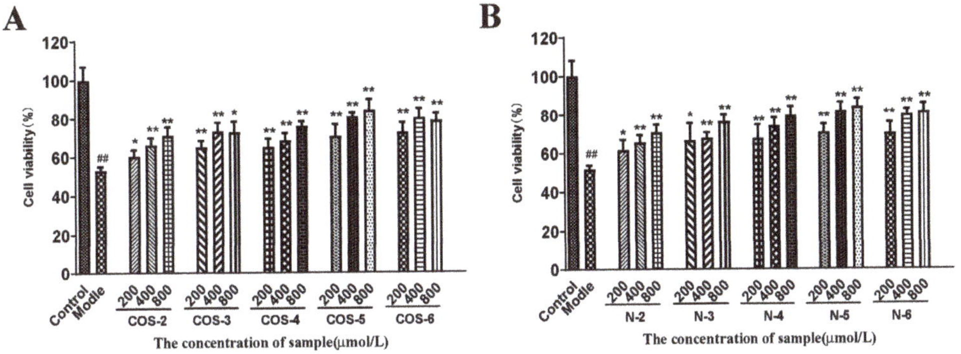

Figure 2. Protective effect of COSs and NACOs against acrolein-induced ARPE-19 cell death. The cells were pretreated with 200, 400, 800 μM COSs (**A**) or NACOs (**B**) for 48 h and then treated with 75 μM acrolein for an additional 24 h. Cell viability was analyzed using the MTT method. Values are mean ± SD of five separate experiments. ## $p < 0.01$ vs. control (no acrolein, no COSs or NACOs); * $p < 0.05$, ** $p < 0.01$ vs. acrolein.

2.3. *Protective Effect of COS–5 and N–5 against Acrolein-Induced Oxidative Stress*

The involvement of oxidative-stress-triggered apoptosis in retinal endothelial cells was considered as the leading cause of AMD [2,36,37]. In this study, RPE cells were stimulated by acrolein to induce oxidative stress. It was evaluated for the capacity of COS–5 and N–5 to prevent oxidative-stress-induced cell death and the imbalance of the antioxidant system. Initially, the effects of COS–5 and N–5 on acrolein-induced ROS generation (Figure S3) and MMP decline (Figure S4) in ARPE-19 cells were evaluated at different concentrations (200, 400, 800 μM). The results showed that there were no significant differences between 400 and 800 μM. Thus, all subsequent experiments were performed with the 400 μM dose. Then, intracellular and mitochondria ROS accumulation, GSH level, and GPx and SOD activities were measured (Figure 3).

ROS are natural by-products of aerobic respiration. ROS can be controlled by various cellular antioxidant compounds and enzymes, and their overproduction would lead to cell death [38]. Compared with the control, intracellular and mitochondria ROS levels were significantly increased to about 270% and 276% after acrolein exposure, respectively (Figure 3A,B). However, pretreatment with COS–5 or N–5 at the concentration of 400 μM reduced acrolein-induced ROS production significantly. GSH is one of the most important endogenous small molecule antioxidants. As shown in Figure 3C, the intracellular GSH level was decreased significantly after acrolein exposure (about 49%). Pretreatment with COS–5 or N–5 could successfully inhibit the decrease in GSH content induced by acrolein, which increased by 39% and 41% ($p < 0.01$), respectively. GSH peroxidase (GPx) and SOD activity was decreased to 30% and 55% after acrolein treatment (Figure 3D,E), respectively. The activities of antioxidant enzymes (GPx and SOD) significantly enhanced after COS–5 or N–5 treatments. These results indicated that the excellent antioxidant activity of COSs and NACOs played a critical role in protecting cells against acrolein-induced oxidative damage.

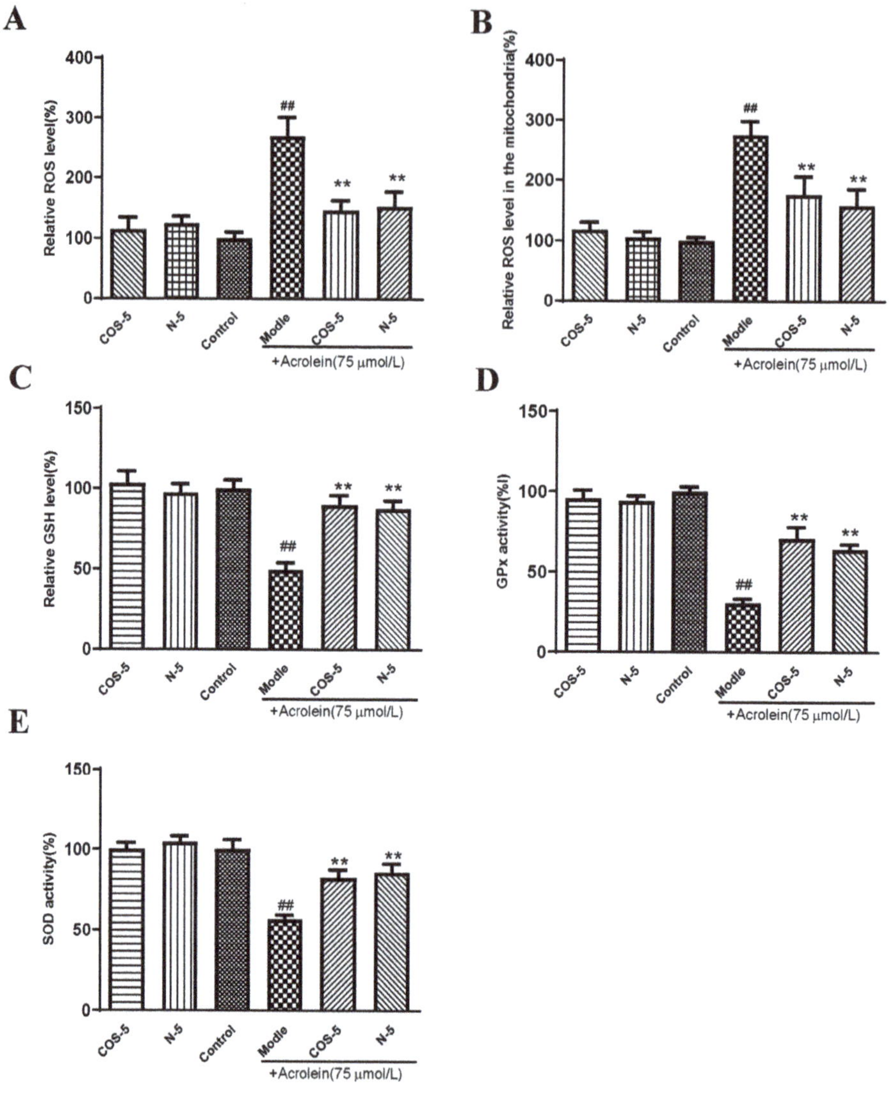

Figure 3. COS–5 and N–5 against acrolein-induced oxidative stress. ARPE-19 cells were treated with 400 μM COS–5 or N–5 for 48 h and then treated with acrolein for an additional 24 h. Cellular ROS generation (**A**), ROS level in mitochondria (**B**), GSH level (**C**), GPx (**D**) and SOD activities (**E**). The data expressed as ratio relative to controls. Values are mean ± SD of five separate experiments. ## $p < 0.01$ vs. control (no acrolein, no COS–5 and N–5); ** $p < 0.01$ vs. acrolein.

In this study, we found that chitooligosaccharides and their derivatives could protect APRE-19 cells from acrolein oxidative damage by improving their antioxidant capacities. However, without acrolein exposure, COS–5 or N–5 pretreatment did not affect these antioxidant biomarkers when compared to control cells (Figure 3). This is an interesting phenomenon. ROS at a low level play important roles as signaling molecules in normal physiology. Navdeep et al. [39] found that the mitochondrial complex III ROS was essential for T cell activation both in vitro and in vivo. It is a huge advantage that the antioxidant activities of N–5 and COS–5 were selective, and they did not affect ROS balance and ROS-mediated signaling pathways in normal cells. The data above showed that COS–5 or N–5 has the potential to be studied further and developed into a novel therapeutic agent for the treatment of AMD.

2.4. COS–5 and N–5 Improved Mitochondrial Function in Acrolein-Treated ARPE-19 Cells

Mitochondria are the main sites of oxidant generation, and are easily affected by oxidants, resulting in mitochondrial dysfunction and apoptosis. We examined mitochondrial function by assaying cellular and mitochondrial ROS production, and mitochondrial membrane potential MMP. The results of cellular (Figure 3A) and mitochondrial ROS production is shown in Figure 3B. MMP is an important index of mitochondrial function, which could be evaluated using a JC-1 fluorescent probe. As shown in Figure 4, MMP was decreased to about 45% by acrolein (75 μM, 24 h), which was consistent with previous reported results [32]. MMP was significantly increased after pretreatment with COS–5 or N–5. Similarly, COS–5 or N–5 did not affect mitochondrial function of normal ARPE-19 cells.

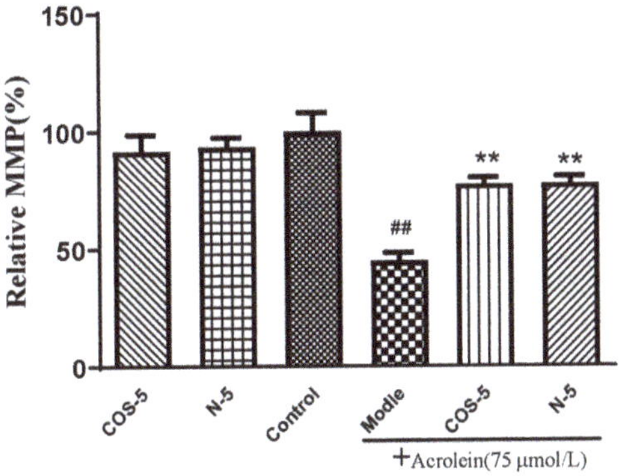

Figure 4. Protective effect of COS–5 and N–5 against acrolein-induced ARPE-19 mitochondrial dysfunction. The cells were pretreated with 400 μM COS–5 or N–5 for 48 h and then treated with 75 μM acrolein for an additional 24 h. The effects of COS–5 or N–5 on mitochondrial membrane potential were tested using the JC-1 method. Data are red/green (590/530 nm) fluorescence ratios. The data are expressed as ratio relative to controls. Values are mean ± SD of five separate experiments. ## $p < 0.01$ vs. control (no acrolein, no COS–5 and N–5); ** $p < 0.01$ vs. acrolein.

Zhou [40] found that COS could entered into cells in a dose-dependent and time-dependent manner, and COS was localized preferentially in the mitochondria. However, it was not reported whether NACOSs could enter into cells. Here, the localization of N–5 in ARPE-19 cells was detected by confocal microscopy using the FITC-labeled N–5 (N5-FITC). After treatment with N5-FITC (100 μM) for 3 h, a green fluorescence was observed around the mitochondria, while nearly no fluorescence was found in control cells (Figure 5), suggesting that N–5 could enter into ARPE-19 cells and localize in the mitochondria. These data indicated that the intracellular localization of chitooligosaccharides was not affected by the introduction of acetyl group into amino. Taken together, the results demonstrated that N–5 could localize in the mitochondria and protect ARPE-19 cells against mitochondrial dysfunction and apoptosis induced by oxidative stress.

2.5. N–5 Promoted Nrf2 Nuclear Translocation and Increased Antioxidant Enzyme Expression

Nuclear transcription factor Nrf2 plays a key role in regulating the expression of phase II detoxification enzymes and antioxidant enzymes. Under normal physiological conditions, Nrf2 was present in the cytoplasm coupled with the negative regulatory protein Kelch Ech-associated protein 1 (Keap1), which interacted with Nrf2 and acted as an adaptor protein, maintaining Nrf2 at a low level and allowing it to be continuously degraded by the proteasome in a ubiquitin-mediated process [41]. When cells were exposed to oxidative stress, Nrf2 in the cytoplasm was released from the negative regulatory protein Keap-1 and translocated to the nucleus, then bonded to an antioxidant response element (ARE). Then, a variety of genes, including glutathione reductase (GR), heme oxygenase-1 (HO-1), catalase (CAT), NAD(P)H Quinone oxidoreductase-1 (NQO-1), and γ-glutamyl cysteine ligase (GCL) were regulated to resist the cell damage caused by oxidative stress [42].

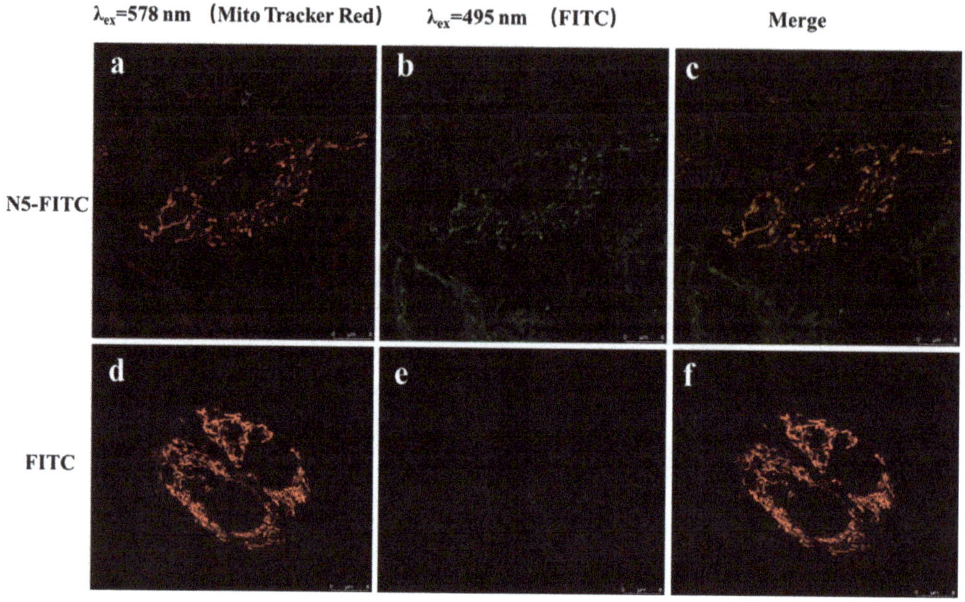

Figure 5. The intracellular localization of N–5 in ARPE-19 cells. The cells are stained with FITC and MitoTracker Red CMXRos. Red: MitoTracker Red CMXRos (**a**,**d**), Green: FITC (**b**,**e**), Merge images (**c**,**f**). Images were captured with confocal microscope. Scale bar: 8 μm.

We determined the effect of oxidative stress induced by acrolein on Nrf2 nuclear translocation in the ARPE-19 cell. Due to the similar activity of N–5 and COS–5, as well as the easy preparation of N–5, we focused on N–5 in subsequent experiments. As Figure 6A,B shows, the level of Nrf2 protein in the nucleus significantly decreased after acrolein damage, similar to a published report [43], while pretreatment with N–5 significantly increased the level of nuclear Nrf2, indicating that N–5 could promote Nrf2 nuclear translocation.

Meanwhile, we detected the effect of N–5 on the transcription of genes downstream of Nrf2. The mRNA expression of HO-1 and NQO-1 were performed via qRT-PCR. As shown in Figure 6C,D, the mRNA levels of HO-1 and NQO-1 were significantly reduced in ARPE-19 cells treated with acrolein, and upregulated significantly when pretreated with N–5. These results suggested that N–5 could activate the Nrf2-ARE pathway in ARPE-19 cells, enhance Nrf2 protein nuclear translocation and upregulate the expression of phase II metabolizing enzymes (such as HO-1 and NQO1) to alleviate acrolein-induced oxidative injury.

Oxidative damage of RPE cells was a major factor in the pathogenesis of AMD, and protecting RPE from oxidative damage and death has become a trend in the treatment and prevention of AMD disease. COS and their derivatives were well-known for their free radical scavenging potential by interrupting radical chain reactions to inhibit oxidative damage [44]. The antioxidant activity of chitosan increased with decreasing Mw [45]. Li et al. [46] reported that COS had strong antioxidant activities such as hydroxyl and superoxide radical scavenging activity and reducing power. Qu [47] found that chitooligosaccharides had a certain radical scavenging activity in vitro, and they protected mice from oxidative stress, increased the activity of SOD, catalase, and GPx significantly in mice on a high-fat diet. However, there are fewer reports on *N*-acetylated oligochitosan with the same repeated unit as chitin. Several high-purity chitosan oligosaccharides and their *N*-acetylated derivatives were prepared in this study, and their protective effect on retinal pigment epithelial cells was studied. Similar to other antioxidants such as curcumin analogs [32], luteolin [48], naringenin [49], or tocopherol [31], chitooligosaccharide monomers also had good protective activity, and COS–5 and N–5 showed the best activities.

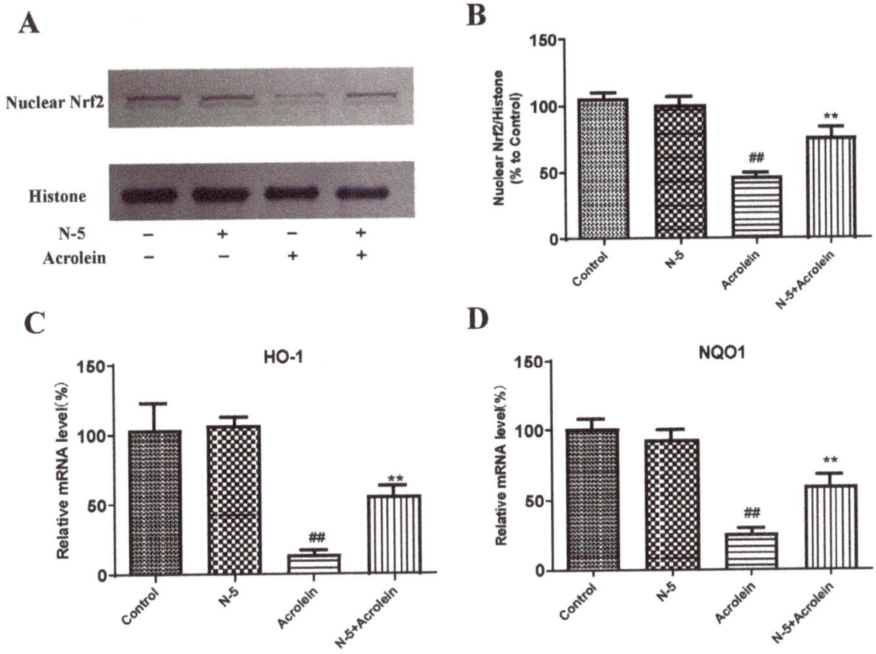

Figure 6. N–5 promoted Nrf2 nuclear translocation and upregulated antioxidant enzyme expressions in the ARPE-19 cell model of acrolein damage. The cells were pretreated with 400 μM N–5 for 48 h and then treated with 75 μM acrolein for an additional 24 h, and mRNA and protein levels were analyzed. Western blot image of nuclear Nrf2 (**A**) and quantification of Western blots (**B**), mRNA expression of HO-1 (**C**) and NQO1 (**D**). The data expressed as ratio relative to controls. Values are mean ± SD of three separate experiments. ## $p < 0.01$ vs. control (no acrolein, no N–5); ** $p < 0.01$ vs. acrolein.

Further studies found that acetyl group introduction did not affect the protective effect of chitooligosaccharides. Subsequent study found that N–5 could enhance the antioxidant capacity of ARPE-19 cells, via reducing ROS production, increasing the GSH level, and enhancing SOD/GPx enzyme activity. In addition, N–5 could localize in mitochondria, increase MMP, reduce mitochondrial dysfunction and cellular damage, and enhance Nrf2 nuclear translocation and the transcription of downstream antioxidant enzyme (HO-1 and NQO1). Interestingly, N–5-mediated antioxidant properties were selective and associated with the oxidative stress state. N–5 does not inhibit ROS production and ROS-mediated signaling pathways in the normal cells. The above results indicated that *N*-acetylated chitooligosaccharides may have a potential application in anti-AMD degenerative diseases.

3. Materials and Methods

3.1. Materials

Chitosan (deacetylation > 95%) was purchased from Jinhu Crust Product Corp (zi bo, Shandong, China). Chitosanase fermented by Renibacter ium sp.QD1 was obtained from the Ocean University of China. Acrolein was purchased from Xiya Reagent (Chengdu, China). MitoTracker Red CM-H_2Xros and Trizol Reagent were purchased from Invitrogen (Foster City, CA, USA). PrimeScript RT-PCR Kit was purchased from TaKaRa (Dalian, China). The reduced glutathione (GSH) assay kit was purchased from the Nanjing Jiancheng Bioengineering Institute (Nanjing, China). The MTT cell proliferation and cytotoxicity detection kits, phenyl methane sulfonyl fluoride (PMSF), reactive oxygen species (ROS) detection kit, mitochondrial membrane potential (MMP) detection kit, BCA protein assay kit, CuZn/Mn-SOD assay kit (WST-8), cellular glutathione peroxidase (GPx) assay kit, Nuclear and Cytoplasmic Protein Extraction kit, PVDF membranes, and BCIP/NBT Alkaline Phosphatase Color Development kit were purchased from the Beyotime Institute of Biotechnology (Shanghai, China). Nrf2 XP Rabbit mAb and Histone H3 XP Rabbit mAb were purchased from Cell signaling technology (Boston, MA, USA). All other reagents were obtained from Sigma-Aldrich (Saint Louis, MO, USA), unless otherwise stated.

3.2. Chitosan Oligosaccharide (COSs) Preparation and Purification

The COSs were prepared via the enzymatic hydrolysis of chitosan and purified with gel filtration chromatography according to a previously reported method [24]. In brief, chitosan (10 g) was added to 80 mL of distilled water, then 1.5 mL of chitosanase solution (10 U/mL) was added. The mixture was stirred at 50 °C for 24 h, and the pH of the reaction mixture was adjusted to 5~6 with HCl solution (4 mol/L) during the hydrolysis process. The hydrolysate was adjusted to pH 8~9 with NaOH solution (1 mol/L) and filtered to remove insoluble parts. The filtrate was concentrated and precipitated by adding a four-fold volume of ethanol at 4 °C overnight. The precipitate was collected via centrifugation for 15 min at 8000 rpm, and then lyophilized to yield powdered products, and identified as a COS mixture.

The COS mixture (200 mg) was dissolved in 2 mL of 0.1 M NH_4HCO_3, and then filtered with a microporous membrane (0.22 μm) to obtain a clear solution. The filtrate was loaded on a Bio Gel P6 column (2.6 × 110 cm) that was connected to an AKTA UPC100 purification system (GE Healthcare, Fairfield, CT, USA) equipped with an online refractive index detector. The column was eluted with 0.1 M NH_4HCO_3 solution at a flow rate 0.5 mL/min. Eluents (8 mL/tube) were collected using a fraction collector to afford the pure dimers, trimers, tetramers, pentamers, and hexamers of the COSs. The COSs were analyzed using the high-performance liquid chromatography (HPLC), mass spectra, nuclear magnetic resonance (NMR) and Fourier-transform infrared spectroscopy (FT-IR) methods [24].

3.3. N-Acetylated Chitooligosaccharide (NACOs) Preparation and Purification

The NACOs were prepared via the acetylation of COSs according to a previously reported method [26]. Briefly, the dried COS mixture (1 g) and $NaHCO_3$ (756 mg) were added to methanol–water solution (8:1; *v*/*v*, 35 mL) with stirring, and 5 mL of acetic anhydride was added dropwise at 0 °C with stirring. After stirring for 4 h at room temperature, the NACO mixture solution was filtered to remove insoluble parts and the reaction completion was monitored using TLC (*n*-propanol:water, 2:1, *v*/*v*). The filtrate was concentrated and lyophilized to obtain the NACO mixture powder.

Then, the NACO mixture (500 mg) was dissolved in 2 mL of water, and filtered with a microporous membrane (0.22 μm). The filtrate was loaded on a graphitization of carbon black column (2.6 × 20 cm) that was connected to an AKTA UPC100 purification system (GE Healthcare, Fairfield, CT, USA). After loading the sample, the column was eluted with the following gradient of water and ethanol with a gradient of solvent B (ethanol) as follows: 0% B for 3 CV (column volume), then up to 60% B over 5 CV. Eluents (10 mL/tube) were collected using a fraction collector and monitored using TLC (*n*-propanol:water, 2:1, *v*/*v*). Pure dimers, trimers, tetramers, pentamers, and hexamers of the NACOs were pooled and lyophilized. The NACO samples were identified via HPLC chromatogram, mass spectra, nuclear magnetic resonance (NMR) and Fourier-transform infrared spectroscopy (FT-IR) analysis.

3.4. MTT Assay for Cell Viability

The ARPE-19 (human retinal pigment epithelial) cell line was purchased from ATCC (CRL2302) and cultured in a DMEM-F12 medium supplemented with 10% fetal bovine serum, 0.348% sodium bicarbonate, 2 mM L-glutamine, 100 μg/mL of streptomycin, and 100 U/mL of penicillin. The cell culture was maintained at 37 °C in a humidified atmosphere of 95% air and 5% CO_2 [50]. ARPE-19 cells were used within 10 generations, and the medium was changed every two days. COSs and NCOSs were dissolved with PBS buffer, filtered through a sterile 0.22 μm filter, and diluted with complete culture medium to different concentrations for the cell experiments.

The ARPE-19 cells were seeded in 96-well plates at 5×10^4 cells per well and incubated overnight. After incubation with different concentrations of COSs or NCOSs for 48 h, the cells were treated with 75 μM acrolein for 24 h. Cell viability was measured via MTT cell proliferation and a cytotoxicity detection kit (Beyotime). After 4 h of incubation with MTT, the solubilization buffer was added to each well and incubated at 37 °C overnight. The optical densities were read at 555 nm using a SpectraMax M5 plate reader (Molecular Devices, Sunnyvale, CA, USA).

3.5. Antioxidant Enzyme Activities, ROS Generation, and Intracellular GSH Levels Assay

The GSH level, superoxide dismutase (SOD) activity, and GPx activity were determined using commercial assay kits [51]. Briefly, cells were placed in 6-well plates at a density of 5×10^5 cells per well. After 12 h, the cells were treated for 48 h with 400 μM of COS–5 or N–5 and then for 24 h with or without 75 μM acrolein. After treatment, the cells were washed twice with PBS, and then the antioxidant enzyme activities and GSH level in the cells were detected.

Moreover, the ROS levels in PRE cells and mitochondria exposed to acrolein were determined using fluorescent probe. In brief, cells were plated in 96-well plates at a density of 2.5×10^4 cells per well for 12 h. ARPE-19 cells were treated with 400 μM of COS–5 or N–5 for 48 h, and then incubated with or without 75 μM acrolein for another 24 h. The ROS level in PRE cells was determined by the 2′, 7′-dichlorofluorescein diacetate (DCFH-DA) method using a SpectraMax M5 plate reader (Molecular Devices, San Jose, CA, USA) at a 488 nm excitation wavelength and a 525 nm emission wavelength [52]. The ROS generation in mitochondria was detected using MitoTracker Red CM-H_2Xros at a 579 nm excitation wavelength and a 599 nm emission wavelength.

3.6. Confocal Imaging

ARPE-19 cells were cultured on glass-bottom cell culture dishes at a density of 2×10^4 cells per well for 12 h. The cells were incubated with 25 nM MitoTracker Red CMXROS at 37 °C for 30 min. Thereafter, the cells washed three times with PBS to remove unbound probes. Then, the cells were incubated with FITC (100 μM) or FITC-labeled N–5 (100 μM) for 3 h at 37 °C. Cellular uptake was terminated by washing the cells three times with PBS. Finally, the cells were observed under a Nikon A1 confocal microscope (Nikon Corporation, Tokyo, Japan). The green fluorescence of FITC was measured at Ex495/Em525, and the red fluorescence of MitoTracker Red CMXRos was measured at Ex578/Em599 [53].

3.7. Mitochondrial Dysfunction Evaluation

Mitochondrial membrane potential (MMP) was detected in live ARPE-19 cells using a cationic fluorescent indicator JC-1, according to the manufacturer's instructions. Briefly, APRE-19 cells were seeded at a density of 2.5×10^4 cells per well in a 96-well plate. After 12 h, the cells were exposed to 400 μmol/mL of N–5 for 48 h. After treatment with 75 μmol/mL of acrolein for 24 h, the cells were treated with JC-1 for 30 min at 37 °C, washed with PBS, and observed under the fluorescence microscope. The $\Delta\psi m$ of ARPE-19 cells in each treatment group was calculated as the fluorescence ratio (590 to 530 nm) [54].

3.8. Western Blot

Western blot was performed as in previously described methods [55] and each Western blot was repeated at least three times. Nuclear proteins were prepared using a Nuclear and Cytoplasmic Protein Extraction Kit, and nuclear Nrf2 was analyzed using Western blot. Briefly, the lysates were homogenized and centrifuged at 13,000 $\times g$ for 15 min at 4 °C. The supernatants were collected, and the protein concentrations were determined using the BCA Protein Assay kit. Equal amounts (20 µg) of each protein sample were loaded on 10% SDS-PAGE gels, electrophoresed, transferred to PVDF membranes, and blocked with 5% non-fat milk. The membranes were incubated with anti-Nrf2 (1:1000) and anti-histone H3 (1:1000) at 4 °C overnight, and then incubated with anti-mouse secondary antibodies at room temperature for 1 h. Protein bands were visualized using a BCIP/NBT Alkaline Phosphatase Color Development Kit. Signals were quantified using ImageJ software (Version 1.52b, NIH, Baltimore, MD, USA), and defined as the ratio of target protein to histone H3.

3.9. Real-Time PCR

Real-time PCR was performed using a previously described method [56]. Total RNA was extracted from the cells using Trizol reagent according to the manufacturer's protocol. Reverse transcription was performed using the PrimeScript RT-PCR Kit followed by semiquantitative real-time PCR using specific primers. The primer sequences are listed in Table 3.

Table 3. Primer sequences.

Primers	Forward	Reverse
HO-1	GGTCCTTACACTCAGCTTTCT	CATAGGCTCCTTCCTCCTTTC
NQO1	AAAGGACCCTTCCGGAGTAA	CCATCCTTCCAGGATTTGAA
β-actin	ACCCTGAAGTACCCCATCGAG	GGATAGCACAGCCTGGATAGCA

3.10. Statistical Analysis

All quantitative experiments were repeated at least 3 times independently. Data are presented as mean ± SD. Data were analyzed by one-way analysis of variance (ANOVA) with Tukey's multiple comparison post hoc test using GraphPad Prism 8.0 Statistics Software (Graphpad Software, Inc., La Jolla, CA, USA). A p value of < 0.05 was considered statistically significant.

4. Conclusions

In conclusion, our study demonstrated that chitosan oligosaccharides (COSs) and their *N*-acetylated chitooligosaccharides (NACOs) exhibited excellent protection effects on acrolein-induced ARPE-19 cell damage. Among the monomers, COS-5 or N-5 pretreatment significantly reduced reactive oxygen species production, raised the intracellular level of GSH and the activity of SOD and GSH-Px, and attenuated the loss of mitochondrial membrane potential. Further study indicated that the N-5 could localize in the mitochondria and promote Nrf2 nuclear transfer and the expression of downstream phase II detoxification enzymes. These results suggest that COSs and NACOs might be promising antagonists against acrolein-induced APRE-19 cell death.

Supplementary Materials: The following supporting information can be downloaded at: https://www.mdpi.com/article/10.3390/md21030137/s1, Figure S1: The cytotoxicity of COSs, NACOs and PACOs in ARPE-19 cell; Figure S2: Effects of COSs and NACOs on the proliferation of ARPE-19 cells; Figure S3: COS-5 and N-5 against acrolein-induced oxidative stress; Figure S4: Protective effect of COS-5 and N-5 against acrolein-induced ARPE-19 mitochondrial dysfunction.

Author Contributions: Conceptualization: C.Y. and C.L.; investigation: C.Y., R.Y. and M.G.; project administration: C.L.; formal analysis: C.Y., R.Y., J.H. and C.L.; data curation: C.Y.; resources: C.Y., R.Y. and M.G.; writing—original draft: C.Y.; writing—review and editing: S.W. and C.L.; supervision: S.W. and C.L.; funding acquisition: S.W. and C.L. All authors have read and agreed to the published version of the manuscript.

Funding: This research was supported in part by programs of the Shandong Major Science and Technology Project (2021ZDSYS22), National Natural Science Foundation of China (U21A20297), Shandong Provincial Natural Science Foundation (ZR2021QH144), National Science and Technology Major Project for Significant New Drugs Development (2018ZX09735004).

Institutional Review Board Statement: Not applicable.

Informed Consent Statement: Not applicable.

Data Availability Statement: Not applicable.

Conflicts of Interest: The authors declare no conflict of interest.

References

1. Wong, W.L.; Su, X.Y.; Li, X.; Cheung, C.M.G.; Klein, R.; Cheng, C.Y.; Wong, T.Y. Global prevalence of age-related macular degeneration and disease burden projection for 2020 and 2040: A systematic review and meta-analysis. *Lancet Glob. Health* **2014**, *2*, E106–E116. [CrossRef]
2. Yan, Y.T.; Ren, Y.F.; Li, X.M.; Zhang, X.X.; Guo, H.Q.; Han, Y.T.; Hu, J.X. A polysaccharide from green tea (*Camellia sinensis* L.) protects human retinal endothelial cells against hydrogen peroxide-induced oxidative injury and apoptosis. *Int. J. Biol. Macromol.* **2018**, *115*, 600–607. [CrossRef]
3. Zhang, X.H.; Bohner, A.; Bhuvanagiri, S.; Uehara, H.; Upadhyay, A.K.; Emerson, L.L.; Bondalapati, S.; Muddana, S.K.; Fang, D.; Li, M.L.; et al. Targeted Intraceptor Nanoparticle for Neovascular Macular Degeneration: Preclinical Dose Optimization and Toxicology Assessment. *Mol. Ther.* **2017**, *25*, 1606–1615. [CrossRef]
4. Handa, J.T.; Rickman, C.B.; Dick, A.D.; Gorin, M.B.; Miller, J.W.; Toth, C.A.; Ueffing, M.; Zarbin, M.; Farrer, L.A. A systems biology approach towards understanding and treating non-neovascular age-related macular degeneration. *Nat. Commun.* **2019**, *10*, 3347. [CrossRef]
5. Felszeghy, S.; Viiri, J.; Paterno, J.J.; Hyttinen, J.M.T.; Koskela, A.; Chen, M.; Leinonen, H.; Tanila, H.; Kivinen, N.; Koistinen, A.; et al. Loss of NRF-2 and PGC-1alpha genes leads to retinal pigment epithelium damage resembling dry age-related macular degeneration. *Redox Biol.* **2019**, *20*, 1–12. [CrossRef]
6. Abd, A.J.; Kanwar, R.K.; Kanwar, J.R. Aged macular degeneration: Current therapeutics for management and promising new drug candidates. *Drug Discov. Today* **2017**, *22*, 1671–1679. [CrossRef]
7. Koskela, A.; Manai, F.; Basagni, F.; Liukkonen, M.; Rosini, M.; Govoni, S.; Dal Monte, M.; Smedowski, A.; Kaarniranta, K.; Amadio, M. Nature-Inspired Hybrids (NIH) Improve Proteostasis by Activating Nrf2-Mediated Protective Pathways in Retinal Pigment Epithelial Cells. *Antioxidants* **2022**, *11*, 1385. [CrossRef]
8. Chuang, C.J.; Wang, M.L.; Yeh, J.H.; Chen, T.C.; Tsou, S.C.; Lee, Y.J.; Chang, Y.Y.; Lin, H.W. The Protective Effects of alpha-Mangostin Attenuate Sodium Iodate-Induced Cytotoxicity and Oxidative Injury via Mediating SIRT-3 Inactivation via the PI3K/AKT/PGC-1 alpha Pathway. *Antioxidants* **2021**, *10*, 1870. [CrossRef]
9. Wen, X.W.; Li, S.; Zhang, Y.F.; Zhu, L.; Xi, X.T.; Zhang, S.Y.; Li, Y. Recombinant human klotho protects against hydrogen peroxide-mediated injury in human retinal pigment epithelial cells via the PI3K/Akt-Nrf2/HO-1 signaling pathway. *Bioengineered* **2022**, *13*, 11767–11781. [CrossRef]
10. Jeung, I.C.; Jee, D.; Rho, C.R.; Kang, S. *Melissa officinalis* L. Extracts Protect Human Retinal Pigment Epithelial Cells against Oxidative Stress-Induced Apoptosis. *Int. J. Med. Sci.* **2016**, *13*, 139–146. [CrossRef]
11. Datta, S.; Cano, M.; Ebrahimi, K.; Wang, L.; Handa, J.T. The impact of oxidative stress and inflammation on RPE degeneration in non-neovascular AMD. *Prog. Retin. Eye Res.* **2017**, *60*, 201–218. [CrossRef] [PubMed]
12. Yao, J.; Bi, H.E.; Sheng, Y.; Cheng, L.B.; Wendu, R.L.; Wang, C.H.; Cao, G.F.; Jiang, Q. Ultraviolet (UV) and Hydrogen Peroxide Activate Ceramide-ER Stress-AMPK Signaling Axis to Promote Retinal Pigment Epithelium (RPE) Cell Apoptosis. *Int. J. Mol. Sci.* **2013**, *14*, 10355–10368. [CrossRef]
13. Nashine, S.; Nesburn, A.B.; Kuppermann, B.D.; Kenney, M.C. Role of Resveratrol in Transmitochondrial AMD RPE Cells. *Nutrients* **2020**, *12*, 159. [CrossRef]
14. Cao, G.F.; Liu, Y.; Yang, W.; Wan, J.; Yao, J.; Wan, Y.S.; Jiang, Q. Rapamycin sensitive mTOR activation mediates nerve growth factor (NGF) induced cell migration and pro-survival effects against hydrogen peroxide in retinal pigment epithelial cells. *Biochem. Biophys. Res. Commun.* **2011**, *414*, 499–505. [CrossRef]
15. Goncalves, I.R.; Brouillet, S.; Soulie, M.C.; Gribaldo, S.; Sirven, C.; Charron, N.; Boccara, M.; Choquer, M. Genome-wide analyses of chitin synthases identify horizontal gene transfers towards bacteria and allow a robust and unifying classification into fungi. *BMC Evol. Biol.* **2016**, *16*, 252. [CrossRef]

16. Chua, E.T.; Shekh, A.Y.; Eltanahy, E.; Thomas-Hall, S.R.; Schenk, P.M. Effective Harvesting ofNannochloropsisMicroalgae Using Mushroom Chitosan: A Pilot-Scale Study. *Front. Bioeng. Biotechnol.* **2020**, *8*, 711. [CrossRef]
17. Ahmad, S.I.; Ahmad, R.; Khan, M.S.; Kant, R.; Shahid, S.; Gautam, L.; Hasan, G.M.; Hassan, M.I. Chitin and its derivatives: Structural properties and biomedical applications. *Int. J. Biol. Macromol.* **2020**, *164*, 526–539. [CrossRef]
18. Bonin, M.; Sreekumar, S.; Cord-Landwehr, S.; Moerschbacher, B.M. Preparation of Defined Chitosan Oligosaccharides Using Chitin Deacetylases. *Int. J. Mol. Sci.* **2020**, *21*, 7835. [CrossRef]
19. Yuan, X.B.; Zheng, J.P.; Jiao, S.M.; Cheng, G.; Feng, C.; Du, Y.G.; Liu, H.T. A review on the preparation of chitosan oligosaccharides and application to human health, animal husbandry and agricultural production. *Carbohydr. Polym.* **2019**, *220*, 60–70. [CrossRef]
20. Tao, W.J.; Sun, W.J.; Liu, L.J.; Wang, G.; Xiao, Z.P.; Pei, X.; Wang, M.Q. Chitosan Oligosaccharide Attenuates Nonalcoholic Fatty Liver Disease Induced by High Fat Diet through Reducing Lipid Accumulation, Inflammation and Oxidative Stress in C57BL/6 Mice. *Mar. Drugs* **2019**, *17*, 645. [CrossRef]
21. Mattaveewong, T.; Wongkrasant, P.; Chanchai, S.; Pichyangkura, R.; Chatsudthipong, V.; Muanprasat, C. Chitosan oligosaccharide suppresses tumor progression in a mouse model of colitis-associated colorectal cancer through AMPK activation and suppression of NF-kappa B and mTOR signaling. *Carbohydr. Polym.* **2016**, *145*, 30–36. [CrossRef]
22. Fang, I.M.; Yang, C.H.; Yang, C.M.; Chen, M.S. Chitosan Oligosaccharides Attenuates Oxidative-Stress Related Retinal Degeneration in Rats. *PLoS ONE* **2013**, *8*, e77323. [CrossRef]
23. Xu, W.; Huang, H.C.; Lin, C.J.; Jiang, Z.F. Chitooligosaccharides protect rat cortical neurons against copper induced damage by attenuating intracellular level of reactive oxygen species. *Bioorg. Med. Chem. Lett.* **2010**, *20*, 3084–3088. [CrossRef]
24. Hao, C.; Gao, L.X.; Zhang, Y.R.; Wang, W.; Yu, G.L.; Guan, H.S.; Zhang, L.J.; Li, C.X. Acetylated Chitosan Oligosaccharides Act as Antagonists against Glutamate-Induced PC12 Cell Death via Bcl-2/Bax Signal Pathway. *Mar. Drugs* **2015**, *13*, 1267–1289. [CrossRef]
25. Chang, S.H.; Wu, C.H.; Tsai, G.J. Effects of chitosan molecular weight on its antioxidant and antimutagenic properties. *Carbohydr. Polym.* **2018**, *181*, 1026–1032. [CrossRef]
26. Morando, M.; Yao, Y.; Martin-Santamaria, S.; Zhu, Z.; Xu, T.; Canada, F.J.; Zhang, Y.; Jimenez-Barbero, J. Mimicking chitin: Chemical synthesis, conformational analysis, and molecular recognition of the beta(1→3) *N*-acetylchitopentaose analogue. *Chemistry* **2010**, *16*, 4239–4249. [CrossRef]
27. Li, K.C.; Liu, S.; Xing, R.G.; Qin, Y.K.; Li, P.C. Preparation, characterization and antioxidant activity of two partially *N*-acetylated chitotrioses. *Carbohydr. Polym.* **2013**, *92*, 1730–1736. [CrossRef]
28. Xiong, C.N.; Wu, H.G.; Wei, P.; Pan, M.; Tuo, Y.Q.; Kusakabe, I.; Du, Y.G. Potent angiogenic inhibition effects of deacetylated chitohexaose separated from chitooligosaccharides and its mechanism of action in vitro. *Carbohydr. Res.* **2009**, *344*, 1975–1983. [CrossRef]
29. Wei, X.L.; Wang, Y.F.; Xiao, J.B.; Xia, W.S. Separation of chitooligosaccharides and the potent effects on gene expression of cell surface receptor CR3. *Int. J. Biol. Macromol.* **2009**, *45*, 432–436. [CrossRef]
30. Liang, C.Y.; Ling, Y.; Wei, F.; Huang, L.J.; Li, X.M. A novel antibacterial biomaterial mesh coated by chitosan and tigecycline for pelvic floor repair and its biological performance. *Regen. Biomater.* **2020**, *7*, 483–490. [CrossRef]
31. Sun, L.J.; Luo, C.; Long, H.A.; Wei, D.Z.; Liu, H.K. Acrolein is a mitochondrial toxin: Effects on respiratory function and enzyme activities in isolated rat liver mitochondria. *Mitochondrion* **2006**, *6*, 136–142. [CrossRef]
32. Feng, Z.H.; Liu, Z.B.; Li, X.S.; Jia, H.Q.; Sun, L.J.; Tian, C.A.; Jia, L.H.; Liu, J.K. alpha-Tocopherol is an effective Phase II enzyme inducer: Protective effects on acrolein-induced oxidative stress and mitochondrial dysfunction in human retinal pigment epithelial cells. *J. Nutr. Biochem.* **2010**, *21*, 1222–1231. [CrossRef]
33. Li, Y.; Zou, X.; Cao, K.; Xu, J.; Yue, T.T.; Dai, F.; Zhou, B.; Lu, W.Y.; Feng, Z.H.; Liu, J.K. Curcumin analog 1, 5-bis (2-trifluoromethylphenyl)-1, 4-pentadieN-3-one exhibits enhanced ability on Nrf2 activation and protection against acrolein-induced ARPE-19 cell toxicity. *Toxicol. Appl. Pharm.* **2013**, *272*, 726–735. [CrossRef]
34. Li, X.; Liu, Z.B.; Luo, C.; Jia, H.Q.; Sun, L.J.; Hou, B.; Shen, W.; Packer, L.; Cotman, C.W.; Liu, J.K. Lipoamide protects retinal pigment epithelial cells from oxidative stress and mitochondrial dysfunction. *Free Radic. Biol. Med.* **2008**, *44*, 1465–1474. [CrossRef]
35. Jin, L.; Abrahams, J.P.; Skinner, R.; Petitou, M.; Pike, R.N.; Carrell, R.W. The anticoagulant activation of antithrombin by heparin. *Proc. Natl. Acad. Sci. USA* **1997**, *94*, 14683–14688. [CrossRef]
36. Wang, K.; Zhu, X.; Zhang, K.; Yao, Y.; Zhuang, M.; Tan, C.Y.; Zhou, F.F.; Zhu, L. Puerarin inhibits amyloid beta-induced NLRP3 inflammasome activation in retinal pigment epithelial cells via suppressing ROS-dependent oxidative and endoplasmic reticulum stresses. *Exp. Cell Res.* **2017**, *357*, 335–340. [CrossRef]
37. Zhu, C.; Dong, Y.C.; Liu, H.L.; Ren, H.; Cui, Z.H. Hesperetin protects against H2O2- triggered oxidative damage via upregulation of the Keap1-Nrf2/ HO-1 signal pathway in ARPE-19 cells. *Biomed. Pharmacother.* **2017**, *88*, 124–133. [CrossRef]
38. Zalewska-Ziob, M.; Adamek, B.; Kasperczyk, J.; Romuk, E.; Hudziec, E.; Chwalinska, E.; Dobija-Kubica, K.; Rogozinski, P.; Brulinski, K. Activity of Antioxidant Enzymes in the Tumor and Adjacent Noncancerous Tissues of Non-Small-Cell Lung Cancer. *Oxidative Med. Cell. Longev.* **2019**, *2019*, 2901840. [CrossRef]
39. Sena, L.A.; Li, S.; Jairaman, A.; Prakriya, M.; Ezponda, T.; Hildeman, D.A.; Wang, C.R.; Schumacker, P.T.; Licht, J.D.; Perlman, H.; et al. Mitochondria Are Required for Antigen-Specific T Cell Activation through Reactive Oxygen Species Signaling. *Immunity* **2013**, *38*, 225–236. [CrossRef]

40. Li, X.; Zhou, C.R.; Chen, X.F.; Zhao, M.Y. Subcellular localization of chitosan oligosaccharides in living cells. *Chin. Sci. Bull.* **2014**, *59*, 2449–2454. [CrossRef]
41. Chu, X.Y.; Liu, Y.M.; Zhang, H.Y. Activating or Inhibiting Nrf2? *Trends Pharmacol. Sci.* **2017**, *38*, 953–955. [CrossRef]
42. Ma, Q. Role of Nrf2 in Oxidative Stress and Toxicity. *Annu. Rev. Pharmacol.* **2013**, *53*, 401–426. [CrossRef]
43. Jia, L.H.; Liu, Z.B.; Sun, L.J.; Miller, S.S.; Ames, B.N.; Cotman, C.W.; Liu, J.K. Acrolein, a toxicant in cigarette smoke, causes oxidative damage and mitochondrial dysfunction in RPE cells: Protection by (R)-alpha-lipoic acid. *Investig. Ophthalmol. Vis. Sci.* **2007**, *48*, 339–348. [CrossRef] [PubMed]
44. Zhao, D.; Wang, J.T.; Tan, L.J.; Sun, C.Y.; Dong, J.N. Synthesis of *N*-furoyl chitosan and chito-oligosaccharides and evaluation of their antioxidant activity in vitro. *Int. J. Biol. Macromol.* **2013**, *59*, 391–395. [CrossRef]
45. Sun, T.; Zhou, D.X.; Mao, F.; Zhu, Y.N. Preparation of low-molecular-weight carboxymethyl chitosan and their superoxide anion scavenging activity. *Eur. Polym. J.* **2007**, *43*, 652–656. [CrossRef]
46. Li, K.C.; Xing, R.G.; Liu, S.; Li, R.F.; Qin, Y.K.; Meng, X.T.; Li, P.C. Separation of chito-oligomers with several degrees of polymerization and study of their antioxidant activity. *Carbohydr. Polym.* **2012**, *88*, 896–903. [CrossRef]
47. Qu, D.F.; Han, J.Z. Investigation of the antioxidant activity of chitooligosaccharides on mice with high-fat diet. *Rev. Bras. Zootec.* **2016**, *45*, 661–666. [CrossRef]
48. Chen, L.; Zhu, Y.Q.; Zhou, J.; Wu, R.; Yang, N.; Bao, Q.B.; Xu, X.R. Luteolin Alleviates Epithelial-Mesenchymal Transformation Induced by Oxidative Injury in ARPE-19 Cell via Nrf2 and AKT/GSK-3 beta Pathway. *Oxidative Med. Cell. Longev.* **2022**, *2022*, 2265725.
49. Chen, W.P.; Ye, Y.X.; Wu, Z.R.; Lin, J.L.; Wang, Y.T.; Ding, Q.; Yang, X.R.; Yang, W.; Lin, B.Q.; Lin, B.Q. Temporary Upregulation of Nrf2 by Naringenin Alleviates Oxidative Damage in the Retina and ARPE-19 Cells. *Oxidative Med. Cell. Longev.* **2021**, *2021*, 4053276. [CrossRef]
50. Shivarudrappa, A.H.; Ponesakki, G. Lutein reverses hyperglycemia-mediated blockage of Nrf2 translocation by modulating the activation of intracellular protein kinases in retinal pigment epithelial (ARPE-19) cells. *J. Cell Commun. Signal.* **2020**, *14*, 207–221. [CrossRef]
51. Li, Y.; Hu, Z.T.; Chen, B.; Bu, Q.; Lu, W.J.; Deng, Y.; Zhu, R.M.; Shao, X.; Hou, J.; Zhao, J.X.; et al. Taurine attenuates methamphetamine-induced autophagy and apoptosis in PC12 cells through mTOR signaling pathway. *Toxicol. Lett.* **2012**, *215*, 1–7. [CrossRef] [PubMed]
52. Xu, Q.L.; Liu, M.Z.; Chao, X.H.; Zhang, C.L.; Yang, H.; Chen, J.H.; Zhao, C.X.; Zhou, B. Acidifiers Attenuate Diquat-Induced Oxidative Stress and Inflammatory Responses by Regulating NF-kappa B/MAPK/COX-2 Pathways in IPEC-J2 Cells. *Antioxidants* **2022**, *11*, 2002. [CrossRef]
53. Wang, X.L.; Jiang, H.; Zhang, N.; Cai, C.; Li, G.Y.; Hao, J.J.; Yu, G.L. Anti-diabetic activities of agaropectin-derived oligosaccharides from Gloiopeltis furcata via regulation of mitochondrial function. *Carbohydr. Polym.* **2020**, *229*, 115482. [CrossRef]
54. Lin, C.W.; Huang, H.H.; Yang, C.M.; Yang, C.H. Protective effect of chitosan oligosaccharides on blue light light-emitting diode induced retinal pigment epithelial cell damage. *J. Funct. Foods* **2018**, *49*, 12–19. [CrossRef]
55. Han, S.X.; Chen, J.J.; Hua, J.J.; Hu, X.J.; Jian, S.H.; Zheng, G.X.; Wang, J.; Li, H.R.; Yang, J.L.; Hejtmancik, J.F.; et al. MITF protects against oxidative damage-induced retinal degeneration by regulating the NRF2 pathway in the retinal pigment epithelium. *Redox Biol.* **2020**, *34*, 101537. [CrossRef]
56. You, L.T.; Peng, H.L.Y.; Liu, J.; Cai, M.R.; Wu, H.M.; Zhang, Z.Q.; Bai, J.; Yao, Y.; Dong, X.X.; Yin, X.B.; et al. Catalpol Protects ARPE-19 Cells against Oxidative Stress via Activation of the Keap1/Nrf2/ARE Pathway. *Cells* **2021**, *10*, 2635. [CrossRef]

marine drugs

Article

Identification and Characterization of a New Cold-Adapted and Alkaline Alginate Lyase TsAly7A from *Thalassomonas* sp. LD5 Produces Alginate Oligosaccharides with High Degree of Polymerization

Chengying Yin [1,2,3,4,†], Jiaxia Sun [1,2,3,4,†], Hainan Wang [1,2,3,4], Wengong Yu [1,2,3,4,*] and Feng Han [1,2,3,4,*]

1 Laboratory for Marine Drugs and Bioproducts of Qingdao Pilot National Laboratory for Marine Science and Technology, Qingdao 266237, China
2 Key Laboratory of Marine Drugs, Ministry of Education, Ocean University of China, Qingdao 266003, China
3 Shandong Provincial Key Laboratory of Glycoscience and Glycoengineering, Ocean University of China, Qingdao 266003, China
4 School of Medicine and Pharmacy, Ocean University of China, Qingdao 266003, China
* Correspondence: yuwg66@ouc.edu.cn (W.Y.); fhan@ouc.edu.cn (F.H.); Tel.: +86-532-82032067 (F.H.)
† These authors contributed equally to this work.

Abstract: Alginate oligosaccharides (AOS) and their derivatives become popular due to their favorable biological activity, and the key to producing functional AOS is to find efficient alginate lyases. This study showed one alginate lyase TsAly7A found in *Thalassomonas* sp. LD5, which was predicted to have excellent industrial properties. Bioinformatics analysis and enzymatic properties of recombinant TsAly7A (rTsAly7A) were investigated. TsAly7A belonged to the fifth subfamily of polysaccharide lyase family 7 (PL7). The optimal temperature and pH of rTsAly7A was 30 °C and 9.1 in Glycine-NaOH buffer, respectively. The pH stability of rTsAly7A under alkaline conditions was pretty good and it can remain at above 90% of the initial activity at pH 8.9 in Glycine-NaOH buffer for 12 h. In the presence of 100 mM NaCl, rTsAly7A showed the highest activity, while in the absence of NaCl, 50% of the highest activity was observed. The rTsAly7A was an endo-type alginate lyase, and its end-products of alginate degradation were unsaturated oligosaccharides (degree of polymerization 2–6). Collectively, the rTsAly7A may be a good industrial production tool for producing AOS with high degree of polymerization.

Keywords: alginate lyase; endo-type; alkaliphilic; polyM-preferred; cold-adaption; high degree of polymerization

Citation: Yin, C.; Sun, J.; Wang, H.; Yu, W.; Han, F. Identification and Characterization of a New Cold-Adapted and Alkaline Alginate Lyase TsAly7A from *Thalassomonas* sp. LD5 Produces Alginate Oligosaccharides with High Degree of Polymerization. *Mar. Drugs* **2023**, *21*, 6. https://doi.org/10.3390/md21010006

Academic Editors: Yuya Kumagai, Hideki Kishimura and Benwei Zhu

Received: 6 December 2022
Revised: 17 December 2022
Accepted: 20 December 2022
Published: 22 December 2022

1. Introduction

Alginate is a natural linear anionic polymer which consists of β-D-mannuronic acid (M) and α-L-guluronic acid (G) linked by β-1,4-glycosidic bonds [1]. It is the only natural marine biological polysaccharide with one carboxyl in each sugar ring [2]. Alginate polymer blocks arrange in three possible ways: poly-α-L-guluronic acid (polyG), poly-β-D-mannuronic acid (polyM), and hetero-polymeric random sequences (polyMG). These characteristics lead to the difference of their high-order structures, so polyM, polyG and their derivatives display different activities [3]. In medical fields, alginates with different arrangement and degree of polymerization (DP) have wide application prospects, including drug delivery and tissue engineering [4–6]. Alginate oligosaccharides (AOS) and their derivatives with different DPs are becoming popular due to their favorable biological activity and water solubility [1]. Most importantly, AOS have been found to play an important role in anti-tumor [7], anti-inflammatory [8], neuroprotective [9], immune regulation [10], anti-obesity [11], antibacterial [12], antioxidant [13,14], anti-diabetic [15] and other aspects [16,17]. These functions of AOS were mostly relevant to gut microbiota. For example,

Zhang et al. proposed that fecal microbiota transplantation (FMT) from AOS-dosed mice improved small intestine function by increasing beneficial microbes [8], and another study showed that GV-971 could suppress neuroinflammation through inhibiting gut dysbiosis to reduce phenylalanine/isoleucine accumulation [9]. In addition, Li et al. determined that unsaturated alginate oligosaccharides (UAOS) obtained by enzyme degradation showed significant anti-obesity effects in a high-fat diet (HFD) mouse model [18], and then they determined that UAOS can attenuate the HFD-induced obesity through modulating gut microbiota by selectively increasing the relative abundance of beneficial intestinal bacteria and decreasing the abundance of inflammogenic bacteria [19]. The different types of AOS had different functions in past studies, including the immuno-stimulatory activity of guluronate oligosaccharide (GOS) [10], the hypoglycaemic and hypolipidaemic activities of oligosaccharide from *S. confusum* (SCO) [15] and the neuroprotective activity of GV-971 (a sodium oligomannate) as mentioned above [9]. It is worth mentioning that UAOS performed significant anti-obesity effects compared with saturated alginate oligosaccharides (SAOS) [18,19].

At present, enzymatic degradation is the most common method to prepare AOS, so the key to producing functional AOS is to find efficient alginate lyases [16,17]. According to amino acid sequence, alginate lyases are divided into 12 polysaccharide lyase families (PL5, 6, 7, 14, 15, 17, 18, 31, 32, 34, 36, 39, 41) in the CAZy database [20]. The PL7 family (http://www.cazy.org/PL7.html, accessed on 11 February 2022) contains the most alginate lyases and is further divided into six subfamilies [21,22]. In addition, based on substrate specificity, it can be classified into polyG-specific, polyM-specific, bifunctional alginate lyase and polyMG-specific alginate lyase [23–25]. Based on the different modes of action, it can also be categorized into endo- and exo-type alginate lyases [26]. Endo-type alginate lyases can cleave the glycosidic bonds in alginate polymer randomly and release unsaturated oligosaccharides (disaccharides, trisaccharides and tetrasaccharides) as the main products. Exo-type alginate lyases cut the alginate chains successively from non-reducing ends to produce monosaccharides.

This study cloned and expressed a new PL7 alginate lyase-encoding gene, *tsaly7A*, from *Thalassomonas* sp. LD5. The recombinant TsAly7A (rTsAly7A) exhibited good properties such as pH stability under alkaline conditions, high activity under low temperature, and wide range of product distribution. These characteristics make rTsAly7A a good industrial production tool for producing AOS with high DPs.

2. Results

2.1. Sequence Analysis of TsAly7A

One predicted alginate lyase gene, *tsaly7A*, was detected and cloned from *Thalassomonas* sp. LD5, composed of 939 bp, encoding 312 amino acid residues. It only contained a catalytic module (CM) as shown in Figure 1A. The original length of *tsaly7A* (*OL-tsaly7A*) had a signal peptide (SP) at the N-terminal end with a length of 17 amino acid residues, a carbohydrate binding module (CBM) at middle with a length of 161 amino acid residues and a CM at C-terminal end (Figure 1A). The theoretical molecular weight of TsAly7A was 34.39 kDa and theoretical pI was 4.57. The sequence data were deposited in GenBank with accession No. OM672104.1. According to the results of Protein BLAST search, the similarity rate between TsAly7A and AlgMsp of PL7 family from *Microbulbifer* sp. 6532A [27] was 71%, indicating that TsAly7A was a new member of PL7. Further phylogenetic analysis proved that TsAly7A belonged to the fifth subfamily of PL7 (Figure 1B).

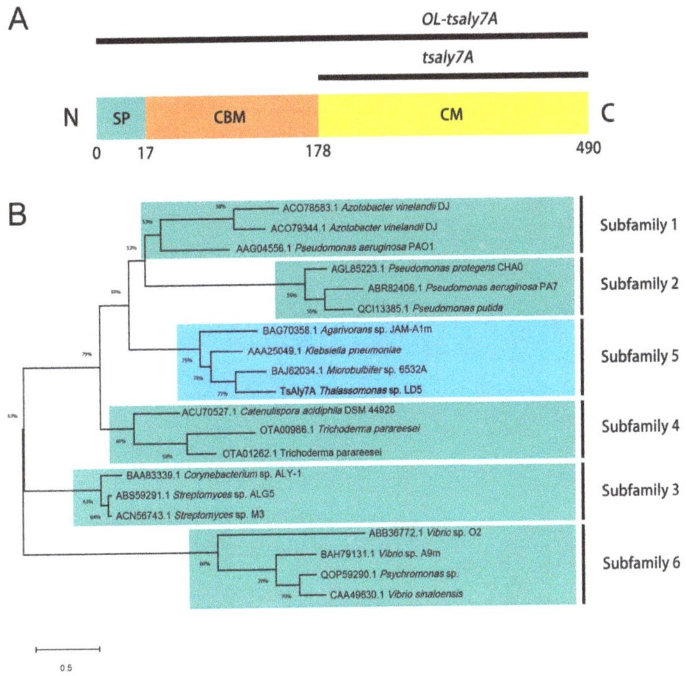

Figure 1. (**A**) Sequence analysis of TsAly7A. Domain structure of *OL-tsaly7A*. (**B**) Phylogenetic tree analysis of TsAly7A. The unrooted phylogenetic tree was constructed by the Maximum Likelihood method and JTT matrix-based model using MEGA X. Bootstrap analysis was computed with 1000 replicates, and bootstrap values below 50% were omitted. TsAly7A was marked with thickening in blue box. Subfamily 1, the first subfamily of PL7.

2.2. Expression and Purification of rTsAly7A

The rTsAly7A was successfully constructed and then expressed in *E. coli* BL21(DE3). By optimizing the induction conditions of rTsAly7A, the yield of rTsAly7A was highest at 18 °C and induced by 0.1 mM IPTG for 24 h (Figure 2A). After 1 L fermentation broth was purified, 13.46 mg pure enzyme of rTsAly7A was finally obtained. Through purification, the specific activity of rTsAly7A was 1536.36 U/mg, and the recovery rate was 31.41%. A single band on SDS-PAGE gel showed the molecular weight of the rTsAly7A was estimated to be about 40 kDa (Figure 2B).

2.3. Biochemical Characterization of the rTsAly7A

The optimum pH of rTsAly7A was 9.1 in Glycine-NaOH buffer (Figure 3A), while the enzyme activity at pH 7.0 was less than 50% of the highest. The enzyme activity of rTsAly7A remained above 80% after 12 h incubation in Na_2HPO_4-NaH_2PO_4 buffer (pH 7.0–8.0) and was most stable at pH 8.9 in Glycine-NaOH buffer for 12 h (Figure 3B), indicating that it was alkaliphilic.

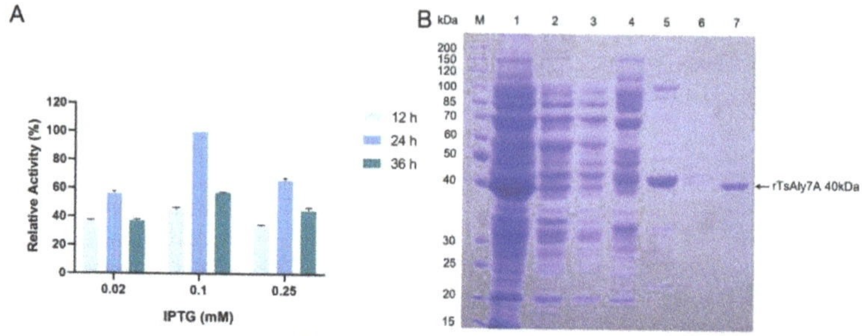

Figure 2. (**A**) Expression and purification of rTsAly7A. Relative enzyme activity of TsAly7A under different induction conditions. (**B**) SDS-PAGE of rTsAly7A. Lane M, protein standard marker; lane 1, crude enzyme; lane 2, flow-through; lane 3, elution by 0 mM imidazole; lane 4, elution by 25 mM imidazole; lane 5, elution by 75 mM imidazole; lane 6, elution by 150 mM imidazole; lane 7, elution by 300 mM imidazole, purified rTsAly7A.

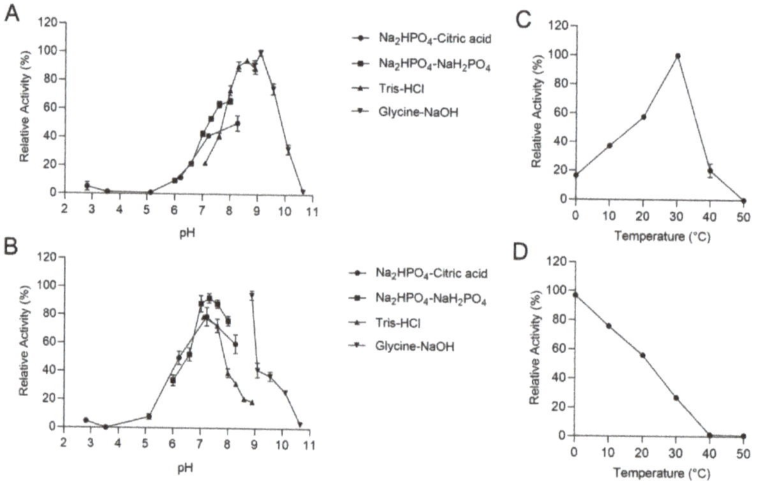

Figure 3. Biochemical properties of rTsAly7A. Optimal pH (**A**), pH stability (**B**), optimal temperature (**C**), thermal stability (**D**) of the rTsAly7A. The relative activity of 100% in (**A**,**C**) was determined at optimal condition. The original activity of 100% in (**B**,**D**) was determined before incubation at optimal condition.

The optimum temperature of rTsAly7A was 30 °C, but the enzyme activity decreased sharply over 30 °C (Figure 3C), whereas it exhibited 16% of highest activity at 0 °C. In addition, after incubation for an hour at 20 °C, it maintained half of the enzyme activity (Figure 3D). Therefore, rTsAly7A is a cold-adapted alginate lyase that can be used at room temperature.

Only Fe^{3+} promoted the enzyme activity by 1.5 times as shown in Figure 4A. The enzyme activity of rTsAly7A was significantly decreased with 1 mM Li^{+}, Cu^{2+}, Co^{2+}, Ba^{2+}, Ca^{2+} and Ni^{2+} (Figure 4A). As for 1mM Zn^{2+}, the enzyme activity of rTsAly7A was mostly lost. In the presence of EDTA, the enzyme activity of rTsAly7A was even completely lost. In addition, it is noteworthy that 1mM Na^{+}, K^{+}, NH_4^{+}, Mg^{2+}, Mn^{2+}, Fe^{2+}, and SDS had no significant effect on rTsAly7A. As shown in Figure 4B, rTsAly7A maintained 50% activity in the absence of NaCl and reached maximum activity in the presence of 100 mM NaCl.

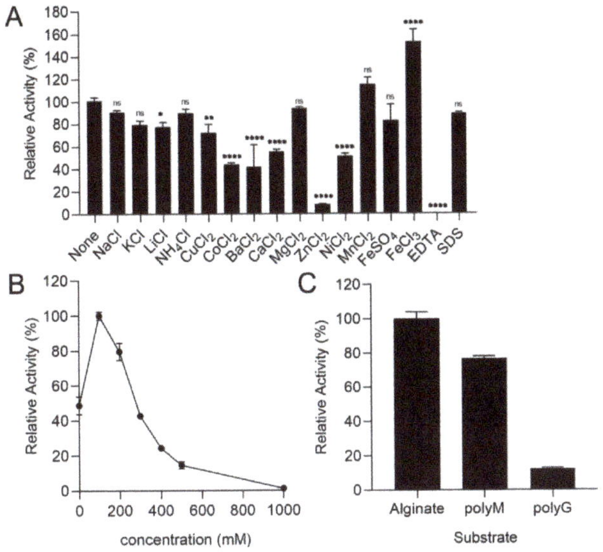

Figure 4. Effects of metal ions, chelator, and surfactant (1 mM) (**A**) and effects of NaCl concentrations (0–1 M) (**B**) on the activity of rTsAly7A. The substrate specificity of rTsAly7A (**C**). The relative activity of 100% was determined at optimal condition. **** for $p < 0.0001$, ** for $p < 0.01$, * for $p < 0.05$, ns for not significant.

2.4. The Substrate Specificity of rTsAly7A

The 0.3% (*w/v*) substrate was prepared under the optimum pH 9.1 and NaCl (100 mM) conditions, and the enzyme activity was determined by using substrate alginate, polyM and polyG, respectively. The degradation ability of polyM was 76% of that of alginate, and the degradation ability of polyG was weak, only 12% of that of alginate (Figure 4C).

2.5. Degradation Mode and End-Products of rTsAly7A

Size-Exclusion Chromatography (SEC) was used to reveal the time-course of alginate degradation by rTsAly7A. At the beginning of the degradation reaction, a large number of products with high DP appeared (Figure 5A). With the extension of degradation time, these products gradually degraded into oligosaccharides with lower DPs. It indicated that rTsAly7A was an endo-type alginate lyase, and some products with low DPs appeared at the initial stage of degradation reaction, indicating that the initial enzymatic reaction speed of the enzyme was very fast.

The SEC results of the final degradation products of rTsAly7A showed five UV absorption peaks at 12.6 mL, 13.2 mL, 13.9 mL, 14.7 mL and 15.6 mL, respectively, with a ratio of 0.24:1.07:1.78:1.16:1 (Figure 5B). The five peaks were collected and analyzed by ESI-MS. The results of mass spectrometry analysis were shown in Figure 5C. There are several obvious nuclear-to-mass ratio peaks in the mass spectrometry results, 351.06, 527.09, 703.12, 879.15 and 1055.18 *m/z* representing molecular peaks $[\Delta DP2{-}H]^-$, $[\Delta DP3{-}H]^-$, $[\Delta DP4{-}H]^-$, $[\Delta DP5{-}H]^-$, and $[\Delta DP6{-}H]^-$, respectively, which correspond to the molecular weights of unsaturated alginate disaccharide, trisaccharide, tetrasaccharide, pentasaccharide and hexasaccharide. Therefore, the final degradation product of rTsAly7A were unsaturated oligosaccharides of DP 2–6.

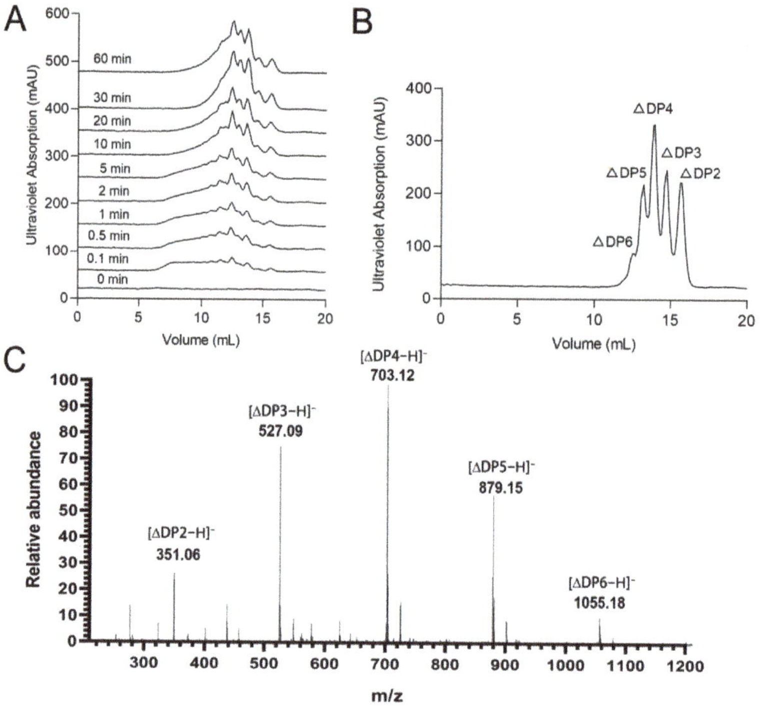

Figure 5. Degradation mode and end-products of rTsAly7A. The time-course of alginate degradation by rTsAly7A (**A**). SEC analysis of end-products of rTsAly7A (**B**). Mass spectra analysis of final product of rTsAly7A (**C**). ΔDP2, unsaturated alginate disaccharide.

3. Discussion

In this study, we characterized an endo-acting, cold-adapted and polyM-preferred alginate lyase TsAly7A from *Thalassomonas* sp. LD5. Notably, different from our previous work on TsAly7B [28], which produced unsaturated oligosaccharides of DP 2–4 as its final products, TsAly7A released DP 2–6 from alginate.

The results reflected that rTsAly7A had a lower optimal temperature (30 °C) and maintained 16% of highest activity at 0 °C, which indicates that rTsAly7A is one cold-adapted alginate lyase. The cold-adapted character of rTsAly7A reveals its adaptation to marine environment in that TsAly7A was cloned from marine bacterium *Thalassomonas* sp. LD5 [29], which was found in the coastal sediments with a temperature of 5 °C. Some cold-adapted alginate lyases had been characterized, but rTsAly7A had some excellent properties in other aspects. For example, AlyS02 from *Flavobacterium* sp. S02, AlyPM from *Pseudoalteromonas* sp. SM0524 and AlgSH17 from *Microbulbifer* sp. SH-1 were all cold-adapted and polyM-preferred alginate lyases [30–32], but AlyS02 and AlyPM could only release the oligosaccharides of DP 2, 3, and their optimal pH was 7.6 and 8.5, respectively. AlgSH17 could release the oligosaccharides of DP 2–6, but it was not really stable as rTsAly7A under alkaline conditions. TsAly7A released unsaturated oligosaccharides of DP 2–6 from alginate and had the highest activity in pH 9.1. In addition, rTsAly7A was stable under alkaline conditions as shown in Figure 3B.

The alkali suitability is one good property in alginate lyase application and alginate oligosaccharide production. Several studies have reported some robust alginate lyase; Alyw203 from *Vibrio* sp. W2 showed outstanding pH stability with a highest activity under alkaline conditions of pH 10.0 [29] and Aly08 from *Vibrio* sp. SY01 held above 80% of its original activity in pH 4.0–10.0 [33]. Similarly, the rTsAly7A showed outstanding pH stability under alkaline conditions, which made it an excellent tool in strict industrial condition.

This study also demonstrated that rTsAly7A had a wide substrate utilization range with a preference for polyM as most alginate lyase from PL7. Similarly, AlyPM and AlgSH17 also preferably degraded polyM [31,32] while AlyS02 preferably degraded polyG [30].

The study of the effect of ions has shown that only Fe^{3+} promoted enzyme activity. However, Li^{+}, Cu^{2+}, Co^{2+}, Ba^{2+}, Ca^{2+} and Ni^{2+} inhibited the enzyme activity of rTsAly7A, which means that it cannot be used with these conditions. Additionally, Zn^{2+} and EDTA showed remarkable inhibitory effects on rTsAly7A, and yet rTsAly7A remained at 89% activity in the presence of SDS, which indicates it may have more extensive use in application. In addition, Na^{+}, K^{+}, $NH_4{}^{+}$, Mg^{2+}, Mn^{2+} and Fe^{2+} had no effect on rTsAly7A. The enzyme activity of rTsAly7A was the highest in the 100 mM NaCl condition and rTsAly7A can maintain a 50% activity without NaCl, which means it would not easily cause equipment corrosion in subsequent industrial production applications without using NaCl.

Therefore, as mentioned above, rTsAly7A is a tool to produce high degree of polymerization oligosaccharides. Studies by Chen et al. showed that the oligosaccharides of DP 5 released by alginate lyase had a remarkable inhibitory effect on the growth of osteosarcoma cells, while DP 2, 3 and 4 had no inhibitory effect [34]. The most common products of alginate lyase were DP 2–4 [30,35,36]. In other words, the oligosaccharides of DP 2–6 released by rTsAly7A may have more new properties can be studied.

4. Materials and Methods

4.1. Strains, Media, Plasmids, and Reagents

Escherichia coli strains BL21 (DE3) and DH5α from TaKaRa (Dalian, China) were cultivated in Luria–Bertani (LB) medium containing Kanamycin (50 μg/mL) when necessary. For the expression of recombinant proteins, plasmid pET-24a (+) was used. The DNA polymerase and DNA Restriction enzyme were from TaKaRa (Dalian, China). TIANamp Bacteria DNA Kit was purchased from TIANGEN BIOTECH (Beijing, China). ClonExpress II One Step Cloning Kit was purchased from Vazyme (Nanjing, China). Qingdao Gather Great Ocean Algae Industry Group Co., Ltd. (Qingdao, China) provided Alginate and polyM, polyG were from Qingdao HEHAI Biotech Co., Ltd. (Qingdao, China).

4.2. Identification, Cloning and Sequence Analysis of TsAly7A

Genomic DNA used as template was extracted from *Thalassomonas* sp. LD5 using TIANamp Bacteria DNA Kit. PCR primers (TsAly7A-F: taagaaggagatatacatatgGTGGTTAATCACTGTGGTGAACTTG, TsAly7A-R: gtggtggtggtggtgctcgagATAGTTATAGCCGGTATGTGAATTGTC) were designed according to the genomic sequence of *Thalassomonas* sp. LD5 to obtain gene Tsaly7A without signal peptide and stop codon. The vector pET-24a (+) was linearized by restriction enzyme *Nde* I and *Xho* I. Then, the gene Tsaly7A was ligated into pET-24a (+) by ClonExpress II One Step Cloning Kit using primers above. The SignalP-5.0 server (http://www.cbs.dtu.dk/services/SignalP/, accessed on 9 December 2020) was used to predict Signal peptide [37]. The recombinant plasmids rTsAly7A were transformed into the *E. coli* DH5α. Theoretical molecular weight and pI were determined using the ProtParam tool (https://web.expasy.org/protparam/, accessed on 9 December 2020) [38]. Multiple sequence alignments and phylogenetic tree construction of TsAly7A were performed using MAGA-X [39–42].

4.3. Expression and Purification of rTsAly7A

According to Zhang et al. [28], protein expression was conducted in *E. coli* BL21 (DE3) strains induced until OD_{600} reached 0.6 with 0.1 mM IPTG for 24 h. The cells were collected, resuspended, and broken up, and then the crude enzymes were extracted from the supernatants according to Zhang et al. [28]. One 1 mL HisTrap™ HP Column (GE healthcare, Stanford, USA) was then used to separate the recombinant proteins from the crude enzyme. SDS-PAGE on a 10% (*w/v*) resolving gel was used to detect the purity and molecular mass of recombinant TsAly7A, and the NCM BCA protein assay kit (NCM Biotech, Suzhou, China) was used to measure the protein content.

4.4. Activity Assay of rTsAly7A

Alginate lyase activity was determined by UV spectrophotometry for its change at 235 nm. Briefly, 900 μL of 0.3% (*w/v*) of alginate substrate (50 mM PB, 100 mM NaCl, pH 9.1) was incubated at 30 °C for 5 min, and then 100 μL of enzyme solution was added. Enzyme boiled at 100 °C for 10 min was used as the control. The A_{235} value was detected by UH5300 UV–visible spectrophotometer (HITACHI, Tokyo, Japan) after being incubated at 30 °C for 10 min. An enzyme activity unit (U) was defined as the amount of enzyme required to increase 0.1 units of UV absorption per minute. These results were repeated 3 times and the average values were indicated along with a standard deviation.

4.5. Biochemical Characterization of rTsAly7A

The enzyme activity was determined at 10–60 °C to find the optimum temperature of rTsAly7A. To determine the thermal stability, the residual activity of the enzyme was determined after incubation at 0–80 °C for 1 h. The substrate was prepared with 50 mM buffers at different pH [Na_2HPO_4-citric acid (pH 2.2–8.0), Na_2HPO_4-NaH_2PO_4 (pH 5.8–8.0), Tris-HCl (pH 7.1–8.9), Glycine-NaOH (pH 8.6–10.6)], and the enzyme activity was measured at the optimum temperature to study the optimum pH value of rTsAly7A. To study its pH stability, the enzyme was incubated in different pH at 0 °C for 12 h, and then its residual activity was determined. As for the effect of sodium chloride on rTsAly7A activity, 0.3% (*w/v*) alginate substrate (50 mM glycine-NaOH, pH 9.1) was prepared by adding different concentrations (0–1 M) of NaCl. To determine the effects of different metal ions and surfactants on TsAly7A, the enzyme activity of rTsAly7A was measured by adding 1 mM different metal ions and SDS at optimal temperature and pH. To determine the substrate specificity of rTsAly7A, 0.3% (*w/v*) of different substrate (polyM, polyG, and alginate) solutions were used to determine the activity of it.

4.6. Degradation Mode and End-Products of rTsAly7A

To clarify the degradation mode of action of rTsAly7A, 1 mL (50 U) enzyme was put in 9 mL alginate substrate [0.3% (*w/v*), 50 mM PB, 100 mM NaCl, pH 9.1] and incubated at 30 °C with progressive time (0, 1, 5, 10, 20, 30 and 60 min, respectively). The reaction was ended by boiling for 10 min. Subsequently, the degradation mode was further detected by fast protein liquid chromatography (FPLC) with a Superdex peptide 10/300 GL column (GE Healthcare, Boston, MA, USA) for separation, 200 mM NH_4HCO_3 at a flow rate of 0.2 mL/min was used as the mobile phase, and UV detector was used to detect A_{235}.

To obtain the final product, rTsAly7A was put in 0.3% (*w/v*) alginate solution to produce a final concentration of 100 U/mL, and then incubated for 12 h at 30 °C. The obtained sample was investigated by gel filtration on Superdex peptide 10/300 GL column. The detection wavelength was 235 nm, the flow rate of the mobile phase (0.2 M NH_4HCO_3) was 0.2 mL/min. In addition, each peak of the final product was collected, and then mixed with acetonitrile 1:1 (*v/v*). After that, its molecular weight was detected by negative-ion electrospray ionization-mass spectrometry (ESI-MS) in the range of 100–2000 *m/z*.

5. Conclusions

In this study, an endo-acting, cold-adapted, and polyM-preferred alginate lyase rTsAly7A from *Thalassomonas* sp. LD5 was detailed. rTsAly7A had a low optimal temperature (30 °C) and remained at 16% of highest activity at 0 °C, which indicated that rTsAly7A is one cold-adapted alginate lyase. Compared with other characterized alginate lyases, its pH stability under alkaline conditions was pretty good in that it can remain at above 90% of activity after incubation at pH 8.9 in Glycine-NaOH buffer for 12 h. rTsAly7A shared the highest activity in the presence of 100 mM and maintained 50% of the highest activity in the absence of NaCl. The SEC results showed rTsAly7A was an endo-type alginate lyase, and its end-products were unsaturated oligosaccharides (degree of polymerization 2–6). Overall, due to the good characteristics, rTsAly7A can be used as a tool enzyme for producing AOS with high degree of polymerization.

Author Contributions: Conceptualization, C.Y., J.S. and F.H.; methodology, J.S.; software, C.Y.; validation, C.Y., J.S. and F.H.; formal analysis, H.W.; investigation, resources and data curation, J.S. and C.Y.; writing—original draft preparation, C.Y.; writing—review and editing, W.Y. and F.H.; visualization, F.H.; supervision, F.H. and W.Y.; project administration, F.H. and W.Y.; funding acquisition, F.H. and W.Y. All authors have read and agreed to the published version of the manuscript.

Funding: This research was funded by the Marine S&T Fund of Shandong Province for Pilot National Laboratory for Marine Science and Technology (Qingdao) (2022QNLM030003-1), Natural Science Foundation of Shandong Province (ZR2019ZD18), and National Key R&D Program of China (2018YFC0311105).

Institutional Review Board Statement: Not applicable.

Informed Consent Statement: Not applicable.

Data Availability Statement: Not applicable.

Conflicts of Interest: The authors declare no conflict of interest.

References

1. Xing, M.; Cao, Q.; Wang, Y.; Xiao, H.; Zhao, J.; Zhang, Q.; Ji, A.; Song, S. Advances in Research on the Bioactivity of Alginate Oligosaccharides. *Mar. Drugs* **2020**, *18*, 144. [CrossRef] [PubMed]
2. Zhang, C.; Wang, W.; Zhao, X.; Wang, H.; Yin, H. Preparation of alginate oligosaccharides and their biological activities in plants: A review. *Carbohydr. Res.* **2020**, *494*, 108056. [CrossRef] [PubMed]
3. Atkins, E.D.T.; Nieduszynski, I.A.; Mackie, W.; Parker, K.D.; Smolko, E.E. Structural Components of Alginic Acid. I. The Crystalline Structure of Poly-B-D-Mannuronic Acid. Results of X-Ray Diffraction and Polarized Infrared Studies. *J. Biopolym.* **1973**, *12*, 1879–1887. [CrossRef] [PubMed]
4. Dhamecha, D.; Movsas, R.; Sano, U.; Menon, J.U. Applications of Alginate Microspheres in Therapeutics Delivery and Cell Culture: Past, Present and Future. *Int. J. Pharm.* **2019**, *569*, 118627. [CrossRef] [PubMed]
5. Rastogi, P.; Kandasubramanian, B. Review of alginate-based hydrogel bioprinting for application in tissue engineering. *Biofabrication* **2019**, *11*, 042001. [CrossRef] [PubMed]
6. Barre, A.; Naudot, M.; Colin, F.; Sevestre, H.; Collet, L.; Devauchelle, B.; Lack, S.; Marolleau, J.-P.; Le Ricousse, S. An Alginate-Based Hydrogel with a High Angiogenic Capacity and a High Osteogenic Potential. *BioRes. Open Access* **2020**, *9*, 174–182. [CrossRef]
7. Zhao, J.; Yao, L.; Nie, S.; Xu, Y. Low-viscosity sodium alginate combined with TiO_2 nanoparticles for improving neuroblastoma treatment. *Int. J. Biol. Macromol.* **2020**, *167*, 921–933. [CrossRef]
8. Zhang, P.; Liu, J.; Xiong, B.; Zhang, C.; Kang, B.; Gao, Y.; Li, Z.; Ge, W.; Cheng, S.; Hao, Y.; et al. Microbiota from alginate oligosaccharide-dosed mice successfully mitigated small intestinal mucositis. *Microbiome* **2020**, *8*, 112. [CrossRef]
9. Wang, X.; Sun, G.; Feng, T.; Zhang, J.; Huang, X.; Wang, T.; Xie, Z.; Chu, X.; Yang, J.; Wang, H.; et al. Sodium oligomannate therapeutically remodels gut microbiota and suppresses gut bacterial amino acids-shaped neuroinflammation to inhibit Alzheimer's disease progression. *Cell Res.* **2019**, *29*, 787–803. [CrossRef]
10. Fang, W.; Bi, D.; Zheng, R.; Cai, N.; Xu, H.; Zhou, R.; Lu, J.; Wan, M.; Xu, X. Identification and activation of TLR4-mediated signalling pathways by alginate-derived guluronate oligosaccharide in RAW264.7 macrophages. *Sci. Rep.* **2017**, *7*, 1663. [CrossRef]
11. Tran, V.C.; Cho, S.-Y.; Kwon, J.; Kim, D. Alginate oligosaccharide (AOS) improves immuno-metabolic systems by inhibiting STOML2 overexpression in high-fat-diet-induced obese zebrafish. *Food Funct.* **2019**, *10*, 4636–4648. [CrossRef]
12. Powell, L.; Pritchard, M.F.; Ferguson, E.; Powell, K.A.; Patel, S.U.; Rye, P.; Sakellakou, S.-M.; Buurma, N.J.; Brilliant, C.; Copping, J.M.; et al. Targeted disruption of the extracellular polymeric network of Pseudomonas aeruginosa biofilms by alginate oligosaccharides. *Npj Biofilms Microbio.* **2018**, *4*, 13. [CrossRef]
13. Feng, W.; Hu, Y.; An, N.; Feng, Z.; Liu, J.; Mou, J.; Hu, T.; Guan, H.; Zhang, D.; Mao, Y. Alginate Oligosaccharide Alleviates Monocrotaline-Induced Pulmonary Hypertension via Anti-Oxidant and Anti-Inflammation Pathways in Rats. *Int. Heart J.* **2020**, *61*, 160–168. [CrossRef]
14. Wang, Y.; Li, L.; Ye, C.; Yuan, J.; Qin, S. Alginate oligosaccharide improves lipid metabolism and inflammation by modulating gut microbiota in high-fat diet fed mice. *Appl. Microbiol. Biotechnol.* **2020**, *104*, 3541–3554. [CrossRef]
15. Yang, C.F.; Lai, S.S.; Chen, Y.H.; Liu, D.; Liu, B.; Ai, C.; Wan, X.Z.; Gao, L.Y.; Chen, X.H.; Zhao, C. Anti-Diabetic Effect of Oligosaccharides from Seaweed Sargassum Confusum Via Jnk-Irs1/Pi3k Signalling Pathways and Regulation of Gut Microbiota. *Food Chem. Toxicol.* **2019**, *131*, 110562. [CrossRef]
16. Mrudulakumari Vasudevan, U.; Lee, O.K.; Lee, E.Y. Alginate Derived Functional Oligosaccharides: Recent Developments, Barriers, and Future Outlooks. *Carbohydr. Polym.* **2021**, *267*, 118158. [CrossRef]
17. Zhang, C.; Li, M.; Rauf, A.; Khalil, A.A.; Shan, Z.; Chen, C.; Rengasamy, K.R.R.; Wan, C. Process and applications of alginate oligosaccharides with emphasis on health beneficial perspectives. *Crit. Rev. Food Sci. Nutr.* **2023**, *63*, 303–329. [CrossRef]

18. Li, S.; He, N.; Wang, L. Efficiently Anti-Obesity Effects of Unsaturated Alginate Oligosaccharides (UAOS) in High-Fat Diet (HFD)-Fed Mice. *Mar. Drugs* **2019**, *17*, 540. [CrossRef]
19. Li, S.; Wang, L.; Liu, B.; He, N. Unsaturated alginate oligosaccharides attenuated obesity-related metabolic abnormalities by modulating gut microbiota in high-fat-diet mice. *Food Funct.* **2020**, *11*, 4773–4784. [CrossRef]
20. Cantarel, B.L.; Coutinho, P.M.; Rancurel, C.; Bernard, T.; Lombard, V.; Henrissat, B. The Carbohydrate-Active EnZymes database (CAZy): An expert resource for Glycogenomics. *Nucleic Acids Res.* **2009**, *37*, D233–D238. [CrossRef]
21. Garron, M.-L.; Henrissat, B. The continuing expansion of CAZymes and their families. *Curr. Opin. Chem. Biol.* **2019**, *53*, 82–87. [CrossRef] [PubMed]
22. Xu, F.; Chen, X.-L.; Sun, X.-H.; Dong, F.; Li, C.-Y.; Li, P.-Y.; Ding, H.; Chen, Y.; Zhang, Y.-Z.; Wang, P. Structural and molecular basis for the substrate positioning mechanism of a new PL7 subfamily alginate lyase from the arctic. *J. Biol. Chem.* **2020**, *295*, 16380–16392. [CrossRef] [PubMed]
23. Han, W.; Gu, J.; Cheng, Y.; Liu, H.; Li, Y.; Li, F. Novel Alginate Lyase (Aly5) from a Polysaccharide-Degrading Marine Bacterium, *Flammeovirga* Sp. Strain My04: Effects of Module Truncation on Biochemical Characteristics, Alginate Degradation Patterns, and Oligosaccharide-Yielding Properties. *Appl. Environ. Microbiol.* **2016**, *82*, 364–374. [CrossRef] [PubMed]
24. Vuoristo, K.S.; Fredriksen, L.; Oftebro, M.; Arntzen, M.; Aarstad, O.A.; Stokke, R.; Steen, I.H.; Hansen, L.D.; Schüller, R.B.; Aachmann, F.L. Production, Characterization, and Application of an Alginate Lyase, Amor_Pl7a, from Hot Vents in the Arctic Mid-Ocean Ridge. *J. Agric. Food Chem.* **2019**, *67*, 2936–2945. [CrossRef] [PubMed]
25. Lee, S.I.; Choi, S.H.; Lee, E.Y.; Kim, H.S. Molecular Cloning, Purification, and Characterization of a Novel Polymg-Specific Alginate Lyase Responsible for Alginate Mg Block Degradation in *Stenotrophomas maltophilia* Kj-2. *Appl. Microbiol. Biotechnol.* **2012**, *95*, 1643–1653. [CrossRef] [PubMed]
26. Xu, F.; Wang, P.; Zhang, Y.-Z.; Chen, X.-L. Diversity of Three-Dimensional Structures and Catalytic Mechanisms of Alginate Lyases. *Appl. Environ. Microbiol.* **2018**, *84*, e02040-17. [CrossRef]
27. Wakabayashi, M.; Sakatoku, A.; Noda, F.; Noda, M.; Tanaka, D.; Nakamura, S. Isolation and characterization of Microbulbifer species 6532A degrading seaweed thalli to single cell detritus particles. *Biogeochemistry* **2011**, *23*, 93–105. [CrossRef]
28. Zhang, Z.; Tang, L.; Bao, M.; Liu, Z.; Yu, W.; Han, F. Functional Characterization of Carbohydrate-Binding Modules in a New Alginate Lyase, Tsaly7b, from *Thalassomonas* sp. Ld5. *Mar Drugs* **2019**, *18*, 25. [CrossRef]
29. Zhang, W.; Xu, J.; Liu, D.; Liu, H.; Lu, X.; Yu, W. Characterization of an Alpha-Agarase from *Thalassomonas* Sp. Ld5 and Its Hydrolysate. *Appl. Microbiol. Biotechnol.* **2018**, *102*, 2203–2212. [CrossRef]
30. Zhou, H.-X.; Xu, S.-S.; Yin, X.-J.; Wang, F.-L.; Li, Y. Characterization of a New Bifunctional and Cold-Adapted Polysaccharide Lyase (PL) Family 7 Alginate Lyase from *Flavobacterium* sp. *Mar. Drugs* **2020**, *18*, 388. [CrossRef]
31. Chen, X.-L.; Dong, S.; Xu, F.; Dong, F.; Li, P.-Y.; Zhang, X.-Y.; Zhou, B.-C.; Zhang, Y.-Z.; Xie, B.-B. Characterization of a New Cold-Adapted and Salt-Activated Polysaccharide Lyase Family 7 Alginate Lyase from *Pseudoalteromonas* sp. SM0524. *Front. Microbiol.* **2016**, *7*, 1120. [CrossRef]
32. Yang, J.; Cui, D.; Ma, S.; Chen, W.; Chen, D.; Shen, H. Characterization of a novel PL 17 family alginate lyase with exolytic and endolytic cleavage activity from marine bacterium *Microbulbifer* sp. SH-1. *Int. J. Biol. Macromol.* **2021**, *169*, 551–563. [CrossRef]
33. Wang, Y.; Chen, X.; Bi, X.; Ren, Y.; Han, Q.; Zhou, Y.; Han, Y.; Yao, R.; Li, S. Characterization of an Alkaline Alginate Lyase with Ph-Stable and Thermo-Tolerance Property. *Mar. Drugs* **2019**, *17*, 308. [CrossRef]
34. Chen, J.; Hu, Y.; Zhang, L.; Wang, Y.; Wang, S.; Zhang, Y.; Guo, H.; Ji, D.; Wang, Y. Alginate Oligosaccharide DP5 Exhibits Antitumor Effects in Osteosarcoma Patients following Surgery. *Front. Pharmacol.* **2017**, *8*, 623. [CrossRef]
35. Zeng, J.; An, D.; Jiao, C.; Xiao, Q.; Weng, H.; Yang, Q.; Xiao, A. Cloning, Expression, and Characterization of a New Ph- and Heat-Stable Alginate Lyase from *Pseudoalteromonas carrageenovora* Asy5. *J. Food Biochem.* **2019**, *43*, e12886. [CrossRef]
36. Chen, Y.; Dou, W.; Li, H.; Shi, J.; Xu, Z. The alginate lyase from *Isoptericola halotolerans* CGMCC 5336 as a new tool for the production of alginate oligosaccharides with guluronic acid as reducing end. *Carbohydr. Res.* **2018**, *470*, 36–41. [CrossRef]
37. Almagro Armenteros, J.J.; Tsirigos, K.D.; Sønderby, C.K.; Petersen, T.N.; Winther, O.; Brunak, S.; Von Heijne, G.; Nielsen, H. SignalP 5.0 improves signal peptide predictions using deep neural networks. *Nat. Biotechnol.* **2019**, *37*, 420–423. [CrossRef]
38. Wilkins, M.R.; Gasteiger, E.; Bairoch, A.; Sanchez, J.C.; Williams, K.L.; Appel, R.D.; Hochstrasser, D.F. Protein Identification and Analysis Tools on the Expasy Server. *Methods Mol. Biol.* **1999**, *112*, 531–552.
39. Felsenstein, J. Confidence Limits on Phylogenies: An Approach Using the Bootstrap. *Evolution* **1985**, *39*, 783–791. [CrossRef]
40. Saitou, N.; Nei, M. The neighbor-joining method: A new method for reconstructing phylogenetic trees. *Mol. Biol. Evol.* **1987**, *4*, 406–425. [CrossRef]
41. Jones, D.T.; Taylor, W.R.; Thornton, J.M. The rapid generation of mutation data matrices from protein sequences. *Comput. Appl. Biosci.* **1992**, *8*, 275–282. [CrossRef] [PubMed]
42. Kumar, S.; Stecher, G.; Li, M.; Knyaz, C.; Tamura, K. MEGA X: Molecular Evolutionary Genetics Analysis across Computing Platforms. *Mol. Biol. Evol.* **2018**, *35*, 1547–1549. [CrossRef] [PubMed]

marine drugs

MDPI

Article

Structural and Biochemical Analysis Reveals Catalytic Mechanism of Fucoidan Lyase from *Flavobacterium* sp. SA-0082

Juanjuan Wang [1,2], Zebin Liu [3,4], Xiaowei Pan [2,4], Ning Wang [2], Legong Li [4], Yuguang Du [3], Jianjun Li [3,*] and Mei Li [2,*]

1 Division of Life Sciences and Medicine, University of Science and Technology of China, Hefei 230027, China
2 National Laboratory of Biomacromolecules, CAS Center for Excellence in Biomacromolecules, Institute of Biophysics, Chinese Academy of Sciences, Beijing 100101, China
3 State Key Laboratory of Biochemical Engineering, Institute of Process Engineering, Chinese Academy of Sciences, Beijing 100190, China
4 College of Life Science, Capital Normal University, Beijing 100101, China
* Correspondence: jjli@ipe.ac.cn (J.L.); meili@ibp.ac.cn (M.L.)

Abstract: Fucoidans represent a type of polyanionic fucose-containing sulfated polysaccharides (FCSPs) that are cleaved by fucoidan-degrading enzymes, producing low-molecular-weight fucoidans with multiple biological activities suitable for pharmacological use. Most of the reported fucoidan-degrading enzymes are glycoside hydrolases, which have been well studied for their structures and catalytic mechanisms. Little is known, however, about the rarer fucoidan lyases, primarily due to the lack of structural information. FdlA from *Flavobacterium* sp. SA-0082 is an endo-type fucoidan-degrading enzyme that cleaves the sulfated fuco-glucuronomannan (SFGM) through a lytic mechanism. Here, we report nine crystal structures of the catalytic N-terminal domain of FdlA (FdlA-NTD), in both its wild type (WT) and mutant forms, at resolutions ranging from 1.30 to 2.25 Å. We show that the FdlA-NTD adopts a right-handed parallel β-helix fold, and possesses a substrate binding site composed of a long groove and a unique alkaline pocket. Our structural, biochemical, and enzymological analyses strongly suggest that FdlA-NTD utilizes catalytic residues different from other β-helix polysaccharide lyases, potentially representing a novel polysaccharide lyase family.

Keywords: fucoidan lyase; polysaccharides; crystal structure; catalytic mechanism

Citation: Wang, J.; Liu, Z.; Pan, X.; Wang, N.; Li, L.; Du, Y.; Li, J.; Li, M. Structural and Biochemical Analysis Reveals Catalytic Mechanism of Fucoidan Lyase from *Flavobacterium* sp. SA-0082. *Mar. Drugs* **2022**, *20*, 533. https://doi.org/10.3390/md20080533

Academic Editors: Yuya Kumagai, Hideki Kishimura and Benwei Zhu

Received: 26 July 2022
Accepted: 17 August 2022
Published: 20 August 2022

1. Introduction

Fucoidans are a class of sulfated, fucose-rich polysaccharides produced by brown algae and certain marine invertebrates [1,2]. The backbone of fucoidans is generally linked via an α-1,3- and/or α-1,4-glycosidic bond and is highly variable in length and monosaccharide composition. In addition to fucose (Fuc), fucoidans also contain galactose (Gal), mannose (Man), glucuronic acid (GlcUA), and other types of monosaccharide [3]. Moreover, the L-fucose residues in fucoidans are usually sulfated at different hydroxyl group positions, including C-2, C-3, and C-4 [4]. The diverse composition in monosaccharides, the variation in sulfate ester pattern and content, and the different branching sites for sugar chains result in considerable structural variation among fucoidans produced by different brown algae [5,6]. Furthermore, the structural complexity of fucoidans is influenced by other factors, including the geographical locations of macroalgal species, the specific time of harvest of brown algae, as well as the methods used for isolation and purification of fucoidans [7].

Fucoidans represent a suitable candidate drug possessing antiviral activity, as they were recently reported to effectively inhibit SARS-CoV-2 [8]. It was shown that fucoidans tightly bind to the S-protein of SARS-CoV-2, thus acting as a decoy that interferes with the binding of the S-protein to the heparin sulfate co-receptor present at the surface of host cells, potentially inhibiting viral infection [8]. In addition to their antiviral activity, fucoidans show antithrombotic, anticoagulant, anti-inflammatory, antitumor, and immunomodulatory effects [9,10]. One report indicated that the sulfate patterns (the sulfate content and the position of the sulfate groups) present on fucoidans are important for their bioactivity [11]. However, native fucoidans are usually characterized by high molecular weight, high viscosity, and irregular structures, considerably hindering their application as therapeutic agents. In contrast, low-molecular-weight fucoidans (LMWFs) are easily absorbed and possess higher bioavailability, rendering these polysaccharides a more promising target for pharmaceutical use [9,12]. Therefore, depolymerization of HMWFs into LMWFs using specific enzymes is a suitable approach, as it preserves the integrity of the specific structure of fucoidans and generates relatively homogeneous degradation products.

Fucoidan-degrading enzymes are promising tools for producing bioactive fucoidan oligosaccharides for a range of biomedical applications [13,14]. Fucoidan-degrading enzymes differ in their mode of action and are usually classified into exo- or endo-enzymes [12]. Exo-fucoidan-degrading enzymes are capable of cleaving fucoidans from the terminus of the sugar chain, usually producing monosaccharides. Endo-fucoidan-degrading enzymes break the glycosidic bond from the middle of the sugar chain to produce oligosaccharides exhibiting different degrees of polymerization [15]. Currently, all fucoidan-degrading enzymes that have been identified act as endo-hydrolases, and are classified into glycoside hydrolases (GHs) family 107 (GH107, endo-α-1,4-L-fucanase (EC 3.2.1.212)), and 168 (GH168, endo-α-(1,3)-L-fucanase (EC 3.2.1.211)) in the Carbohydrate Active enZymes database (CAZy database, http://www.cazy.org, accessed on 1 July 2022) [16,17]. The marine bacterium *Flavobacterium* sp. SA-0082 was earlier reported to produce a novel type of extracellular endo-fucoidan lyase that cleaves the sulfated fucoglucuronomannan from *Kjellmaniella crassifolia* (Kj-fucoidan) [18,19]. Two genes that encode for putative fucoidan lyase have been identified in the genome of this marine bacterium (*Flavobacterium* sp. SA-0082), and their gene products were termed FdlA and FdlB [19]. These two enzymes are 56% identical at the amino acid sequence level. The enzymatic activity of FdlA is higher than that of FdlB when acting on Kj-fucoidan [20].

Earlier studies carried out biochemical characterization and enzymatic analysis for native FdlA, demonstrating that the optimal conditions for catalytic activity of FdlA are a temperature of 40 °C, slightly alkane pH of pH 7.5, as well as the presence of NaCl at 0.4 M concentration [12,21]. Previous studies found that polysaccharides lacking sulfated fucose are not cleaved by native FdlA, indicating that the sulfated fucoses of fucoidans are important components for their recognition and cleavage by the lyase [19]. The final products of Kj-fucoidan cleaved by FdlA were identified as three types of trisaccharides, characterized by an identical backbone structure termed $\Delta^{4,5}$Glc*p*UAβ1-2L-Fuc*p*α1-3D-Man*p*. Nevertheless, these trisaccharide molecules possess different numbers of sulfate groups and/or different sulfation positions, namely monosulfated (Molecular weight (Mw) 564 Da, Fuc*p*(3-*O*-sulfate)), disulfated (Mw 644 Da, Fuc*p*(3-*O*-sulfate)α1-3D-Man*p*(6-*O*-sulfate)), and trisulfated (Mw 724 Da, Fuc*p*(2,4-*O*-disulfate)α1-3D-Man*p*(6-*O*-sulfate)) trisaccharides (Scheme 1), with the monosulfated form being the major degradation product [21]. Based on the structures of the final products, it can be deduced that FdlA acts on the α-1,4-linkage between D-mannose and D-glucuronic acid in Kj-fucoidan, which possesses a branched sulfated fucose linked on the C-3 hydroxyl group of D-mannose [5,21]. However, despite the extensive body of biochemical and enzymological analysis, the precise catalytic mechanisms responsible for FdlA activity remain elusive.

To date, FdlA has not been classified into any enzyme family in the CAZy database. However, as it acts as a uronic acid-containing polysaccharide lyase, it presumably belongs to the family of polysaccharide lyases (PL). At present, 42 PL families have been identified in the CAZy database, and are grouped into six classes based on their overall folding, namely into the right-handed parallel β-helix class (termed β-helix henceforth), the $(\alpha/\alpha)_n$ barrel class, the β-jelly roll class, the β-propeller class, the β-sandwich and β-sheet class, as well as the triple-stranded β-helix class [22]. Members from the same PL family show high sequence similarity and possess essentially conserved catalytic residues. However,

FdlA exhibits low amino acid sequence homology with all these PL members, rendering it impossible to classify FdlA into the existing PL families without information about its structure and key catalytic residues [5,23].

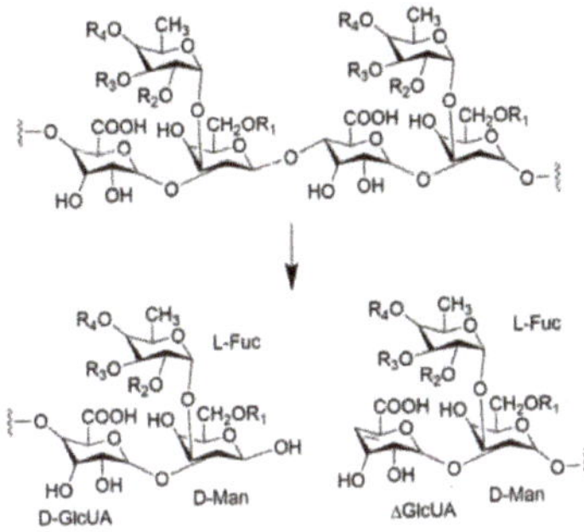

Sulfate Residue(s)	R_1	R_2	R_3	R_4	MW
1	-H	-H	$-SO_3H$	-H	564
2	$-SO_3H$	-H	$-SO_3H$	-H	644
3	$-SO_3H$	$-SO_3H$	-H	$-SO_3H$	724

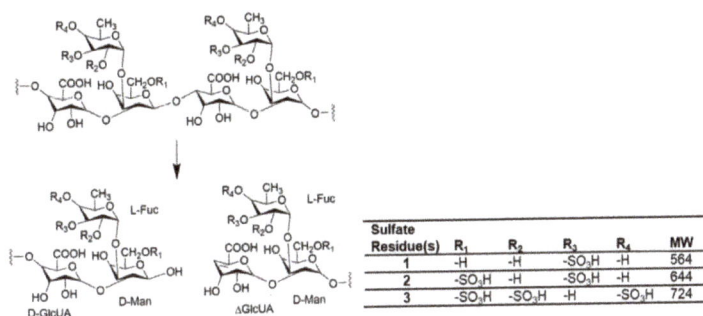

Scheme 1. Enzymatic reaction catalyzed by FdlA to digest Kj-fucoidan and yield three types of trisaccharides.

Despite possessing different folds, all PLs degrade uronic acid-containing polysaccharides via a β-elimination mechanism, utilizing Brønsted base and acid to cleave the scissile glycosidic bond [24]. This reaction process yields a new non-reducing end with an unsaturated bond in the sugar products. The catalytic mechanisms of PLs are generally divided into two groups based on the neutralizers used for the C-5 carboxyl group: (i) His/Tyr β-elimination and (ii) metal ion (usually Ca^{2+})-assisted β-elimination. In the former type, amino acid residues are used as a neutralizer, and a histidine and a tyrosine usually act as Brønsted base and acid, respectively. In the latter, a metal ion serves as a neutralizer, and an arginine and a lysine commonly act as Brønsted base and acid, respectively [25]. One previous report found that metal ions are unable to stimulate FdlA activity [19], suggesting that FdlA adopts the His/Tyr β-elimination mechanism for catalysis. However, the key residues for catalysis and their locations in FdlA remain unclear.

While previously obtained structural and enzymatic data provide important information for understanding the structure and function of fucoidan hydrolases and polysaccharide lyases, the overall folding and the catalytic mechanism of fucoidan lyases remain to be elucidated. Here, we report crystal structures and enzymological characterization of wild type (WT) and eight single mutants of the catalytic N-terminal domain (NTD) of FdlA, revealing its unique substrate binding pocket and identifying the key catalytic residues. Our results provide detailed structural information on fucoidan lyase and therefore should facilitate a deeper understanding of the catalytic mechanisms used by uronic polysaccharide lyases.

2. Results

2.1. Purification and Biochemical Characterization of FdlA-NTD

As shown in Figure S1, the full-length FdlA from *Flavobacterium* sp. SA-0082 contains 697 amino acid residues including a secretory signal peptide (Met1–Thr24). Based on the conserved domain database (CDD), the C-terminal region (residue 472–697) of FdlA contains an F5/8 type C domain (known as the discoidin domain) and a por secretion tail (known as a secretion system C-terminal sorting domain) [26,27], thus it may not be related to FdlA lyase activity, while its NTD is likely to constitute the catalytic domain of FdlA. This assumption was supported by sequence alignment of FdlA and FdlB, another fucoidan lyase from *Flavobacterium* sp. SA-0082. This result showed that both enzymes contain an N-terminal domain with a high sequence identity of approximately 75% (Figure S1).

As the full-length FdlA tends to aggregate when expressed in *E. coli*, we constructed a truncated version of FdlA solely consisting of the NTD (FdlA-NTD, residue 25–471), and successfully expressed and purified the truncated recombinant enzyme (Figure S2A,B). Size exclusion chromatography indicated that this FdlA-NTD form exists in solution as monomers. Circular dichroism (CD) analysis showed that FdlA-NTD is stable at temperatures below 35 °C for at least 120 min, while its secondary structure starts to change at 40 °C following a short incubation of 10 min (Figure S2C). This observation suggested that FdlA-NTD is characterized by low heat resistance. Furthermore, our FdlA-NTD form exhibited superior pH stability under neutral and alkaline pH conditions, preserving its secondary structure at pH 6.0–11.0, even after extended incubation of 17 h (Figure S2D).

2.2. *Enzymatic Properties of FdlA-NTD*

We next evaluated the activity of FdlA-NTD under various conditions by measuring the 232 nm absorption of the products of Kj-fucoidan degraded by FdlA-NTD (Figure 1), according to a previously described method [19]. FdlA-NTD shows relatively high salt tolerance, displaying the highest activity in the presence of 0.5 M NaCl (Figure 1A). The optimal pH and temperature for catalytic activity of FdlA-NTD were pH 7.5 and 40 °C after 1 min-incubation (Figure 1B,C). However, we found that FdlA-NTD activity was greatly decreased after incubation at 40 °C for 5 min and its enzymatic activity was almost completely lost following 30 min-incubation (Figure 1D). Our enzymatic data were consistent with the CD results obtained for FdlA-NTD (Figure S2C). On the basis of these findings, we next performed all enzyme reactions under the optimal conditions but at room temperature (25 °C) instead of 40 °C.

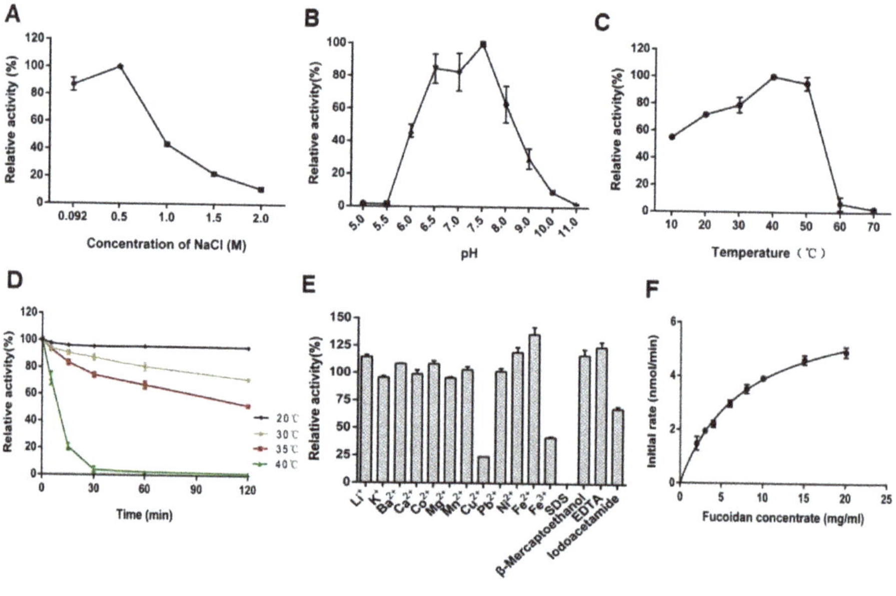

Figure 1. Biochemical and enzymatic characterization of FdlA-NTD using Kj-fucoidan as the substrate. (**A**) Effects of NaCl on FdlA-NTD activity. (**B**) Effects of pH on FdlA-NTD activity. (**C**) Effects of temperature on FdlA-NTD activity. (**D**) The kinetics of the thermal inactivation of FdlA-NTD at 20 °C (black diamond), 30 °C (yellow circle), 35 °C (red square) and 40 °C (green triangle). (**E**) Effects of metal ions and chemical reagents on FdlA-NTD activity. (**F**) The catalytic kinetics of FdlA-NTD. Error bars represent standard deviation (n = 3 independent experiments).

Enzymes of the PL family are commonly found to be associated with metal ions, especially Ca^{2+}. These ions participate in the catalytic step through a metal-dependent β-elimination mechanism. One earlier study demonstrated that native FdlA does not require metal ions for catalysis [19]; therefore, we tested the effect of metal ions and a variety of chemical reagents on the enzymatic activity of FdlA-NTD. As shown in Figure 1E, most metal ions, including Ca^{2+} and Ba^{2+}, failed to affect the catalytic activity of FdlA-NTD, while Cu^{2+} and Fe^{3+} greatly inhibited the catalytic activity of FdlA-NTD. A small number of chemical reagents, including EDTA, slightly stimulated FdlA-NTD activity. Together, these results strongly suggested that the activity of FdlA-NTD, similar to that of the native full-length protein, is independent of metal ions [19]. On the basis of these findings, we concluded that the truncated FdlA-NTD possesses identical enzymatic properties as its full-length native protein, and it may adopt the His/Tyr elimination mechanism for catalysis.

We next determined the kinetic parameters of the catalytic reaction of recombinant FdlA-NTD with Kj-fucoidan concentrations ranging from 0.2 to 2% (*w*/*v*) for 1 min, under the optimized conditions (Figure 1F), using the Lineweaver-Burk equation [28]. The kinetic values obtained were only the apparent parameters, as saturation of Kj-fucoidan towards FdlA-NTD was not reached, even at an almost saturated concentration of Kj-fucoidan. The calculated apparent Km and kcat values of FdlA-NTD towards Kj-fucoidan were 7.7 $\pm$ 0.5 mg/mL and 59.0 $\pm$ 4.3 s^{-1}, respectively, resulting in the kinetic efficiency (kcat/Km) of 7.66 $\pm$ 0.011 mL/mg/s.

2.3. Analysis of Degradation Products of the FdlA-NTD

To identify the degradation products of FdlA-NTD, we purified its degraded oligosaccharide products through high-performance liquid chromatography (HPLC) before characterizing these products by mass spectrometry (MS) (Figure 2). Analysis of the primary MS of peak at *m/z* 563.146 (Figure 2B). The molecular weight was consistent with a monosulfated trisaccharide, the major trisaccharide product previously reported for native FdlA [21]. Further analysis of the secondary MS of the peak at *m/z* 563.146 identified the exact structure of the degradation product as $\triangle^{4,5}$Glc*p*UAβ1-2(L-Fuc*p*(3-*O*-sulfate)α1-3)D-Man*p*, matching well with the previously the digested products showed that the major degradation product corresponded to the reported monosulfated trisaccharide product.

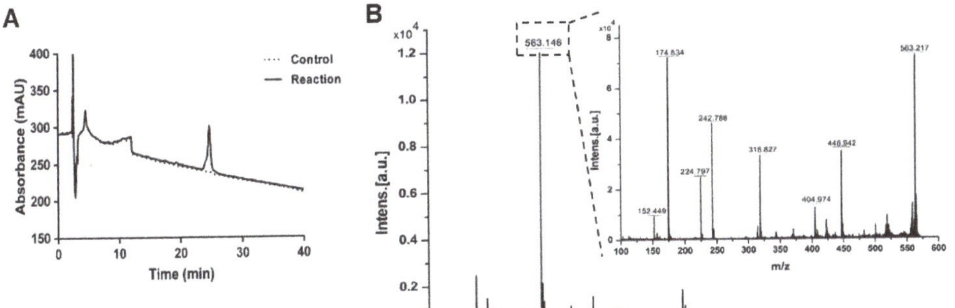

Figure 2. Identification of products of the Kj-fucoidan digested by FdlA-NTD. (**A**) The HPLC purification of Kj-fucoidan products degraded by FdlA-NTD. (**B**) Mass spectrum (negative ESI-MS) of the products of Kj-fucoidan cleaved by FdlA-NTD. The secondary MS result is shown in the inset.

2.4. Overall Structure of FdlA-NTD

We solved the crystal structure of FdlA-NTD WT at 1.3 Å resolution using the single-wavelength anomalous diffraction (SAD) method (Table S1). In the FdlA-NTD structure, two molecules are present in an asymmetric unit and adopt nearly identical conformations, with a root-mean-squares deviation (RMSD) of 0.11 Å for all Cα atoms (Figure S3).

FdlA-NTD forms a right-handed parallel β-helix (Figure 3A), one type of the six PL classes, shaping like a fish skeleton with a dimension of 67 Å $\times$ 22 Å $\times$ 47 Å. Here, we adopted the nomenclature of Yoder and Yurnak in describing the β-helix structure [29]. The β-helix fold comprises three parallel β-sheets, PB1, PB2, and PB3, together with three turns (T) linking two β-strands, T1 (between PB1 and PB2), T2 (between PB2 and PB3), and T3 (between PB3 and PB1). In most β-helix proteins, PB1 and PB2 form an antiparallel β

sandwich, while PB3 is positioned nearly perpendicular to PB2. The regular β helix unit can be regarded as one coil with a specific order of PB1-T1-PB2-T2-PB3-T3 (Figure 3A).

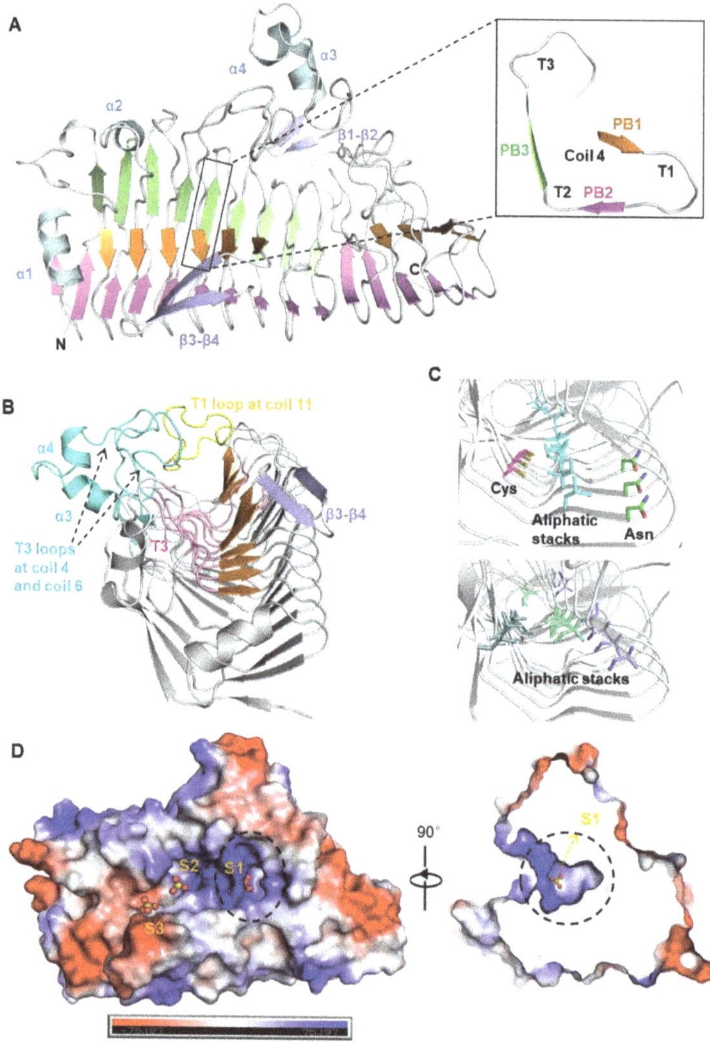

Figure 3. Overall structure of FdlA-NTD. (**A**) Cartoon representation of FdlA-NTD. The PB1 (orange), PB2 (violet), PB3 (green), and accessory elements, including four α helices (α1–α4, light cyan) and two pairs of antiparallel strands (β1–β2 and β3–β4, slate) are indicated. Coil 4 as a representative coil of β-helix structure was shown in the inset. (**B**) The groove formed by PB1 (orange) and T3 (light pink), and enclosed by α3–α4, β1–β2 and T3 loops from coils 4 and 6 (cyan) at one side, β3–β4 (slate) at the opposite side, and the T1 loop from coil 11 (yellow) at the C-terminal end. (**C**) The unusual cysteine ladder as well as four aliphatic stacks and a short asparagine ladder located inside the β-helix structure of FdlA-NTD. The residues constitute various ladders and stacks are shown as sticks, and in different colors for carbon atoms. (**D**) Electrostatic surface representation of FdlA-NTD (blue and red represent the positive and negative charge, respectively). Three sulfate groups in the 'groove-pocket' region are shown in ball-and-stick mode. S1 is located in the alkaline pocket at the C-terminal end of the groove (marked by dotted circle).

The FdlA-NTD molecule contains 13 coils, with coils 1–6 being complete, while the other coils lacking either PB1 or PB3. The T3 loops at coils 1–9 together with the adjacent PB1 sheets form a 30-Å long concave groove at the surface of the β-helix (Figure 3B). PB2s and PB3s are located at the bottom face of the β-helix, beneath PB1s and T3s, respectively, supporting the shape of the groove from below.

In addition, FdlA-NTD possesses several accessory elements, including four α-helices (α1–α4) and two pairs of antiparallel strands (β1–β2 and β3–β4) (Figure 3A). The α1 is an amphipathic helix lying at the N-terminal end of the β-helix, with the hydrophobic region facing towards the β-helical interior. Two helices (α3 and α4) as well as one pair of antiparallel strands (β1–β2) are located at the T3 loop of coil 5. Together with the long flexible T3 loops at coil 4 and coil 6, these fragments form a side wall at one side of the groove, while the other pair of antiparallel strands (β3–β4) inserts into the T1 loop of coil 6, and shapes the opposite side-wall of the groove. At the C-terminal end, the groove is sealed by the T1 loop, which is located in coil 11 and protrudes upwards (Figure 3B). This structural arrangement suggests that these accessory elements play a pivotal role in encircling the elongated groove, and this semi-open groove presumably constitutes the substrate binding site for FdlA-NTD.

2.5. Structural Elements for FdlA-NTD Stabilization

A β-helix fold usually contains a number of characteristic residues whose side-chains are stacked or aligned either within the interior, or sometimes at the exterior space, of the β-helix [29–31]. These residues greatly contribute to the stabilization of β-helix proteins and are generally divided into three types: asparagine ladders, aliphatic stacks (comprising mainly residues Val, Ile, and Leu), and aromatic stacks [32]. When analyzing the FdlA-NTD structure, we identified four aliphatic stacks and one short asparagine ladder (Figure 3C). The longest aliphatic stack on PB2 is located opposite the other three shorter aliphatic stacks lying on PB1 and PB3, and contains 12 hydrophobic residues located on coils 2–13, almost spanning across the entire molecule. In addition to these common stacks and ladders, we also found an unusual cysteine ladder composed of five cysteine residues (Cys168, Cys192, Cys267, Cys290, Cys309) that are located at the T2-PB3 juncture of coils 4–8 (Figure 3C), beneath the potential substrate binding groove. Together, these stacks and ladders stabilize the β-helix folding of FdlA-NTD.

2.6. FdlA Uses a Unique Positively-Charged 'Groove-Pocket' for Substrate Binding

Enzymes belonging to five PL families (PL1, PL3, PL6, PL9, and PL31) adopt right-handed parallel β-helix folding, similar to FdlA-NTD. We compared our FdlA-NTD structure with lyase structures selected from each of the five families (PL1-pectate lyase: 2ewe [30]; PL3-pectate lyase: 4z04 and 4ew9 [33]; PL6-alginate lyase: 6itg and 6a40 [34]; PL9- pectate lyase: 5olq and 5olr [35]; PL31-alginate lyase: 6kfn [36]), and found that FdlA-NTD failed to superimpose well with these PLs (r.m.s.d of 2.5–3.6 Å for all Cα atoms). Besides this, FdlA-NTD exhibits low sequence homology (lower than 15%) and possesses non-conserved catalytic residues with all other structurally characterized PL proteins (Figure S4).

One common feature of all these β-helix PLs is that they possess a surficial groove that was previously shown to be the substrate binding groove of these PLs [30,33–36]. However, the T1 and T3 loops of these enzymes exhibit a wide range of lengths and adopt different conformations, resulting in the different sizes and shapes of these grooves (Figure S4). These structural variations may facilitate specific substrate recognition, in agreement with the fact that these enzymes differ in their substrate selectivity.

In contrast to other PL enzymes, which form a planar groove, FdlA-NTD extends its C-terminal part of the surficial groove into a deep pocket, measuring 11 Å × 13 Å × 8 Å (Figure 3D). The region comprising the deep pocket and the C-terminal part of the groove (between coil 5 and coil 9) is characterized by a strong positive charge (Figure 3D), which is unfavorable for metal binding due to the electrostatic repulsion. This feature is in agreement with the results of our enzymatic assays, showing that FdlA-NTD catalysis is independent of metal ions. In agreement with this result, the β-helix PLs (from PL1, PL3, PL9, and PL31) adopting metal-dependent elimination mechanism possesses an acidic active region (Figure S4), which presumably stabilizes the binding of metal ions.

Moreover, we observed several bulbs of non-protein densities in the 'groove-pocket' region, and modeled these densities as three sulfate groups (S1–S3) (Figures 3D and S5A), based on the density shape and the fact that high concentration of sulfate ammonium was added in the crystallization reagent. One sulfate S1 is located in the alkaline pocket (Figure 3D), strongly indicating that the positively charged pocket facilitates the attraction and interaction with the negative charged sulfate groups of fucoidans, explaining the previous observation that FdlA can only cleave fucoidans containing sulfated fucoses. We docked a monosulfated trisaccharide into the FdlA-NTD structure and found that the alkaline pocket can well accommodate the trisaccharide (Figure S5B), thus the pocket may act as an anchor to grasp the bent sugar chain tightly into the 'groove-pocket' region. Compared with a planar groove, the 'groove-pocket' mode is more suitable for the branched polysaccharide chain and thus may play an essential role in substrate recognition and stabilization. Such a structural design can be very efficient in the degradation of high molecular weight polysaccharides with branched chains.

2.7. Enzyme-Substrate Docking Model Reveal the Catalytic Site

As we failed to obtain the structures of FdlA-NTD in complex with substrate or product or their analogues, we then docked [37] representative substrate oligosaccharides, namely hexasaccharide (HS), nonasaccharide (NS), and dodecasaccharide (DS) (($\triangle^{4,5}$GlcpUAβ1-2(L-Fucp(3-O-sulfate)α1-3)D-Manp)-α1-4GlcpUAβ1-2(L-Fucp(3-O-sulfate)α1-3)D-Manp)$_{1\text{-}3}$, into the FdlA-NTD structure, and established three docking models, namely FdlA-NTD-HS, FdlA-NTD-NS, and FdlA-NTD-DS (Figure 4). When we analyzed the FdlA-NTD-HS model, we observed that one trisaccharide unit is accommodated in the alkaline pocket, while another trisaccharide unit is bound within the groove. In FdlA-NTD-NS and FdlA-NTD-DS, models of FdlA-NTD binding to longer oligosaccharides, we found that the first trisaccharide unit is deeply inserted inside the pocket, and the second trisaccharide is positioned at the opening of the pocket. The remaining one or two trisaccharide units are located within the groove (Figure 4A). These results confirmed our hypothesis that the alkaline pocket is responsible for binding a trisaccharide unit of the sugar substrate. Interestingly, the sulfate groups of different substrates are not located at the same position within the alkaline pocket, which is probably because the entire pocket is positively charged, thus enabling the sulfate group of trisaccharides to bind at multiple sites. This observation also explains the finding of a previous study, showing that the native FdlA is able to degrade fucoidans of different sulfated levels and produce three types of trisaccharides [21].

Previous results suggested that the site within the oligosaccharides that is attacked by FdlA is the glycosidic O (C-4 oxygen) atom between two neighboring trisaccharide units [21]. Our docking models showed that these oligosaccharides contain two trisaccharides located at similar positions, independent of their length. The glycosidic O atom between the two units can be well superimposed among three docking models (Figure 4A), suggesting this C-4 oxygen atom represents the cleaved site. According to the nomenclature of sugar-binding subsites proposed by Davies et al. [38], the monosaccharides are numbered as the subsite +1, +2, +3, +n, starting from the cleaved site to the reducing end of the polysaccharides, and −1, −2, −3, −n to the non-reducing end of the polysaccharides. The proceeding of β-elimination catalysis requires neutralization of the C-5 carboxyl group at +1 subsite. The carboxyl groups in the three docking models are also located at similar places. In addition, both glycosidic O atoms between −1 and +1 subsites and the carboxyl group at +1 subsite are hydrogen bonded with Tyr242 (Figure 4A), implying the essential role of Tyr242 for FdlA-NTD catalysis. Tyr242 in the substrate binding groove is located at the edge of the alkaline pocket (Figure 4A). This arrangement, together with our observation that the pocket is able to accommodate a trisaccharide unit (Figure S5B), strongly suggests that Tyr242 directly participates in cleaving the substrate to produce trisaccharides, and the alkaline pocket assists in orientating the polysaccharide substrate into a position close to Tyr242. This suggestion is in line with findings from our enzymatic analysis that the cleaved products of FdlA-NTD are exclusively trisaccharides (Figure 2).

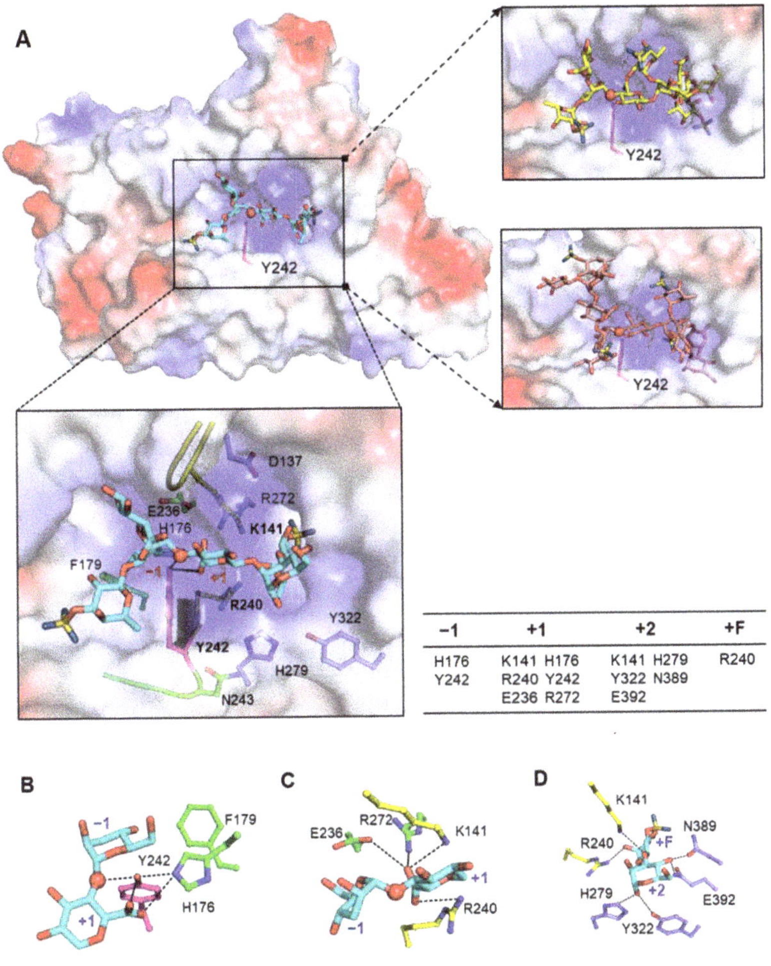

Figure 4. Docking models of FdlA-NTD with three types of oligosaccharides. (**A**) Docking models of FdlA-NTD with hexasaccharide (FdlA-NTD-HS, cyan), nonasaccharide (FdlA-NTD-NS, yellow), and dodecasaccharide (FdlA-NTD-DS, deep salmon). Oligosaccharides are shown as sticks, the glycosidic O atom at the putative cleavage site is highlighted as a red ball. Residue Tyr242 is shown as magenta sticks and indicated. The bottom box shows the residues of FdlA-NTD potentially interacting with HS in the FdlA-NTD-HS docking model. Residues are shown as sticks in different colors according to their locations. Residues close to Tyr242 (His176, Phe179, Glu236, and Asn243) are shown as green sticks for carbon atoms, residues shaping the alkaline pocket (Asp137, Arg272, His279, and Tyr322) are shown as blue sticks for carbon atoms, residues Lys141 and Arg240 near the +1 subsite are shown as yellow sticks for carbon atoms. Residues involved in the interaction with different subsites of HS are listed. (**B**) The potential interactions between Tyr242, His176, and HS. Glycosidic O atom (red ball) and carboxyl group at +1 subsite are hydrogen-bonded with Tyr242. (**C**) Interactions between residues of FdlA-NTD and the C-5 carboxyl group at +1 subsite of HS. (**D**) Interactions between residues of FdlA-NTD and the +2 and +F subsites of HS.

2.8. Residues Essential for Enzymatic Activity of FdlA-NTD

Based on our crystal structure and docking models, we selected 11 residues potentially essential for FdlA-NTD activity (Figure 4), and generated 12 single mutants, by replacing each of the 11 residues with alanine as well as mutating Tyr242 to phenylalanine (Figure S2B). We first measured the enzymatic activity of 12 mutants (Figure 5A) and found that eight of them (D137A, K141A, H176A, F179A, E236A, R240A, Y242A, and Y242F) almost completely abolished their activities, H279A mutant retained approximately 65% of the activity compared with WT, while mutations of Asn243, Arg272, and Tyr322 to Ala only negligibly affect their activities. These results are consistent with our docking models, which showed that Asn243, Arg272, and Tyr322 are located slightly distant from the substrate compared with other residues (Figure 4A). Circular dichroism (CD) spectra showed that all inactive mutants possess similar secondary structures to the wild-type protein (Figure 5B), indicating that the loss of activity of these mutants is due to the residue mutations, but not protein conformational changes.

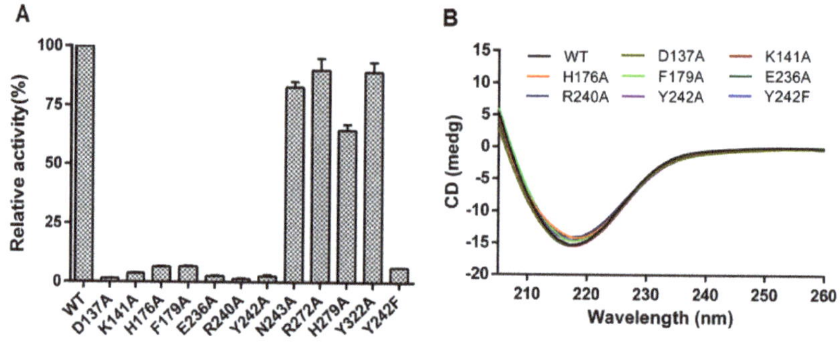

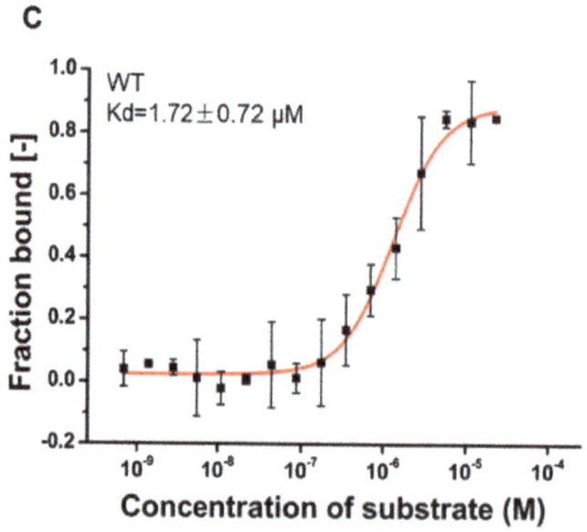

Enzyme	Kd (μM)
WT	1.72 ± 0.72
D137A	5.90 ± 2.44
K141A	1.12 ± 0.42
H176A	2.56 ± 0.64
F179A	1.42 ± 0.22
E236A	1.10 ± 0.45
R240A	1.28 ± 0.27
Y242A	0.47 ± 0.27
Y242F	3.20 ± 1.41

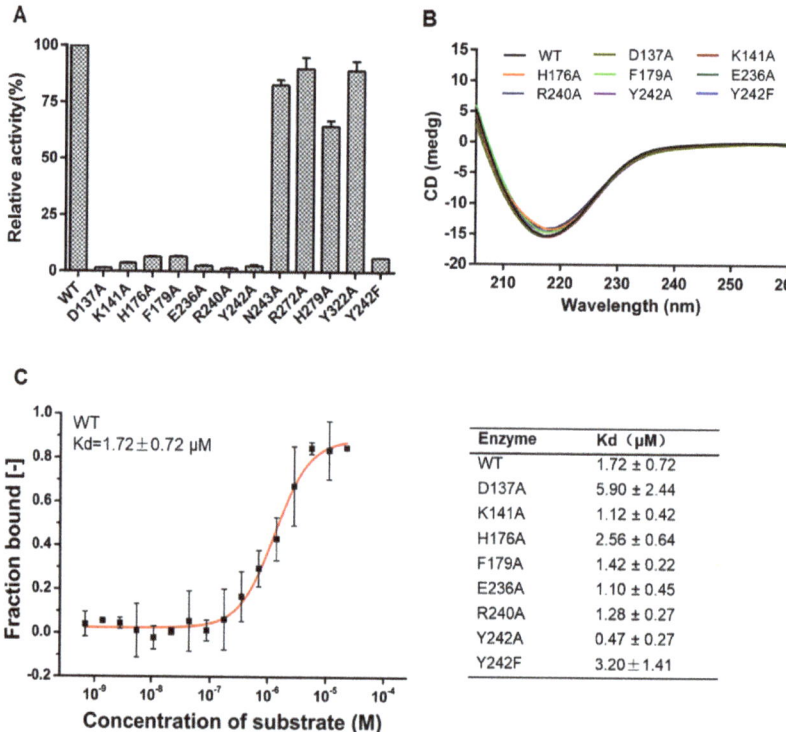

Figure 5. Characterization of FdlA-NTD mutants. (**A**) Enzymatic activities of the WT and mutant forms of FdlA-NTD towards Kj-fucoidan. (**B**) CD spectra of the WT and mutant forms of FdlA-NTD. (**C**) Binding affinity of FdlA-NTD (wild type and inactive mutants) with the substrate (Kj-fucoidan). The representative result of WT with Kj-fucoidan is shown.

To assess whether these mutations affect the interaction between FdlA-NTD and the polysaccharide substrate, we next measured the binding affinity of FdlA-NTD (wild type and inactive mutants) with the substrate (Kj-fuoicdan) using the MicroScale Thermophoresis (MST) method (Figures 5C and S6). We found that the inactive FdlA-NTD mutants exhibited similar K_d values as the wild-type form. These binding assay data clearly demonstrated that while our inactive mutants lost their catalytic activity, they maintained their substrate binding ability. This experimental observation is in agreement with the fact that the substrate of FdlA-NTD is a type of high molecular weight macromolecule, hence it may form multiple interactions with the protein. Thus, a single mutation of the enzyme does not significantly affect its binding affinity with the substrate.

2.9. Crystal Structures of FdlA-NTD Mutants

To analyze the potential function of these residues, we further solved 11 crystal structures of FdlA-NTD mutants (eight inactive and three active mutants) except for H279A, which yielded no crystals (Figure S7, Table S1). The overall structures and the putative active region of the three active mutants (N243A, R272A, and Y322A) are nearly identical to that of the WT (Figure 6A, R272A as a representative), well explaining how full activities of these mutants were maintained. Furthermore, we found that the inactive mutants failed to exhibit significant structural changes compared with the wild type, which is consistent with our CD results (Figure 5B). However, we identified changes around the potential active site in several inactive mutants (Figure 6), implying the potential roles of these residues in catalysis.

Mutation of Y242A resulted in a large structural change at the potential active site (Figures 6B and S7A), with a 3 Å shift of Asn243, which narrows the substrate groove in the mutant structure. However, the Y242F mutant, which also lost its catalytic activity, possesses a potential active site nearly identical to the wild-type form (Figures 6C and S7B). This result highlighted the importance of the hydroxyl group of the Tyr242 side chain. In our docking models of FdlA-NTD with fuco-oligasaccharide, the hydroxyl group of Tyr242 side chain is located within a hydrogen bond distance with the glycosidic O atom between −1 and +1 subsites (Figure 4A), thus allowing Tyr242 to donate a proton to glycosidic O atom and function as a catalytic acid. This suggestion was supported by a previous report showing that a conserved tyrosine residue in β-helix PL31 family members serves as the Brønsted acid [36].

Brønsted base is responsible for proton extraction from C-5 atom in β-elimination reaction [39]. Two positively charged residues Lys141 and Arg240 have their side chains pointing closely to the C-5 atom at the +1 subsite (Figure 4C), hence are potential candidates for a catalytic base. Our structures showed that the K141A mutant possesses an active site almost identical to the WT (Figures 6D and S7C), similar to the Y242F mutant. In contrast, the R240A mutant exhibits visible structural changes around the active site. Specifically, the Try242 residue was rotated approx. 90 degrees, and shifted toward Ala240 (Figures 6E and S7D). As it constitutes the catalytic acid, the hydroxyl group of the Tyr242 side chain is essential for the enzymatic activity, and its improper positioning may severely affect the catalysis of the enzyme. These structures suggested that the loss of activity of the R240A mutant may be due to the shift of the Tyr242 side chain. In contrast, Lys141 possibly functions as a catalytic base by capturing a proton from the C-5 atom at +1 subsite.

Similar to R240A, the mutant form F179A also exhibited a structural rearrangement around the active site, with a 3.8 Å shift of the Tyr242 side chain towards Ala179 (Figures 6F and S7E). Residue His176 is located close to Tyr242, and the H176A mutation shows a slight influence on the Tyr242 side chain conformation (Figures 6G and S7F). Therefore, mutation of Phe179 and His176 possibly results in the dysfunction of Tyr242 and hence loss of the catalytic activity of FdlA-NTD. In addition, His176 forms a hydrogen bond (2.8 Å) with the hydroxyl group of Tyr242 side chain in WT (Figure 4B), implying another possibility that it might play a role in providing a proton to Tyr242 to facilitate the catalytic reaction.

In the WT structure, both Asp137 and Glu236 form hydrogen bonds with Arg272, while Arg272 participates in the shaping of the alkaline pocket (Figure 6H–J). In both D137A and E236A mutant structures, the side chain of Arg272 switches to the opposite direction compared with that in WT due to the loss of the acidic residue (Arg272 in E236A mutant also exhibits an alternative conformation similar to that in WT), and partially occupies the deep substrate pocket (Figures 6J and S7G,H). These results suggest that the steric hindrance of Arg272 in the two mutants may interfere with the substrate fully entering the pocket and hence the correct positioning of the glycosidic O atom, thus resulting in the complete loss of activities of D137A and E236A mutants. This hypothesis is supported by the fact that the R272A mutation does not significantly affect the enzymatic activity, as this mutant form possesses an identical active site (Figure 6A) hence a similar pocket compared to that of the WT form.

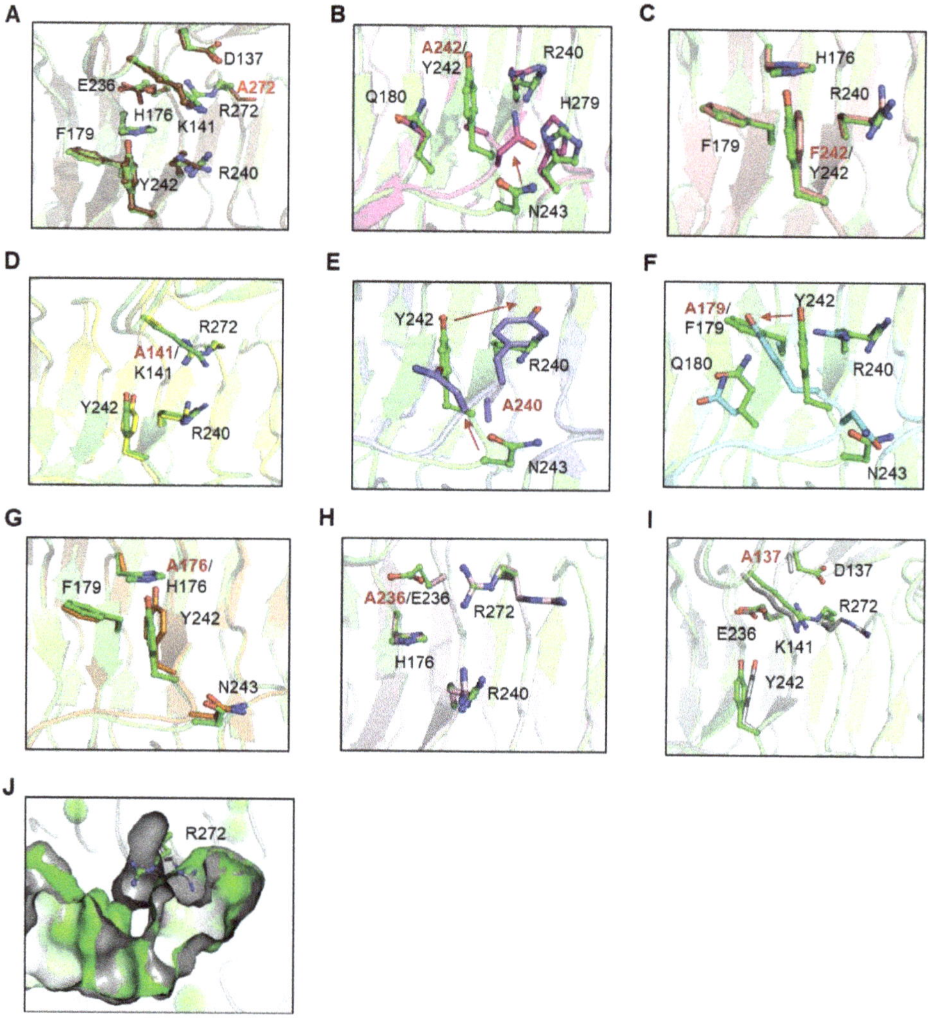

Figure 6. Comparison between the active sites of the inactive mutants and WT of FdlA-NTD. (**A–I**) Comparison of mutants R272A (**A**), Y242A (**B**), Y242F (**C**), K141A (**D**), R240A (**E**), F179A (**F**), H176A (**G**), D236A (**H**), D137A (**I**) with WT. Key residues are shown as sticks. The carbon atoms are shown in green for WT in (**A–I**), brown for R272A in (**A**), magenta for Y242A in (**B**), pink for Y242F in (**C**), yellow for K141A in (**D**), slate for R240A in (**E**), cyan for F179A in (**F**), orange for H176A in (**G**), light pink for D236A in (**H**) and gray for D137A in (**I**). Residues are labeled with the mutated residues labeled in red. (**J**) The side chain of Arg272 (gray stick) in D137A mutant (grey surface) partially occupies the deep substrate pocket present in WT (green surface).

3. Discussion

In this study, we purified recombinant FdlA-NTD and identified its cleaved product of Kj-fucoidan as the monosulfated trisaccharide, which is the same as the major product of native FdlA [21]. However, native FdlA produced two additional types of trisaccharides using Kj-fucoidan as substrate, all of which contained an identical backbone with the monosulfated trisaccharide product but carried a different number of sulfate groups. One possible explanation for this observation is that the substrate (Kj-fucoidan) that FdlA and FdlA-NTD cleave exhibits slightly different structures, resulting in different product profiles for FdlA-NTD and FdlA. The Kj-fucoidan used in the previous study was isolated from brown algae harvested in the sea of Hokkaido, Japan. In contrast, the Kj-fucoidan used in our work was obtained from brown algae growing near Dalian, China. Despite being harvested from the same species, the different geographical locations of brown algae may result in the production of fucoidan characterized by different structures/sulfated levels [4], which may account for the small discrepancy of the enzymatic products between the present work and the earlier report.

We performed an enzymatic assay on FdlA-NTD and identified its optimal catalytic conditions. In addition, we showed that the sulfhydryl reagent (iodoacetamide) reduces the activity of FdlA-NTD (Figure 1E). An earlier report showed similar results for native FdlA, implying that FdlA constitutes a sulfhydryl enzyme [19]. However, our crystal structure of FdlA-NTD suggested that it is not a sulfhydryl enzyme, as the five cysteine residues are actually located beneath the hypothetical substrate binding groove (Figure 3C). Thus, the cysteine residues may not directly participate in the catalysis, but rather help to stabilize the groove from the bottom by forming the cysteine ladder. Therefore, the inhibition of FdlA/FdlA-NTD by sulfhydryl reagents may be due to the conformational disturbance upon the modification of the cysteine ladder.

FdlA-NTD possibly belongs to the β-helix PL family; however, its unique structural features, as well as the non-conserved nature of its catalytic residues compared with other known PLs with β-helix fold suggested that FdlA constitutes a novel β-helix PL family hitherto not identified. In addition, FdlA may use unique catalytic residues functioning as Brønsted base and acid for the β-elimination catalysis. While it remains considerably challenging to unambiguously identify residues responsible for proton abstraction and transfer without structures of FdlA-NTD in complex with substrates or products, we were able to infer from our crystal structures and docking models that Tyr242 and Lys141 serve as the potential Brønsted acid and base, respectively.

Our biochemical data demonstrated that FdlA-NTD lyase favors the β-elimination catalytic mechanism independent of metal ions, and thus is likely to use positively charged amino acid residues to neutralize the negative charge of the substrate. Usually, more than one residue functions as a neutralizer in PLs [40], thus the potential neutralizer residues are difficult to identify, since mutation of a single neutralizer residue may not greatly affect its activity. Based on our structural and docking models, several positively charged residues such as Arg240, His176, and Lys141, located near the +1 subsite, potentially serve as neutralizers in FdlA-NTD, weakening the negative charge of the C-5 carboxyl group at +1 subsite, and making the C-5 proton susceptible to the attack by a Brønsted base.

On the basis of our structure and biochemical analysis of wild-type and mutant proteins combined with docking models, we propose the following model describing the catalytic process of FdlA (Figure 7). First, the substrate binds in the groove of the enzyme and the binding is stabilized through multiple interactions. One trisaccharide unit is inserted into the deep alkaline pocket, which is critical for substrate recognition and the proper positioning of the cleaved glycosidic bond. Next, the positively charged residues including Arg240 and His176, which are located near the +1 subsite, neutralize the C-5 carboxyl group of D-GlcUA at +1 subsite, thus reducing the pKa of the C-5 proton, making it more susceptible to the attack by a base. Subsequently, abstraction of the proton occurs on C-5, a process that is presumably accomplished by Lys141, leading to the formation of an enolate intermediate. The hydroxyl group of the Tyr242 side chain is directed to the glycosidic oxygen of the scissile bond where it may function as a Brønsted acid to break the glycosidic bond between −1 and +1 subsites, generating a 4,5-unsaturated sugar at the new non-reducing end of the product. Lastly, a new catalytic cycle is repeated after the cleaved products leave the putative active site.

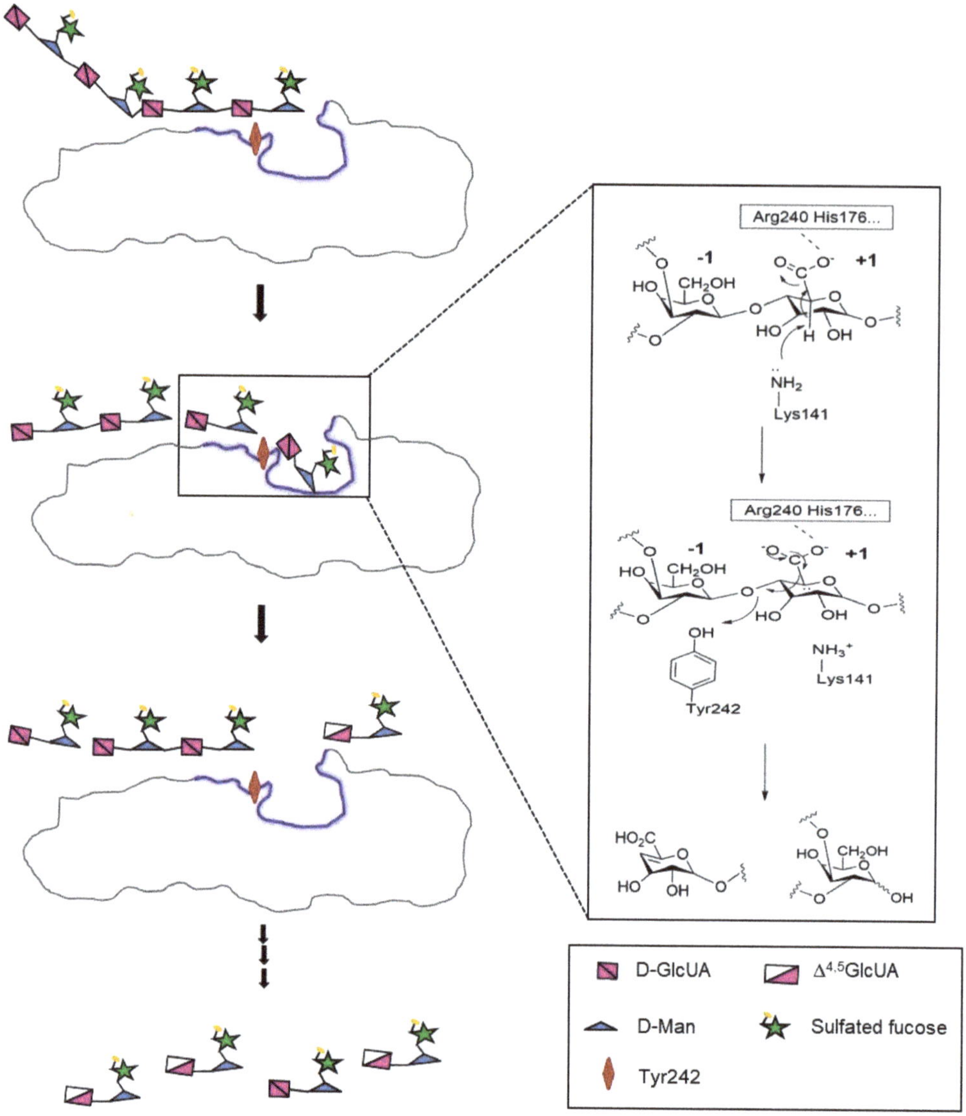

Figure 7. Proposed catalytic model of FdlA-NTD towards Kj-fucoidan. Schematic of the FdlA-NTD and kj-fucoidan were shown. The positively-charged region of the 'groove-pocket' of FdlA-NTD was colored blue. During catalysis, the positively charged residues (such as Arg240 and His176) stabilize the negatively charged carboxylate group at +1 subsite, thus facilitating the depriving of the proton at the C-5 position (+1 subsite) by a catalytic base (possibly Lys141). Tyr242 may serve as a catalytic acid to donate a proton, then the glycosidic bond between −1 and +1 subsites are broken and generate a 4,5-unsaturated sugar at the new non-reducing end of the product.

4. Materials and Methods

4.1. Materials

Unless specified, all chemicals are of analytical grade and were purchased from Sigma (St. Louis, DE, USA) or Aladdin (Shanghai, China). *Escherichia coli* Trans10 and BL21 (DE3) were purchased from TransGen Biotech (Beijing, China). Crystallization screen commercial kits were purchased from Hampton Research (Aliso Viejo, CA, USA). Ni^{2+}-NTA column,

Superdex™ 200 10/300 GL, and DEAE Sepharose Fast Flow were purchased from GE Life Sciences and GE Healthcare ((Chicago, IL, USA). Fucoidan from *Kjellmaniella crassifolia* used in this experiment was given by Professor Qiukuan Wang of Dalian Ocean University (Dalian, China).

4.2. Cloning, Expression, and Purification

The codon-optimized sequence of full-length FdlA encoding a fucoidan lyase (fucoglucuronomannan lyase) from *Flavobacterium* sp. SA-0082 (GenBank™ accession number AAO00510.1) was synthesized by Shanghai Sangon Biotech Co. Ltd. (Shanghai, China). Sequence analysis showed that the NTD of FdlA is likely the catalytic domain. Therefore, the cDNA encoding FdlA-NTD (residue 25–471) without signal peptide was cloned into pET28a between the *Nde* I and *XhoI* I restriction sites, with an N-terminal 6 × his tag. All point mutations of FdlA-NTD were generated through the QuickChange site-directed mutagenesis method (Stratagene Ltd., La Jolla, CA, USA) by overlap-PCR [41].

The above plasmids were transformed into *Escherichia coli* BL21 (DE3) and the clones were cultured in Lucia-Bertani (LB) medium containing 25 μg/mL Kannamycin at 37 °C until the OD_{600nm} reached 0.6–0.8. Isopropyl β-D-1-thiogalactopyranoside (IPTG) was then added at a final concentration of 1 mM and the cells were cultured at 18 °C for an additional 18 h. The cells were harvested and resuspended in lysis buffer (20 mM Hepes pH 7.5, 400 mM NaCl, 5% glycerol, 10 mM imidazole). After sonication, the cell lysate was centrifuged at 18,000 rpm for 30 min at 4 °C and the supernatant was loaded onto the Ni^{2+}-NTA affinity column. The target protein was eluted by imidazole of 300 mM concentration and further purified through size-exclusion chromatography (Superdex™ 200 10/300 GL colume) in a buffer containing 20 mM Hepes pH 7.5, 100 mM NaCl, 5% glycerol. The purity of the enzyme was analyzed via SDS-PAGE in 12% polyacrylamide gels.

To obtain the selenomethionine (SeMet)-labeled FdlA-NTD ($FdlA\text{-}NTD^{SeMet}$), the protein was expressed in *E. coli* B834 (DE3). The cells grown overnight in LB medium were harvested when the OD_{600nm} reached 0.6–0.8 and then transferred into M9 medium supplemented with various amino acids (60 mg/liter L-SeMet, 100 mg/liter L-lysine, L-threonine, L-phenylalanine; 50 mg/liter L-leucine, L-isoleucine, L-valine). The cells were incubated at 37 °C for 40 min, then cooled to 16 °C for 30 min and IPTG was added. Finally, the culture was incubated at 16 °C for 18 h. The purification steps of $FdlA\text{-}NTD^{SeMet}$ were the same as those of the native protein described above.

4.3. Crystallization, Data Collection, and Structure Determination

Crystals were grown at 18 °C through the sitting-drop vapor diffusion method by mixing 0.7 μL of the protein solution (14 mg/mL) with an equal volume of various reservoir solutions. FdlA-NTD crystals were formed in a reservoir solution containing 0.1 M CAPS, pH 10.5, 0.2 M Li_2SO_4, 2 M $(NH_4)_2SO_4$, 1% (*v*/*v*) Pluronic F-68 at 18 °C. Crystals of $FdlA\text{-}NTD^{SeMet}$ were obtained under the same conditions without Pluronic F-68. Crystals of mutants D137A and E236A were grown in a reservoir solution containing 0.1 M Tris, pH 8.5, 0.2 M Li_2SO_4, 30% (*w*/*v*) polyethylene glycol (PEG) 4000, and crystals of mutant R240A were grown in a reservoir solution containing 0.1 M Hepes sodium, pH 7.5, 10% (*v*/*v*) 2-Propanol, 20% PEG 4000. Other mutants were crystallized under the same conditions as wild-type.

The crystals were cryoprotected by adding 20% (*v*/*v*) glycerol to each crystallization solution. The X-ray diffraction data of FdlA-NTD and various mutants were collected at beamlines BL17U1, BL18U1, BL19U1, and BL02U1 of the Shanghai Synchrotron Radiation Facility (SSRF) in China [42,43]. All diffraction data were processed using the program HKL2000 [44]. Data collection statistics are shown in Table S1.

The initial phase of FdlA-NTD was solved by single-wavelength anomalous diffraction (SAD) method using Autosol in the Phenix program (version 1.15.2) [45]. The structural model was automatically built through AutoBuild in the Phenix program. Structures of FdlA-NTD mutants were determined by molecular replacement (MR) method through

Phaser-MR in the Phenix program using the WT FdlA-NTD structure as the initial model. All structures were refined through Refine in Phenix program and Coot (version 8.6.1) [46] alternately. The statistics of structural refinement were summarized in Table S1.

4.4. Circular Dichroism

CD spectra were recorded by Chirascan Plus (Applied Photophysics Ltd., London, UK) and used to evaluate the structural stability of FdlA-NTD by detecting its secondary structural change under different conditions. Protein was diluted to a final concentration of 0.2 mg/mL. The pH stability was estimated by measuring the CD spectra of protein incubated in Britton-Robinson (B & R) buffer systems at different pH (5.0–12.0) for 17 h at room temperature. For thermal stability, FdlA-NTD was incubated at different temperatures for 120 min in a buffer containing 50 mM sodium phosphate buffer (pH 7.5), and the CD spectra were recorded starting at 5 min.

4.5. Enzymatic Activity Assay

Fucoidan from *Kjellmaniella crassifolia* was used as the substrate of FdlA-NTD enzyme assay. *Kjellmaniella crassifolia* was cultured along the coast of Dalian, China and Kj-fucoidan was extracted following the extraction procedure reported in earlier literature [19,21]. The standard reaction mixture (200 μL) of enzymatic assay consists of 1% (*w*/*v*) Kj-fucoidan and appropriately diluted enzyme solution. The lyase activity of FdlA-NTD toward Kj-fucoidan was measured by monitoring the increase of 232 nm absorbance, which was caused by the production of 4, 5-unsaturated glucuronic acid-containing oligosaccharides, in the mixture. The extinction coefficient of the 4, 5-unsaturated bond at 232 nm was assumed as 5.5 L/(mmol·cm). One unit of the enzyme was defined as the amount of enzyme needed to catalyze the production of 1 μmol unsaturated oligosaccharides per minute, and the activity of one-milligram enzyme was defined as the specific activity of FdlA-NTD. Absorption at 232 nm was measured continuously at room temperature for 10min using a U-3900 UV-Visible spectrophotometer (Hitachi High-tech, Tokyo, Japan). Each measurement was repeated at least two times.

4.6. Biochemical Characterization of FdlA-NTD

To determine the optimal catalytic pH of FdlA-NTD, B & R buffer systems (pH 5.0–12.0) were used at a concentration of 50 mM for the reaction using 1% (*w*/*v*) Kj-fucoidan as the substrate. To determine the optimal temperature, reactions were performed at different temperatures, ranging from 10 °C to 70 °C. All enzymatic reactions under different temperatures were incubated for 1min, and then the reaction mixtures were boiled to stop the catalysis. To determine the thermal inactivation of FdlA-NTD, the reaction system was pre-incubated at 20 °C, 30 °C, 35 °C, and 40 °C, respectively, for varied time intervals (5 min to 120 min) at pH 7.5, and then chilled on ice for at least 10 min. The activities were measured under standard conditions (pH 7.5, 40 °C for 1 min). To determine the optimal NaCl concentration, the activity of FdlA-NTD was measured under standard conditions with different NaCl concentrations (0.092 M–2 M).

The effects of metal ions or chemical reagents (1 mM) on the catalytic activity of FdlA-NTD were determined by adding 1 mM of various metal ions or chemical reagents [$Pb(CH_3COO)_2$, $NiSO_4$, $MnSO_4$, $CuSO_4$, $BaCl_2$, $CoCl_2$, $CaCl_2$, $MgCl_2$, $FeSO_4$, $Fe_2(SO_4)_3$, KCl, LiCl, SDS, EDTA, β-mercaptoethanol, iodoacetamide] to the standard enzyme assay system as above. Since phosphate in B & R buffer might impact the assay, 50 mM Tris-HCl (pH 7.5) was used instead. The system without supplying metal ions or chemical reagents was used as the control.

Kinetic parameters were determined under initial rate conditions using non-linear regression analysis of the Michaelis–Menten equation. The lyase activity was measured at room temperature using Kj-fucoidan as substrate at concentrations ranging from 0.2 to 2% (*w*/*v*) in a 50 mM B & R buffer (pH 7.5) after being incubated for 60 s.

4.7. Analysis of Degradation Products

The molecular weight (MW) of Kj-fucoidan is within a range since it is a mixture of heterogeneous polysaccharides. To estimate the average MW of Kj-fucoidan, the samples were analyzed by High-Performance Gel Permeation Chromatography (HPGPC) with TSK GEL GMPWXL column, and the polysaccharides were eluted with mobile phase containing double distilled water at a flow rate of 0.5 mL/min and detected by Evaporative Light-scattering Detector (Acchrom, Beijing, China). The average MW of Kj-fucoidan was estimated as 80 kDa.

High-performance liquid chromatography (HPLC) analysis was used to purify the degradation products of Kj-fucoidan cleaved by FdlA-NTD. FdlA-NTD was incubated with 1% (*w*/*v*) Kj-fucoidan in 50 mM sodium phosphate buffer (pH 7.5) for 3 h at 37 °C, and the enzyme was then inactivated by heating in a water bath at 100 °C for 10 min. The reaction mixture was centrifuged at 12,000 rpm for 10 min, and the supernatant was subjected to high-performance liquid chromatography analysis. HPLC analysis was performed on an Acchrom S6000 HPLC system (Acchrom Technologie, Dalian, China) and the separation was performed on an Acchrom XAmide column (4.6 mm × 250 mm, 5 μm, Acchrom Technologies, Dalian, China). The mobile phase consisted of water (A), acetonitrile (B), and ammonium formate (C) with the following elution gradients: mobile phase A from 0 to 40%, mobile phase B from 90% to 50%, and mobile phase C at 10% within 40 min, at a flow rate of 1.5 mL/min and a column temperature of 40 °C. The enzymatic digestion products were detected at 232 nm with a UV detector.

Mass spectrometric (MS) analysis was used to identify the degradation products of FdlA-NTD. The purified enzymatic digestion products were mixed with the matrix DHB and analyzed by a matrix-assisted laser resolved ionization-time of flight mass spectrometer (UltraflextremeTM MALDI-TOF/TOF, Brucker, Karlsruhe, Germany) in reflection mode.

4.8. Microscale Thermophoresis Assay

Microscale thermophoresis (MST) assay was performed on NT.115 Monolith instrument from NanoTemper Technologies using standard treated capillaries (NanoTemper, Munich, Germany). The purified wild-type and mutant proteins (10 μM) were labeled using a Protein Labeling Kit RED-NHS 2nd Generation. The substrate Kj-fucoidan (45 μM) was prepared in a ligand buffer containing 25 mM Hepes pH 7.5, 100 mM NaCl, and done two-fold dilution in series. For the MST assay, 150 nM labeled protein was incubated with a series of substrates in a ligand buffer containing 0.05% Tween-20 for 5 min in NT.115 capillaries separately. Each capillary containing the mixed enzyme and substrate was tested by Monolish NT.115 at 25 °C, 20% excitation power, and medium MST power. Thermophoresis data were analyzed by MO. Affinity Analysis software (version 2.3, NanoTemper) [47]. Each measurement was repeated at least two times.

4.9. Molecular Docking

Molecular docking analysis of FdlA-NTD with various oligosaccharides (substrates) was performed to identify the amino acid residues potentially critical for the active site formation and catalysis of FdlA-NTD. The structural coordinates of oligosaccharide molecules containing a sulfate group were built with a CHARMM-GUI server online (http://www.charmm-gui.org/, accessed on 15 July 2021) [48] and converted into mol2 format by Open Bable tool for Ledock program (version 1.0) [37,49]. A root-mean-squares deviation (RMSD) value and the number of binding poses were set to 1 and 500, respectively. All docked results were sorted by score energy ranking. The docking results ranking on the top of the list were chosen for analysis in the next step.

5. Conclusions

FdlA from *Flavobacterium* sp. SA-0082 is the first fucoidan lyase reported so far. Here, we determined the atomic-resolution crystal structures of the FdlA N-terminal catalytic domain. In addition, we performed extensive biochemical and enzymatic analysis on the wild-type and mutant forms of FdlA-NTD, revealing key residues essential for the catalysis. Compared with other β-helix PLs, FdlA-NTD possesses a similar overall folding, but considerably different active site and key residues that potentially serve as the catalytic acid and base in β-elimination reaction. Moreover, we revealed that FdlA-NTD uses a unique 'groove-pocket' for substrate binding and the alkaline pocket is suitable to accommodate a trisaccharide unit, thus rationalizing the observation that the final product of FdlA-NTD is exclusively trisaccharide. Together, our work identified the unique structural and catalytic features of FdlA-NTD, providing novel insights into the mode of action of PLs, and enriching our knowledge on the fucoidan-degrading enzymes. Our results may further aid the applied research in designing mutated forms of FdlA-NTD that would be used in producing specific products for industrial use.

Supplementary Materials: The following supporting information can be downloaded at: https://www.mdpi.com/article/10.3390/md20080533/s1, Figure S1: Sequence alignment of FdlA and FdlB; Figure S2: Purification and characterization of FdlA-NTD; Figure S3: Structural superposition of two molecules in an asymmetric unit of FdlA-NTD crystal structure; Figure S4: Comparison of FdlA-NTD with representative members of other β-helix PL families; Figure S5: The sulfate groups and docked trisaccharide in the 'groove-pocket' region of FdlA-NTD; Figure S6: The MST curves of inactive mutants of FdlA-NTD with the substrate (Kj-fucoidan); Figure S7: Electron density maps of the mutated site in inactive mutants; Table S1: Diffraction data and refinement statistics of WT and mutants of FdlA-NTD.

Author Contributions: Investigation, J.W., Z.L., X.P. and N.W.; writing—original draft preparation, J.W.; writing—review and editing, M.L. and J.L.; supervision, M.L. and J.L.; project administration, L.L., Y.D., M.L. and J.L.; funding acquisition, M.L. and J.L. All authors have read and agreed to the published version of the manuscript.

Funding: This research was funded by the Strategic Priority Research Program of CAS, grant number XDB27020106 and the National Natural Science Foundation of China, grant numbers 21877114 and 31930064.

Institutional Review Board Statement: Not applicable.

Informed Consent Statement: Not applicable.

Data Availability Statement: Atomic coordinates and crystallographic structure factors have been deposited in the protein data bank under accession codes: 7XZF (WT), 7XZ7 (D137A), 7XZ8 (K141), 7XZE (H176A), 7XZD (F179A), 7XZ9 (E236A), 7XZC (R240A), 7XZB (Y242A), 7XZA (Y242F). All other data supporting the finding in this study are available from the corresponding authors upon reasonable request.

Acknowledgments: We thank Q, Wang from Dalian Ocean University for kindly providing the Kj-fucoidan. We thank Y. Chen, Z. Yang, and B. Zhou from IBP, CAS for MST experiment; L. Niu, X. Ding, and M. Zhang from IBP, CAS for mass spectrometry; J. Li from IBP, CAS for CD assay; X. Zhao for the assistance in sample preparation. We are grateful to the staff at the Shanghai Synchrotron Radiation Facility (Shanghai, China) for technical support during diffraction data collection. We thank Torsten Juelich (University of Chinese Academy of Sciences) for linguistic assistance during the preparation of the article.

Conflicts of Interest: The authors declare no conflict of interest.

References

1. Li, B.; Lu, F.; Wei, X.; Zhao, R. Fucoidan: Structure and Bioactivity. *Molecules* **2008**, *13*, 1671–1695. [CrossRef] [PubMed]
2. Yu, L.; Ge, L.; Xue, C.; Chang, Y.; Zhang, C.; Xu, X.; Wang, Y. Structural study of fucoidan from sea cucumber *Acaudina molpadioides*: A fucoidan containing novel tetrafucose repeating unit. *Food Chem.* **2014**, *142*, 197–200. [CrossRef] [PubMed]
3. Anastyuk, S.D.; Shevchenko, N.M.; Nazarenko, E.L.; Dmitrenok, P.S.; Zvyagintseva, T.N. Structural analysis of a fucoidan from the brown alga *Fucus evanescens* by MALDI-TOF and tandem ESI mass spectrometry. *Carbohydr. Res.* **2009**, *344*, 779–787. [CrossRef] [PubMed]

4. Ale, M.T.; Mikkelsen, J.D.; Meyer, A.S. Important Determinants for Fucoidan Bioactivity: A Critical Review of Structure-Function Relations and Extraction Methods for Fucose-Containing Sulfated Polysaccharides from Brown Seaweeds. *Mar. Drugs* **2011**, *9*, 2106–2130. [CrossRef] [PubMed]
5. Cao, H.; Mikkelsen, M.; Lezyk, M.; Bui, L.; Tran, V.; Silchenko, A.; Kusaykin, M.; Pham, T.; Truong, B.; Holck, J.; et al. Novel Enzyme Actions for Sulphated Galactofucan Depolymerisation and a New Engineering Strategy for Molecular Stabilisation of Fucoidan Degrading Enzymes. *Mar. Drugs* **2018**, *16*, 422. [CrossRef]
6. Zayed, A.; El-Aasr, M.; Ibrahim, A.-R.S.; Ulber, R. Fucoidan Characterization: Determination of Purity and Physicochemical and Chemical Properties. *Mar. Drugs* **2020**, *18*, 571. [CrossRef]
7. Usov, A.I.; Bilan, M.I. Fucoidans—Sulfated polysaccharides of brown algae. *Russ. Chem. Rev.* **2009**, *78*, 785–799. [CrossRef]
8. Kwon, P.S.; Oh, H.; Kwon, S.J.; Jin, W.; Zhang, F.; Fraser, K.; Hong, J.J.; Linhardt, R.J.; Dordick, J.S. Sulfated polysaccharides effectively inhibit SARS-CoV-2 in vitro. *Cell Discov.* **2020**, *6*, 50. [CrossRef]
9. Luthuli, S.; Wu, S.; Cheng, Y.; Zheng, X.; Wu, M.; Tong, H. Therapeutic Effects of Fucoidan: A Review on Recent Studies. *Mar. Drugs* **2019**, *17*, 487. [CrossRef]
10. Wijesekara, I.; Pangestuti, R.; Kim, S.-K. Biological activities and potential health benefits of sulfated polysaccharides derived from marine algae. *Carbohydr. Polym.* **2011**, *84*, 14–21. [CrossRef]
11. Kusaykin, M.; Bakunina, I.; Sova, V.; Ermakova, S.; Kuznetsova, T.; Besednova, N.; Zaporozhets, T.; Zvyagintseva, T. Structure, biological activity, and enzymatic transformation of fucoidans from the brown seaweeds. *Biotechnol. J.* **2008**, *3*, 904–915. [CrossRef] [PubMed]
12. Kusaykin, M.I.; Silchenko, A.S.; Zakharenko, A.M.; Zvyagintseva, T.N. Fucoidanases. *Glycobiology* **2016**, *26*, 3–12. [CrossRef] [PubMed]
13. Furukawa, S.-I.; Fujikawa, T.; Koga, D.; Ide, A. Purification and Some Properties of Exo-type Fucoidanases fromVibriosp. N-5. *Biosci. Biotechnol. Biochem.* **2014**, *56*, 1829–1834. [CrossRef]
14. Lahrsen, E.; Liewert, I.; Alban, S. Gradual degradation of fucoidan from *Fucus vesiculosus* and its effect on structure, antioxidant and antiproliferative activities. *Carbohydr. Polym.* **2018**, *192*, 208–216. [CrossRef] [PubMed]
15. Silchenko, A.S.; Rasin, A.B.; Zueva, A.O.; Kusaykin, M.I.; Zvyagintseva, T.N.; Rubtsov, N.K.; Ermakova, S.P. Discovery of a fucoidan endo-4O-sulfatase: Regioselective 4O-desulfation of fucoidans and its effect on anticancer activity in vitro. *Carbohydr. Polym.* **2021**, *271*, 118449. [CrossRef]
16. Vuillemin, M.; Silchenko, A.S.; Cao, H.T.T.; Kokoulin, M.S.; Trang, V.T.D.; Holck, J.; Ermakova, S.P.; Meyer, A.S.; Mikkelsen, M.D. Functional Characterization of a New GH107 Endo-α-(1, 4)-Fucoidanase from the Marine Bacterium Formosa haliotis. *Mar. Drugs* **2020**, *18*, 562. [CrossRef]
17. Zueva, A.O.; Silchenko, A.S.; Rasin, A.B.; Kusaykin, M.I.; Usoltseva, R.V.; Kalinovsky, A.I.; Kurilenko, V.V.; Zvyagintseva, T.N.; Thinh, P.D.; Ermakova, S.P. Expression and biochemical characterization of two recombinant fucoidanases from the marine bacterium *Wenyingzhuangia fucanilytica* CZ1127(T). *Int. J. Biol. Macromol.* **2020**, *164*, 3025–3037. [CrossRef]
18. Sakai, T.; Kimura, H.; Kato, I. A marine strain of flavobacteriaceae utilizes brown seaweed fucoidan. *Mar. Biotechnol.* **2002**, *4*, 399–405. [CrossRef]
19. Sakai, T.; Kimura, H.; Kato, I. Purification of Sulfated Fucoglucuronomannan Lyase from Bacterial Strain of *Fucobacter marina* and Study of Appropriate Conditions for Its Enzyme Digestion. *Mar. Biotechnol.* **2003**, *5*, 380–387. [CrossRef]
20. Takayama, M.; Koyama, N.; Sakai, T.; Kato, I. Enzymes Capable of Degrading a Sulfated-Fucose-Containing Polysaccharide and Their Encoding Genes. U.S. Patent No. US 6,489,155 B1, 3 December 2002.
21. Sakai, T.; Kimura, H.; Kojima, K.; Shimanaka, K.; Ikai, K.; Kato, I. Marine Bacterial Sulfated Fucoglucuronomannan (SFGM) Lyase Digests Brown Algal SFGM into Trisaccharides. *Mar. Biotechnol.* **2003**, *5*, 70–78. [CrossRef]
22. Lombard, V.; Bernard, T.; Rancurel, C.; Brumer, H.; Coutinho Pedro, M.; Henrissat, B. A hierarchical classification of polysaccharide lyases for glycogenomics. *Biochem. J.* **2010**, *432*, 437–444. [CrossRef] [PubMed]
23. Xu, F.; Wang, P.; Zhang, Y.-Z.; Chen, X.-L.; Zhou, N.-Y. Diversity of Three-Dimensional Structures and Catalytic Mechanisms of Alginate Lyases. *Appl. Environ. Microbiol.* **2018**, *84*, e02040-17. [CrossRef] [PubMed]
24. Garron, M.-L.; Cygler, M. Uronic polysaccharide degrading enzymes. *Curr. Opin. Struct. Biol.* **2014**, *28*, 87–95. [CrossRef] [PubMed]
25. Garron, M.L.; Cygler, M. Structural and mechanistic classification of uronic acid-containing polysaccharide lyases. *Glycobiology* **2010**, *20*, 1547–1573. [CrossRef] [PubMed]
26. Baumgartner, S.; Hofmann, K.; Chiquet-Ehrismann, R.; Bucher, P. The discoidin domain family revisited: New members from prokaryotes and a homology-based fold prediction. *Protein. Sci.* **1998**, *7*, 1626–1631. [CrossRef]
27. Veith, P.D.; Nor Muhammad, N.A.; Dashper, S.G.; Likić, V.A.; Gorasia, D.G.; Chen, D.; Byrne, S.J.; Catmull, D.V.; Reynolds, E.C. Protein Substrates of a Novel Secretion System Are Numerous in the Bacteroidetes Phylum and Have in Common a Cleavable C-Terminal Secretion Signal, Extensive Post-Translational Modification, and Cell-Surface Attachment. *J. Proteome Res.* **2013**, *12*, 4449–4461. [CrossRef]
28. Hayakawa, K.; Guo, L.; Terentyeva, E.A.; Li, X.-K.; Kimura, H.; Hirano, M.; Yoshikawa, K.; Nagamine, T.; Katsumata, N.; Ogata, T.; et al. Determination of specific activities and kinetic constants of biotinidase and lipoamidase in LEW rat and *Lactobacillus casei (Shirota)*. *J. Chromatogr. B* **2006**, *844*, 240–250. [CrossRef]

29. Yoder, M.D.; Lietzke, S.E.; Jurnak, F. Unusual structural features in the parallel beta-helix in pectate lyases. *Structure* **1993**, *1*, 241–251. [CrossRef]
30. Scavetta, R.D.; Herron, S.R.; Hotchkiss, A.T.; Kita, N.; Keen, N.T.; Benen, J.A.; Kester, H.C.; Visser, J.; Jurnak, F. Structure of a plant cell wall fragment complexed to pectate lyase C. *Plant Cell* **1999**, *11*, 1081–1092. [CrossRef]
31. Huang, W.; Matte, A.; Li, Y.; Kim, Y.S.; Linhardt, R.J.; Su, H.; Cygler, M. Crystal structure of chondroitinase B from Flavobacterium heparinum and its complex with a disaccharide product at 1.7 A resolution. *J. Mol. Biol.* **1999**, *294*, 1257–1269. [CrossRef]
32. Petersen, T.N.; Kauppinen, S.; Larsen, S. The crystal structure of rhamnogalacturonase A from Aspergillus aculeatus: A right-handed parallel beta helix. *Structure* **1997**, *5*, 533–544. [CrossRef]
33. Alahuhta, M.; Taylor, L.E., II; Brunecky, R.; Sammond, D.W.; Michener, W.; Adams, M.W.; Himmel, M.E.; Bomble, Y.J.; Lunin, V. The catalytic mechanism and unique low pH optimum of *Caldicellulosiruptor bescii* family 3 pectate lyase. *Acta Crystallogr. D Biol. Crystallogr.* **2015**, *71*, 1946–1954. [CrossRef] [PubMed]
34. Lyu, Q.; Zhang, K.; Shi, Y.; Li, W.; Diao, X.; Liu, W. Structural insights into a novel Ca^{2+}-independent PL-6 alginate lyase from Vibrio OU02 identify the possible subsites responsible for product distribution. *Biochim. Biophys. Acta (BBA) Gen. Subj.* **2019**, *1863*, 1167–1176. [CrossRef] [PubMed]
35. Luis, A.S.; Briggs, J.; Zhang, X.; Farnell, B.; Ndeh, D.; Labourel, A.; Baslé, A.; Cartmell, A.; Terrapon, N.; Stott, K.; et al. Dietary pectic glycans are degraded by coordinated enzyme pathways in human colonic Bacteroides. *Nat. Microbiol.* **2017**, *3*, 210–219. [CrossRef]
36. Itoh, T.; Nakagawa, E.; Yoda, M.; Nakaichi, A.; Hibi, T.; Kimoto, H. Structural and biochemical characterisation of a novel alginate lyase from *Paenibacillus* sp. str. FPU-7. *Sci. Rep.* **2019**, *9*, 14870. [CrossRef]
37. Wang, Z.; Sun, H.; Yao, X.; Li, D.; Xu, L.; Li, Y.; Tian, S.; Hou, T. Comprehensive evaluation of ten docking programs on a diverse set of protein–ligand complexes: The prediction accuracy of sampling power and scoring power. *Phys. Chem. Chem. Phys.* **2016**, *18*, 12964–12975. [CrossRef]
38. Davies, G.J.; Wilson, K.S.; Henrissat, B. Nomenclature for sugar-binding subsites in glycosyl hydrolases. *Biochem. J.* **1997**, *321*, 557–559. [CrossRef]
39. Xu, F.; Chen, X.-L.; Sun, X.-H.; Dong, F.; Li, C.-Y.; Li, P.-Y.; Ding, H.; Chen, Y.; Zhang, Y.-Z.; Wang, P. Structural and molecular basis for the substrate positioning mechanism of a new PL7 subfamily alginate lyase from the arctic. *J. Biol. Chem.* **2020**, *295*, 16380–16392. [CrossRef]
40. Dong, F.; Xu, F.; Chen, X.-L.; Li, P.-Y.; Li, C.-Y.; Li, F.-C.; Chen, Y.; Wang, P.; Zhang, Y.-Z. Alginate Lyase Aly36B is a New Bacterial Member of the Polysaccharide Lyase Family 36 and Catalyzes by a Novel Mechanism With Lysine as Both the Catalytic Base and Catalytic Acid. *J. Mol. Biol.* **2019**, *431*, 4897–4909. [CrossRef]
41. Kokoska, R.J.; McCulloch, S.D.; Kunkel, T.A. The Efficiency and Specificity of Apurinic/Apyrimidinic Site Bypass by Human DNA Polymerase η and *Sulfolobus solfataricus* Dpo4. *J. Biol. Chem.* **2003**, *278*, 50537–50545. [CrossRef]
42. Wang, Q.-S.; Zhang, K.-H.; Cui, Y.; Wang, Z.-J.; Pan, Q.-Y.; Liu, K.; Sun, B.; Zhou, H.; Li, M.-J.; Xu, Q.; et al. Upgrade of macromolecular crystallography beamline BL17U1 at SSRF. *Nucl. Sci. Tech.* **2018**, *29*, 68. [CrossRef]
43. Zhang, W.-Z.; Tang, J.-C.; Wang, S.-S.; Wang, Z.-J.; Qin, W.-M.; He, J.-H. The protein complex crystallography beamline (BL19U1) at the Shanghai Synchrotron Radiation Facility. *Nucl. Sci. Tech.* **2019**, *30*, 170. [CrossRef]
44. Otwinowski, Z.; Minor, W. Processing of X-ray diffraction data collected in oscillation mode. *Methods Enzymol.* **1997**, *276*, 307–326.
45. Adams, P.D.; Grosse-Kunstleve, R.W.; Hung, L.W.; Ioerger, T.R.; McCoy, A.J.; Moriarty, N.W.; Read, R.J.; Sacchettini, J.C.; Sauter, N.K.; Terwilliger, T.C. PHENIX: Building new software for automated crystallographic structure determination. *Acta Crystallogr. D Biol. Crystallogr.* **2002**, *58*, 1948–1954. [CrossRef]
46. Emsley, P.; Cowtan, K. Coot: Model-building tools for molecular graphics. *Acta Crystallogr. Sect. D Biol. Crystallogr.* **2004**, *60*, 2126–2132. [CrossRef]
47. Scheuermann, T.H.; Padrick, S.B.; Gardner, K.H.; Brautigam, C.A. On the acquisition and analysis of microscale thermophoresis data. *Anal. Biochem.* **2016**, *496*, 79–93. [CrossRef] [PubMed]
48. Park, S.J.; Lee, J.; Qi, Y.; Kern, N.R.; Lee, H.S.; Jo, S.; Joung, I.; Joo, K.; Lee, J.; Im, W. CHARMM-GUI Glycan Modeler for modeling and simulation of carbohydrates and glycoconjugates. *Glycobiology* **2019**, *29*, 320–331. [CrossRef]
49. O'Boyle, N.M.; Banck, M.; James, C.A.; Morley, C.; Vandermeersch, T.; Hutchison, G.R. Open Babel: An open chemical toolbox. *J. Cheminform.* **2011**, *3*, 33. [CrossRef]

marine drugs

MDPI

Article

Biochemical Characterization and Elucidation of the Hybrid Action Mode of a New Psychrophilic and Cold-Tolerant Alginate Lyase for Efficient Preparation of Alginate Oligosaccharides

Shengsheng Cao [1], Li Li [1], Benwei Zhu [1,2,]* and Zhong Yao [1,2]

1 College of Food Science and Light Industry, Nanjing Tech University, Nanjing 211816, China
2 Suqian Advanced Materials Industry Technology Innovation Center of Nanjing Tech University, Suqian 223800, China
* Correspondence: zhubenwei@njtech.edu.cn

Abstract: Alginate lyases with unique biochemical properties have irreplaceable value in food and biotechnology industries. Herein, the first new hybrid action mode *Thalassotalea algicola*-derived alginate lyase gene (TAPL7A) with both psychrophilic and cold-tolerance was cloned and expressed heterologously in *E. coli*. With the highest sequence identity (43%) to the exolytic alginate lyase AlyA5 obtained from *Zobellia galactanivorans*, TAPL7A was identified as a new polysaccharide lyases family 7 (PL7) alginate lyase. TAPL7A has broad substrate tolerance with specific activities of 4186.1 U/mg, 2494.8 U/mg, 2314.9 U/mg for polyM, polyG, and sodium alginate, respectively. Biochemical characterization of TAPL7A showed optimal activity at 15 °C, pH 8.0. Interestingly, TAPL7A exhibits both extreme psychrophilic and cold tolerance, which other cold-adapted alginate lyase do not possess. In a wide range of 5–30 °C, the activity can reach 80–100%, and the residual activity of more than 70% can still be maintained after 1 h of incubation. Product analysis showed that TAPL7A adopts a hybrid endo/exo-mode on all three substrates. FPLC and ESI-MS confirmed that the final products of TAPL7A are oligosaccharides with degrees of polymerization (Dps) of 1–2. This study provides excellent alginate lyase candidates for low-temperature environmental applications in food, agriculture, medicine and other industries.

Keywords: alginate lyase; biochemical characterization; endo/exolytic; psychrophilic; cold-tolerant

Citation: Cao, S.; Li, L.; Zhu, B.; Yao, Z. Biochemical Characterization and Elucidation of the Hybrid Action Mode of a New Psychrophilic and Cold-Tolerant Alginate Lyase for Efficient Preparation of Alginate Oligosaccharides. *Mar. Drugs* **2022**, *20*, 506. https://doi.org/10.3390/md20080506

Academic Editor: Hitoshi Sashiwa

Received: 13 July 2022
Accepted: 3 August 2022
Published: 5 August 2022

1. Introduction

Alginate is a structural polysaccharide in the cell wall of *Phaeophyta*, such as *Saccharin japonica* and *Undaria pinnatifida* [1]. Alginate consists of β-D-mannuronate (M) and its C5 epimer α-L-guluronate (G) randomly combined by 1,4 glycosidic bonds [1]. Alginate has been widely used in food, agriculture, medicine, materials and other industrial fields because of its excellent properties. For example, alginates can be used as food stabilizers and thickeners to improve the stability of ice cream [2]. As the products of alginate lyase degradation of alginate, alginate oligosaccharides (AOS) have the advantages of outstanding solubility and high bio-availability under the same biochemical activity as polysaccharide. Alginate oligosaccharides have probiotic properties and can regulate the intestinal micro-ecological balance by promoting the proliferation of *Bifidobacterium* [3]. In addition, AOS can promote the growth of crop roots, while polysaccharides did not show a corresponding effect [4].

As one of the modifying enzymes of alginate, alginate is degraded to low molecular oligosaccharides by alginate lyase by a β-elimination mechanism. Alginate lyases are mainly derived from marine bacteria (*Pseudomonas*, *Vibrio*), soil bacteria (*Klebsiella*, *Azotobacter*), viruses (*Chlorella vius*), fungi (*Corollospora intermedia*) and other microorganisms; marine algae (*Laminaria japonica*); marine echinoderms and mollusks (*Haliotis discus hannai*) [5].

According to the CAzy database, alginate lyases are classified into 14 polysaccharide lyase (PL) families, including PL5, PL6, PL7, PL8, PL14, PL15, PL17, PL18, PL31, PL32, PL34, PL36, PL39 and PL41 families. In addition, alginate lyases can be classified into polyG-lyase (EC4.2.2.11), polyM-lyase (EC4.2.2.3) and bifunctional lyase because of the difference in substrate specificity [6]. According to the action mode, endo-alginate lyase degrades the substrate to oligosaccharides with a degree of polymerization of 2 or more, while exo-alginate degrades the substrate to monosaccharides. In recent years, alginate lyases with both endo- and exo-activities have been gradually characterized, and their simple and clear product distributions have attracted extensive attention in tailoring special AOS [7]. However, the commercial application of alginate lyases is largely limited by low activity and poor adaptability to industrial environments [8]. Most of the alginate lyases with mixed endo/exo-mode belong to the PL17 family, and only Alg2951 derived from *Alteromonas portus* HB161718^T belongs to the PL7 family. To meet the environmental conditions for industrial applications, the discovery of extreme alginate lyases such as thermophilic and salt-tolerant enzymes have received extensive attention. Among them, cold-adapted enzymes have gradually attracted widespread attention in industrial applications [9]. Biocatalysis at lower temperatures reduces the instability of some biologically active substances. Therefore, with the biocatalytic degradation process of alginate from brown-algae at lower temperatures, more active substances can be retained [10]. The use of alginate lyases with high activity and catalytic efficiency at low temperature can reduce energy consumption and cost in the process of producing bioethanol from brown algae crops. The inactivation of mesophilic and hyperthermic enzymes requires higher temperatures and consumes more energy. Low temperature cannot only effectively prevent the reproduction of harmful microorganisms, but also selectively inactivate the alginate lyase by raising the temperature slightly to achieve the purpose of terminating the reaction [9,11]. Alginate lyases with excellent biochemical properties at low temperature have potential in industrial applications such as food, medicine and biotechnology.

The cold-adapted alginate lyases found so far are concentrated in the PL6, PL7, PL15 and PL17 families [7,12–14]. However, most of these characterized cold-adapted alginate lyases have good stability at low temperature, but lose more specific activity, and the optimal temperature is not lower than 20 °C. In relation to the PL7 family, there are dozens of alginate lyases that have been biochemically characterized, including some structural resolved, such as AlyA5 isolated from *Z. galactanivorans* and VxAly7D isolated from *Vibrio xiamenensis* QY104 [15,16]. The alginate lyases of the PL7 family have broad substrate specificities, and different enzymes have different modes of action. However, it is difficult for the discovered enzymes to have both high activity at low temperature and cold-tolerance, such as Aly3C derived from *Psychromonas* sp. C-3, AlyL1 derived from *Agarivorans* sp. L11 [13,17].

Herein, a cold-tolerant and psychrophilic PL7 family alginate lyase (TAPL7A) from *Thalassotalea algicola* was firstly cloned and expressed in *Escherichia coli*. We investigated the enzymatic properties and product distribution of TAPL7A, in detail. Its optimal temperature is 15 °C and optimal pH is 8.0. This enzyme is the first PL7 family alginate lyase with high activity and stability below 0–30 °C. Furthermore, TAPL7A adopts a hybrid endo/exo-mode to degrade three substrates into oligosaccharides with degrees of polymerization of 1–2 at low temperature, with a preference for polyM. This work provides a new psychrophilic and cold-tolerant alginate lyase for the preparation of alginate oligosaccharides, and provides new data for the study of the structure and functional mechanism of psychrophilic enzymes.

2. Results

2.1. Sequence Analysis of Gene TAPL7A

We first cloned and analyzed the gene of alginate lyase TAPL7A from *Thalassotalea algicola* in this study. The open reading frame (ORF) of TAPL7A, consisting of 1041 bp of nucleotides, encoded a putative alginate lyase composed of 347 amino acids with a theoretical molecular mass of 36.76 kDa. The isoelectric point (*p*I) of TAPL7A is 6.17. TAPL7A containing a 16-residue signal peptide (Met1-Ala16). Based on the results of the conserved domain analysis, TAPL7A contains only an alginate_lyase2 domain of 214 amino acids (Phe28-Arg343) (Figure 1a). TAPL7A has the highest identity of 43% with AlyA5 from *Zobellia galactanivorans* (GenBank accession no. CAZ98266.1) [15], which indicates that TAPL7A is a new member of the PL7 family. In order to study the relationship between the amino-acid sequence and structure function of TAPL7A, 11 structurally resolved alginate lyases from the PL7 family were selected for sequence alignment (Figure 1b). It is evident that TAPL7A contains conserved regions such as "QIH", "YFKAGVYNQ" and "(R/E)(S/T/N) EL", which form the active center in PL7 family alginate lyases and play a role in substrate recognition and catalysis [13]. The two catalytic residues His, Tyr and two neutralization residues Arg, Gln predicted to be involved in the catalytic process based on sequence alignment were also conserved in PL7 alginate lyases.

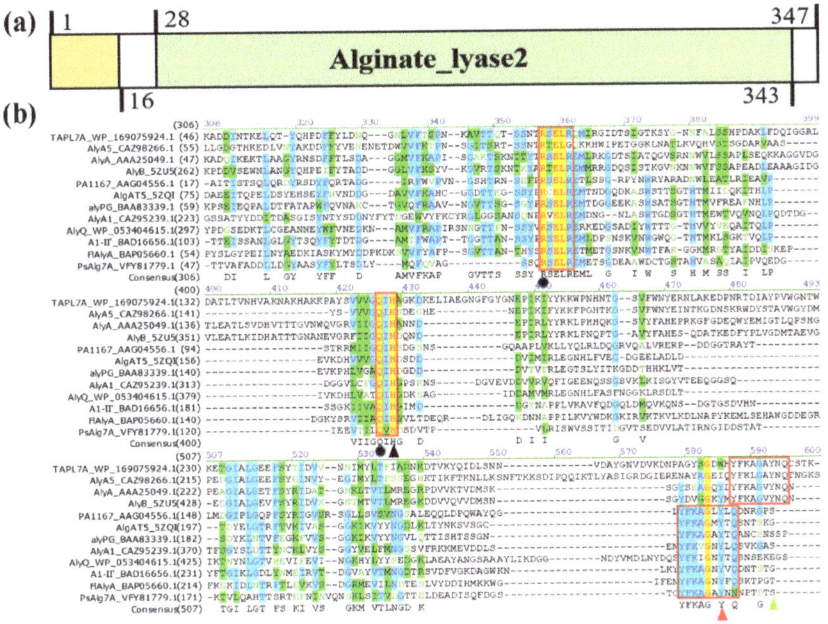

Figure 1. The domain analysis and multiple amino-acid sequence alignment of TAPL7A and other alginate lyases of PL7 family. (**a**) The domain of TAPL7A. (**b**) AlyA5 (CAZ98266.1) from *Zobellia galactanivorans* Dsij^T. AlyA (AAA25049.1) from *Klebsiella pneumoniae subsp.* aerogenes, AlyB (5ZU5) from *Vibrio splendidus*, PA1167 (AAG04556.1) from *Pseudomonas aeruginosa* PAO1, AlgAT5 (5ZQI) from *Defluviitalea*, alyPG (BAA83339.1) from *Corynebacterium* sp. ALY-1, AlyA1 (CAZ95239.1) from *Zobellia galactanivorans* Dsij^T, AlyQ (WP_053404615.1) from *Persicobacter* sp. CCB-QB2, A1-II′ (BAD16656.1) from *Sphingomonas* sp. A1, FlAlyA (BAP05660.1) from *Sphingomonas* sp. A1, PsAlg7A (VFY81779.1) from *Paradendryphiella salina*. Shaded yellow indicates identical and similar amino-acid residues in alginate lyase. The red boxes indicate the positions of the three conserved regions. Black triangles are catalytic bases, red triangles and green triangles represent catalytic acids of PL7 lyase in different red boxes, respectively. Black circles indicate the neutralization residues.

According to the CAZy database, the PL7 family is subdivided into 5 subfamilies 1, 2, 3, 4, 5 based on sequence similarity. In recent years, some PL7 enzymes with low sequence similarity to other enzymes in the database have been classified into a new subfamily 6 [13]. To further identify the evolutionary relationship of TAPL7A, 12 sequences from 5 subfamilies, 1 eukaryotic origin and 5 unclassified sequences were selected to construct a phylogenetic tree according to the CAZy database. It was found that TAPL7A clusters with representative enzymes of subfamily 5 (Figure 2), thus TAPL7A is considered as a new member of the subfamily 5. The results are also consistent with sequence homology. Several alginate lyases have been characterized in subfamily 5, but their substrate specificity is not limited by the subfamily. For example, AlyA (GenBank accession no. AAA25049.1) from *Klebsiella pneumoniae subsp. aerogenes* prefers polyG [18], AlyA5 (GenBank accession no. CAZ98266.1) from *Zobellia galactanivorans* Dsij^T prefers polyMG [15], and Alg7D (GenBank accession no. ABD81807.1) from *Saccharophagus degradans* 2–40 prefers polyM [19]. Therefore, the substrate specificity of TAPL7A cannot be predicted based on sequence alignment and phylogenetic-tree analysis alone, although it shares the highest identity with AlyA5.

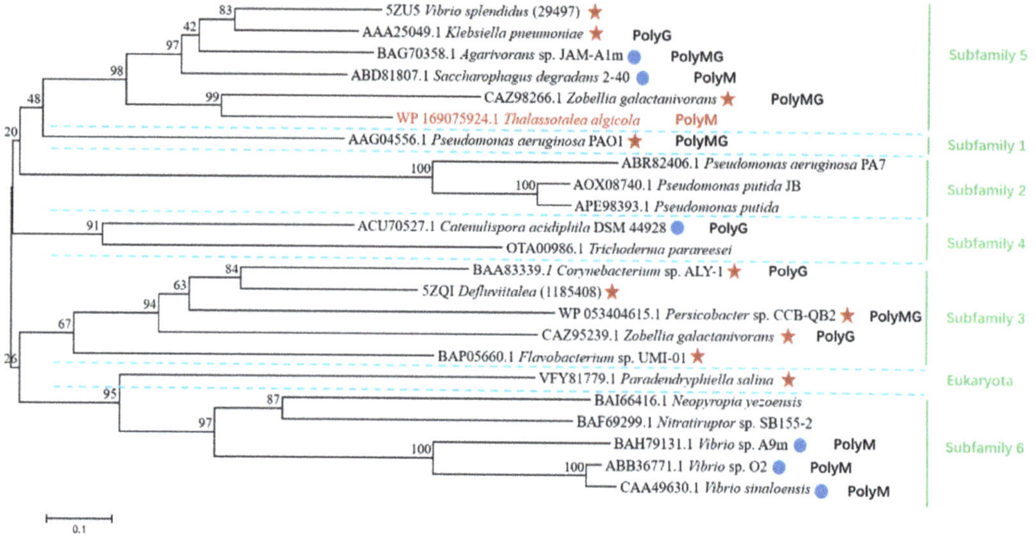

Figure 2. Phylogenetic analysis of TAPL7A with other alginate lyases of PL7 family. Subfamilies are separated by blue dotted lines according to the CAZy database. Enzymes for structure-solved are indicated by red five-pointed stars. Characterized enzymes are indicated by blue circles. PloyMG, PolyM, and PolyG represent the specific substrates of each enzyme, respectively. The red font is TAPL7A. The green vertical lines and fonts on the right represent the various subfamilies and PsAlg7A of eukaryotic origin.

2.2. Cloning and Expression of TAPL7A

After heterologous expression, most of the recombinant proteins aggregated in the sonicated bacterial pellet in the form of body proteins (Figure 3, Line 1 and line 2). After renaturation of the body proteins with reference to the method of Singh et al. [20], the active crude enzyme solution was obtained. Recombinant TAPL7A was purified by Ni-NTA Sepharose affinity chromatography. The target protein expression and purification were verified by SDS-PAGE analysis. As shown in Figure 3 (Line 3), it can be observed that the band of the target protein TAPL7A is clearly located between 35 kDa and 40 kDa, which is consistent with the predicted molecular mass of 36.76 kDa. The molecular mass of PL7 family alginate lyases mainly depend on their modular domains. The molecular weight of single-domain PL7 lyases is concentrated between 25–40 kDa, such as AlyA5 [15]. There are also alginate lyases of the PL7 family that contain, in addition to the catalytic domain, one or two carbohydrate-binding domains (CBMs) involved in substrate binding and regulation of product distribution [21,22].

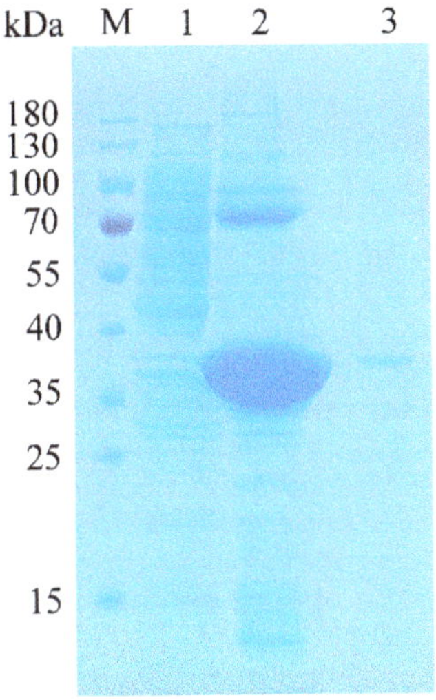

Figure 3. SDS-PAGE analysis of the molecular mass and purification effect of TAPL7A. Lane M protein: restrained marker (Thermo Scientific, USA); lane 1: the supernatant of *E. coli*-pET21a-TAPL7A; lane 2: induced cell lysate of *E. coli*-pET21a-TAPL7A; lane 3: renatured purified TAPL7A.

2.3. Substrate Specificity and Enzymatic Kinetics of TAPL7A

Three substrates (0.5% *w/v* sodium alginate, 0.5% *w/v* poly M and 0.5% *w/v* poly G) were used to perform activity assays and determine the substrate specificity of TAPL7A. The recombinant TAPL7A showed higher activity towards polyM (4186.1 U/mg) than that to polyG (2494.8 U/mg) and sodium alginate (2314.9 U/mg) (Table 1). Thus, TAPL7A is a new PL7 alginate lyase with a preference for polyM and can degrade polyG and sodium alginate with the same activity.

Table 1. Substrate specificity and kinetics of TAPL7A.

Substrate	Activity	K_m (mM)	V_{max} (μmol/s)	k_{cat} (s^{-1})
Alginate	2314.9 U/mg	0.26	0.0648	14.305
PolyM	4186.1 U/mg	3.43	0.0622	13.730
PolyG	2494.8 U/mg	1.89	0.07412	16.362

The kinetic parameters (K_m and V_{max}) of TAPL7A towards polyM, polyG and sodium alginate were calculated according to hyperbolic regression analysis as shown in Table 1. The K_m values of TAPL7A towards polyM, polyG, and sodium alginate were 3.43 mM, 1.89 mM and 0.26 mM, respectively. TAPL7A is considered to have the strongest affinity for the M-M blocks. It suggested that TAPL7A exhibited the higher catalytic efficiency towards G-block than that towards M-block and MG-block. Although the activities of TAPL7A on polyG and sodium alginate are only half of that on polyM, the catalytic efficiency are higher. It is speculated that the isoleucine (I) in the conserved motif "QIH" residue recognizes substrates, and that alginate lyases containing the "QIH" motif generally show a preference for polyG or polyMG blocks [23], similar to AlyA5, which has the highest identity to TAPL7A, and is a polyMG-preferred enzyme [15].

2.4. Effect of Temperature and pH on TAPL7A

TAPL7A exhibits surprising psychrophilicity, showing maximum activity at 15 °C and retaining more than 80% of its maximum activity between 5–30 °C (Figure 4c). In addition, the optimal incubation temperature for TAPL7A was 15 °C, and more than 70% of the residual activity was maintained after incubation at 5–30 °C for 1 h (Figure 4c).

In general, the optimal temperature below 35 °C and maintaining more than 50% of the maximum activity at 20 °C can be referred to as cold-adapted enzymes (Table 2). Several cold-adapted alginate lyases have been reported with optimal temperatures no lower than 20 °C [13,17,23–26]. This psychrophilic and highly cold-tolerant property of TAPL7A is rare among the cold-adapted alginate lyases. To the best of our knowledge, TAPL7A is currently the alginate lyase with the lowest optimal temperature 15 °C [27]. In order to highlight the excellent cold adaptation of TAPL7A, several cold-adapted enzymes were compared (Table 2). Characterized, cold-adapted alginate lyases exhibit either high activity at low temperature with poor cold tolerance, or strong cold tolerance with low activity at low temperature. For example, AlyL1 derived from *Agarivorans* sp. L11 has better cold resistance, but when the temperature is lower than 15 °C, its activity is only 20–50% of the maximum activity [28]. The thermophilic mechanism of thermophilic enzymes is currently thought to be their more compact conformation and rigid structure (such as disulfide bonds) [29]. Compared to thermostable enzymes, cold-adapted enzymes have highly flexible structural features. The high flexibility also comes with a stability trade-off, leading to thermal instability and, in the case of a few studies, cold instability [9,11]. The possible relatively loose structure of TAPL7A explains its low activity and instability in the environment at temperatures above 30 °C (Figure 4c). It is evident that compared to other cold-adapted enzymes, TAPL7A has more potential for industrial applications in low temperature environments (Table 2).

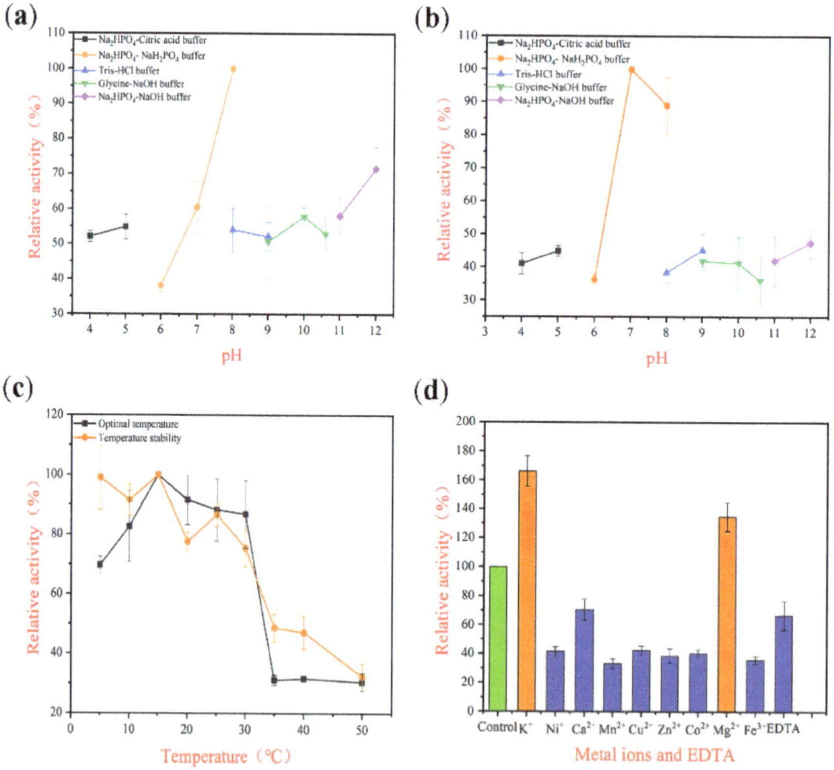

Figure 4. Biochemical characterization of TAPL7A. (**a**) The optimal pH of TAPL7A. (**b**) The pH stability of TAPL7A. (**c**) The optimal temperature and temperature stability of TAPL7A. (**d**) The effects of metal ions and EDTA on activity of TAPL7A. Orange represents metal ion activation; blue represents metal ion inhibition.

The optimal pH of TAPL7A is 8.0 (Figure 4a). Furthermore, TAPL7A maintained more than 50% of the maximum activity at pH 4.0–5.0 and pH 7.0–12.0, and maintained a high residual activity after incubation at the same pH environment (Figure 4a). The enzyme was mostly stable at pH 7.0–8.0 (Figure 4b). Most of the cold-adapted alginate lyases maintain high activity in the pH range near neutral, but their activity decreases sharply in the acidic and strongly alkaline range. For example, the enzymatic activity and stability of TsAly7B dropped below 40% of the maximum activity in environments below pH 6.0 and above pH 9.0 [22]. In contrast, TAPL7A has good pH adaptability.

2.5. *Effect of Metal Ions on TAPL7A*

The effect of metal ions on enzyme activity was also investigated (Figure 4d). K^+ and Mg^{2+} can activate the activity of TAPL7A, while Ni^+, Ca^{2+}, Mn^{2+}, Zn^{2+}, Cu^{2+}, Co^{2+} and Fe^{3+} inhibit the activity of TAPL7A. In marine environments, the activity of alginate lyases including TAPL7A are normally activated by K^+ and Na^+, such as AlgNJ04 from *Vibrio* sp. NJ-04 [30]. Both divalent/trivalent metal ions other than Mg^{2+} and the metal ion chelator EDTA inhibited the activity of TAPL7A. The effect of metal ions on TAPL7A activity is similar to that of Alg2951 from *Alteromonas portus* HB161718^T [31].

Table 2. Properties of TAPL7A and partially characterized cold-adapted alginate lyases.

Enzyme	PL Family	Organism	Optimal Temperature (°C)/pH	Activity/Residual Activity at 5–15 °C	Degree of Polymerization of the Product (DP)	Mode of Action	Refs.
TAPL7A	PL7	*Thalassotalea algicola*	15/8.0	80–100%/90–100%	1–2	Endo+Exo	This study
Alyw201	PL7	*Vibrio* sp. W2	35/8.0	No data-60%/No data-90%	2–6	Endo	[23]
AlyC3	PL7	*Psychromonas* sp. C-3	20/8.0	58–92%/No data	1–3	Endo	[13]
AlyL1	PL7	*Agarivorans* sp. L11	40/8.6	20–54.5%/80–95%	2–3	Endo	[17]
TsAly7B	PL7	*Thalassomonas* sp. LD5	30/7.6	10–40%/60–80%	2–4	Endo	[22]
AlyPM	PL7	*Pseudoalteromonas* sp. SM0524	30/8.5	19–45%/90–100%	2–4	Endo	[26]
AlgB	PL7	*Vibrio* sp. W13	30/8.0	No data	2–5	Endo	[32]
A9mT	PL7	*Vibrio* sp. A9mT	30/7.5	No data/60–75%	No data	No data	[33]
Alg2951	PL7	*Alteromonas portus* HB161718^T	25/8.0	40–70%/100%	1, 3	Endo+Exo	[31]
AlyGC	PL6	*Glaciecola chathamensis*	30/7.0	50–60%/No data	1	Exo	[12]
AlgSH17	PL17	*Microbulbifer* sp. SH-1	30/7.0	No data	1, 2–6	Endo+Exo	[7]

2.6. *Effect of NaCl on TAPL7A*

Adapted to the marine environment, many alginate lyase enzymes are salt tolerance or/and salt activated [24,26,34]. For instance, the activity of AlgM4 from *Vibrio weizhoudaoensis* M0101 was significantly enhanced approximately 7-folds by 1.0 M NaCl [34]. Salt tolerance of TAPL7A was observed at NaCl concentrations of 0.1–1.0 M, taking the activity at 0 M NaCl as 100%. As shown in Figure 5, recombinant TAPL7A showed activity at 0 M NaCl, while increasing concentrations of NaCl (0–1.0 M) exhibited an increase and then a decrease in activity. The enzyme activity was increased 3-folds in the presence of 0.4 M NaCl. The activity of TAPL7A increased rapidly at NaCl concentrations in the range of 0–0.4 M and started to decrease slowly at concentrations above 0.4 M. Thus, TAPL7A is a new salt-activated alginate lyase. An amount of 0.4 M NaCl is comparable to the salt concentration of the optimal growth environment of *Thalassotalea algicola* [35]. The activity of TAPL7A at 1 M NaCl concentration was still higher than 0 M, which may indicate that its adaptation to salt concentration fluctuations varies with the salt concentration of the original growth environment of the strain. Similarly, AlyC3 derived from *Psychromonas* sp. C-3 has similar adaptations to environmental salt concentrations [13]. Several salt-activated alginate lyases have been found to have different mechanisms of salt tolerance. The salt activation of AlyPM derived from *Pseudoalteromonas* sp. SM0524 is due to its affinity for the substrate being enhanced by NaCl [26], while the salt activation of AlgM4 is due to the fact that its secondary structure can be altered by NaCl, possibly enhancing its substrate affinity and resistance to thermal denaturation [34]. The salt activation mechanism of TAPL7A requires further study.

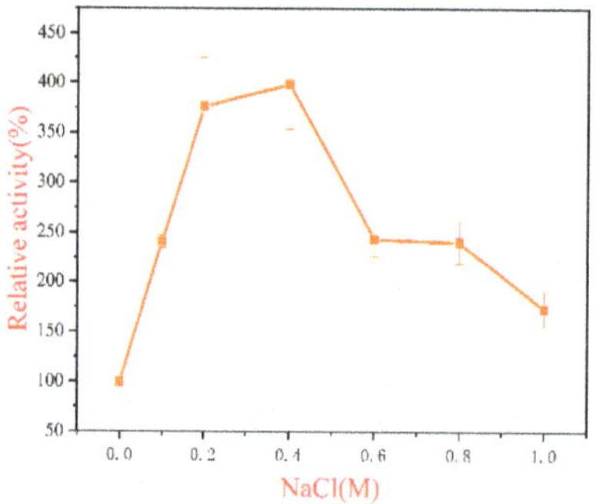

Figure 5. Effect of NaCl on TAPL7A.

2.7. Products Distribution and Action Pattern of TAPL7A

The degradation products of TAPL7A were analyzed by FPLC over a time gradient of 0–48 h (Figure 6). In the early stage of the reaction, the three substrates were mainly degraded to trisaccharides by TAPL7A. As the reaction progresses, trisaccharides are gradually degraded into disaccharides and monosaccharides. The verification of the composition of the degradation products was undertaken using ESI-MS (Figure 7). When sodium alginate, polyM and polyG are used as substrates, oligomers of DP1, 2 and 3 (Signals of 175.02 m/z [ΔDP1-H]$^-$, 351.05 m/z [ΔDP2-H]$^-$, and 527.01 m/z [ΔDP3-H]$^-$) are released as end products (Figure 7a–c). Consistent with the FPLC results, a signal of the monosaccharide conversion product 4-deoxy-L-erythron-5-hexoseuloseuronate acid (DEH) was also detected in the ESI-MS spectrum. Therefore, in the reaction process of TAPL7A, endo-activity is mainly used in the early stage, and exo-activity is mainly used in the later stage. It can be seen from the above results that TAPL7A can efficiently degrade three substrates into monosaccharide and disaccharide with a mixed endo/exo-mode. The product distribution of endo-lyase of the PL7-5 subfamily is concentrated in DP2-5, while the exo-lyase is concentrated in DP1 and 2. For example, endo-lyase AlyL2 derived from *Agarivorans* sp. L11 [28] and exo-lyase AlyA5 derived from *Zobellia galactanivorans* [15].

AOS is an excellent material for food, medicine and agricultural applications, and the difference in its degree of polymerization and structural composition will also lead to different effects. The unsaturated monosaccharide 4-deoxy-L-erythron-5-hexoseuloseuronate acid (DEH) produced by exo-lyases can be non-enzymatically converted to KDG for bioethanol production [36]. The AOS produced by the degradation of substrates by Alg2951 with the same endo/exo-mode of action has excellent antioxidant capacity [31]. Therefore, TAPL7A is an excellent tool enzyme for the production of high value-added AOS with low energy consumption and acid-base stability.

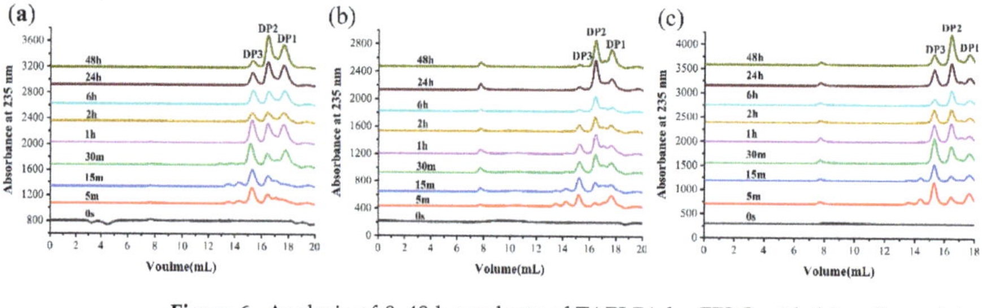

Figure 6. Analysis of 0–48 h products of TAPL7A by FPLC with (**a**) sodium alginate, (**b**) polyM, (**c**) polyG. The eluents were detected by measuring the absorbance at 235 nm.

(a)

(b)

(c)

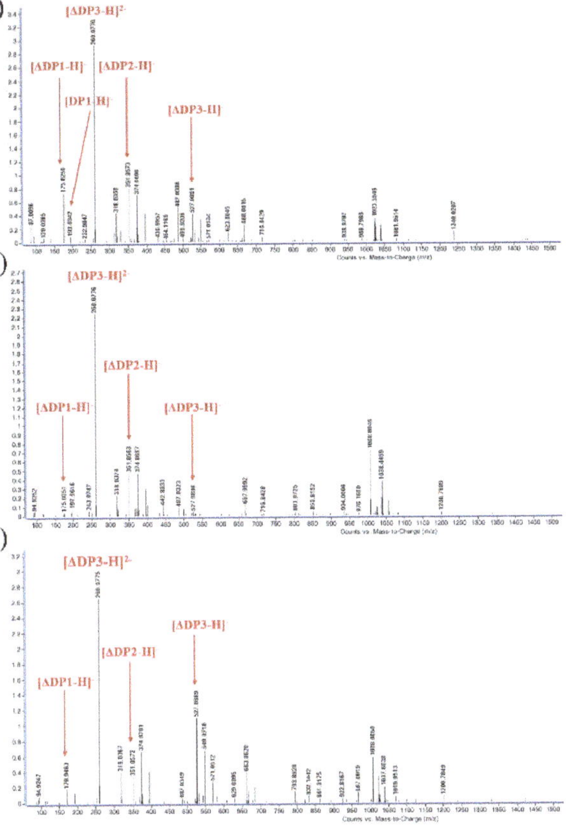

Figure 7. Analysis of 48 h product composition of TAPL7A by ESI-MS with (**a**) sodium alginate, (**b**) polyM, (**c**) polyG as substrates; The oligo-uronates are commonly described by their degree of polymerization (DPx). Oligo-uronates with the unsaturated terminal uronate are denoted in this study as ΔDPx, and such an oligomer would be ΔDP1.

2.8. Molecular Modeling

Most of the characterized PL7 family alginate lyases are endo-lyase with a wide range of substrate specificities. The mode of action and substrate preference of enzymes of the PL7 family are complex, such as the bifunctional endo-lyase PA1167 [37], the bifunctional exo-lyase VxAly7D [16], and the mixed endo/exo Alg2951 [31]. Therefore, structural studies of the PL7 family provide useful information on the mode of substrate recognition and depolymerization. The structure of the alginate lyase AlyA5 derived from *Zobellia galactanivorans* (PDB ID: 4BE3) was used as a template to construct a structural model of TAPL7A with 100% confidence using the online URL PHYRE2 (Figure 8a). The overall structure of TAPL7A is typical of the PL7 β-sandwich jelly roll-fold [15]. TAPL7A has 16 anti-parallel β-strands to form the main structure, of which three conserved motifs "(R/E) (S/T/N) EL", "QIH" and "YFKAGVYNQ" are located at β-4, β-7 and β-15, respectively. These three chains make up the catalytic cavity. Catalytic residues His160 and Tyr300 of TAPL7A predicted based on sequence alignment are displayed in the homology model (Figure 8a). The relatively loose structure of TAPL7A and the greater opening of the flexible loops can be seen from the structural alignment of TAPL7A (green structure) with AlyA5 (blue structure) (Figure 8b). This may also be evidence of TAPL7A psychrophilic and cold tolerance.

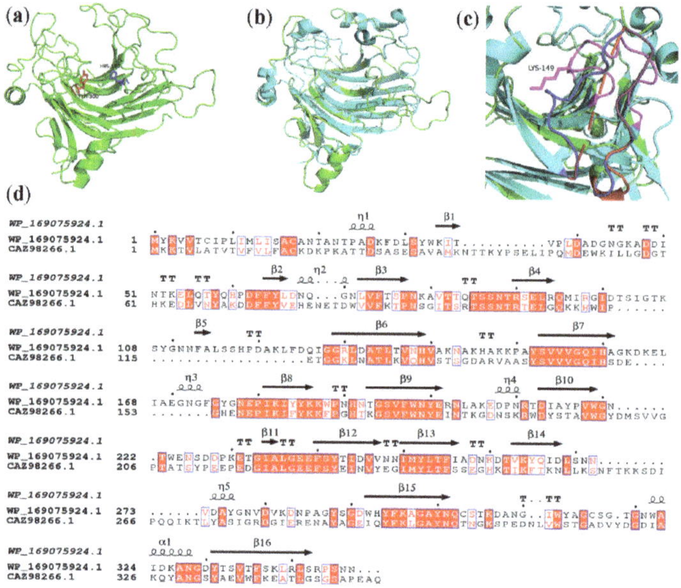

Figure 8. (**a**) Overall structure of TAPL7A; (**b**) The structural comparison of TAPL7A (green) and AlyA5 (cyan); (**c**) Comparison of loops at the ends of catalytic groove of TAPL7A (red and purple) and AlyA5 (blue); (**d**) Structure-based sequence alignment of TAPL7A and AlyA5. Conservative amino acids are highlighted by the red background and similar amino acids are highlighted by the red letters. α-helices are displayed as squiggles, β-strands are rendered as arrows, strict β-turns as TT letters. This figure has been generated using the program ESPRIPT 3.0.

Most of the PL7 family lyases have multiple flexible loops in their domains, which play a role in structural stability and mechanism of action. The structural determinants responsible for the exolytic activity of AlyA5 are three large additional loops, Trp197-Asp217, Ser257-Glu284 and Gly304-Asp318, which close the catalytic groove of the concave β-sheet at one end (Figure 8b) [15]. The structural basis of polyM-specific FlAlyA indicates that two flexible loops linked by hydrogen bonds above its catalytic cleft are involved in controlling the substrate specificity [38]. Comparing the structures of FlAlyA and AlyA5, it can be found that there are two to three flexible loops above their active clefts that play a role in substrate binding. However, the active cleft end of FlAlyA is unblocked, unlike AlyA5, which is blocked by three flexible loops. Structural alignment indicated that the loop blocked at the end of the catalytic groove in AlyA5 (blue loop Trp197-Asp217 in Figure 8c,d) was missing 7 amino acids at the corresponding position in TAPL7A (red putative loop Trp219-Thr232 in Figure 8c,d) and could not form a loop, so that the catalytic groove of TAPL7A was opened. As for one of the possible reasons for the exo-lyase activity, the loop His139-Ser153 in TAPL7A that extends into the catalytic groove but does not block the catalytic groove (purple loop Figure 8c,d). Only Tyr152 and Ser153 of this loop are conserved in AlyA5, but the remaining positions are replaced by other residues (His139-Ala151). In particular, the hydrophobic Ala138 at the top of this loop in AlyA5 is replaced by a basic Lys149 in TAPL7A, which may form hydrogen bonds with the substrate. Further research is needed, and structural elucidation will help to understand how the hybrid mode of action works.

3. Discussion

The ocean, which makes up 71% of the surface of the world, is a veritable treasure trove. In this treasure trove, marine enzymes represent an essential resource. Marine enzymes may have different characteristics from enzymes of terrestrial origin and show excellent potential applications in biological and industrial technologies. The special environment of the ocean may create special enzymes adapted to the industrial environment, such as heat-, salt- and base-tolerant enzymes. The potential of marine enzymes for biotechnology and industrial applications has been shown in numerous studies [39–45]. For example, thermostable proteases of marine origin have the potential to be used commercially in protein processing and in the production of protein hydrolysates in the detergent industry [46]. It is foreseeable that marine enzymes will become an important tool in various industrial fields in the future.

Alginate lyase is a key enzyme in the marine environment, which plays an important role in alginate degradation. Although hundreds of alginate lyases have been reported, only a few of them have specific properties. In this study, we report, for the first time, on both cold-adapted and cold-tolerant alginate lyase and their hybrid mode for efficient preparation of alginate oligosaccharides. TAPL7A is a new member of the PL7-5 subfamily and shares the highest homology of 43% with the alginate lyase AlyA5. TAPL7A has a typical PL7 family β-sandwich jelly roll-fold. The conserved motifs "QIH", "YFKAGVYNQ" and "(R/E) (S/T/N) EL" of PL7 family alginate lyases may play a catalytic and substrate binding role in TAPL7A. TAPL7A has an optimal pH of 8.0 and also has a wide range of pH adaptability and pH stability. The enzyme maintains 80–100% activity between 5–30 °C. Moreover, 70–100% of the activity can be retained after incubation at 5–30 °C for 1 h. To the best of our knowledge, this enzyme has the lowest optimal temperature (15 °C) and better cold adaptability among the alginate lyases found so far. In the presence of 0.4 M NaCl in the solution system, the activity of TAPL7A increased 3-fold compared with the absence of NaCl. Meanwhile, 0.4 M (2% *w*/*v*) NaCl is also the optimal salt concentration for *Thalassotalea algicola* growth [35]. The salt concentration-activated mechanism of TAPL7A may be adapted to the changes in the growth environment of *Thalassotalea algicola*. K^+ and Mg^{2+} activate the activity of TAPL7A, while Ni^+, Ca^{2+}, Mn^{2+}, Zn^{2+}, Cu^{2+}, Co^{2+} and Fe^{3+} inhibit its activity.

In addition, the enzyme has a unique hybrid endo/exo-mode. TAPL7A preferentially degrades polyM, but also has half the degradation activity of polyM for alginate and polyG. Early in the reaction, the three substrates can be degraded into alginate oligosaccharides with a degree of polymerization of DP1-3, and the trisaccharides can be degraded into monosaccharides and disaccharides with the progress of the reaction. Although we do not have the detailed crystal structure of TAPL7A, based on homologous model and sequence alignment, we speculate that one of the factors affecting its unique degradation pattern is the flexible loops (His139-Ser153) above its catalytic cleft. For example, Qin et al. studied the structural basis of the alginate lyase FlAlyA and confirmed that the flexible loops near the active cleft of the PL7 family lyase have an important impact on substrate binding and mode of action [38]. In regard to the excellent psychrophilic and cold tolerance of TAPL7A, we speculate that it is due to its relatively loose overall structure. A more in-depth study of TAPL7A, especially the structural basis, will provide a solid foundation for the analysis and understanding of cold-adaptive mechanisms and endo/exolytic patterns. With the growing demand for high value-added alginate oligosaccharides, alginate lyases with their special degradation mechanism and product distribution will become the first choice. At the same time, psychrophilic and cold-tolerant alginate lyases will consume less capacity during the production of alginate oligosaccharides, reducing costs and retaining more biological activity. In conclusion, TAPL7A is a potentially promising tool for tailoring alginate oligosaccharides at low temperature.

4. Materials and Methods

4.1. Materials

Sodium alginate was provided by Sigma-Aldrich (M/G ratio 77/23 isolated from *Macrosystis pyrifera*, viscosity $\geq$ 2000 Cp, St. Louis, MO, USA). PolyM and polyG with average DPs of 39 (purity: about 95%; M/G ratio: 3/97 and 97/3; average molecular weight: 7200 Da) were purchased from Qingdao BZ Oligo Biotech Co., Ltd. (Qingdao, China). All other chemicals and reagents were of analytical grade. In this study, *E. coli*

DH5α was used as the host for plasmid construction and *E. coli* BL21 (DE3) was used as the host for gene expression. E. coli was incubated at 37 °C in Luria–Bertani (LB) broth or LB broth agar plates (LB broth supplemented with 1.5% *w*/*v* agar) that both contained 100 μg/mL ampicillin.

4.2. Sequence Analysis of Gene TAPL7A

The theoretical molecular weight (Mw) and isoelectric point (*p*I) of TAPL7A were calculated online at the online website Compute *p*I/Mw tool of Expasy (https://web.expasy.org/compute_pi/, accessed on 10 September 2021). Signal peptides predicted by the online website SignalP-6.0 (https://services.healthtech.dtu.dk/service.php?SignalP-6.0, accessed on 23 September 2021). The alignment of protein sequences of TAPL7A and other enzymes was performed with ESPript program (https://espript.ibcp.fr/ESPript/ESPript/index.php, accessed on 29 September 2021). The conserved domains were analyzed by Simple Modular Architecture Research Tool (SMART) (http://www.ebi.ac.uk/Tools/pfa/iprscan/, accessed on 15 October 2021) [47]. According to the protein sequences of PL7 family enzymes, the phylogenetic tree was constructed through the Molecular Evolutionary Genetics Analysis (MEGA) Program version 5.05.

4.3. Cloning, Expression and Purification of TAPL7A

According to the genomic sequence information of *Thalassotalea algicola*, a pair of specific primers with *Nde* I and *Xho* I (TAPL7A-F: CGCCATATGTGCGCGAACACCGC-GAACAC, TAPL7A-R: CCGCTCGAG TGAGCCGCCCGAGCAACAAC) was designed. The expression vector was pET-21a (+) plasmid and *E. coli* BL21 (DE3) was used as the expression host. The recombinant strain was incubated at 37 °C until OD600 was 0.4–0.6, and expression of the recombinant enzyme was induced at 22 °C for 36 h after the addition of 0.1 mM IPTG. Referring to the method of Singh et al., 8 M urea was used to dissolve the inclusion body proteins in the precipitate of the disrupted bacterial solution, and the renatured body proteins were obtained by dialysis [20,48]. According to the method of zhu et al., the renatured TAPL7A was purified by a Ni-NTA Sepharose column (GE Healthcare, Uppsala, Sweden), and the TAPL7A before and after purification was verified by 12% (*w*/*v*) sodium dodecyl sulfate polyacrylamide gel electrophoresis (SDS-PAGE) [49]. Protein concentration was determined by a protein quantitative analysis kit (Beyotime Institute of Biotechnology, Nantong, China).

4.4. Substrate Specificity and Enzymatic Kinetics of TAPL7A

Purified TAPL7A (50 μL) was reacted with 150 μL of each of the three substrates (sodium alginate, polyM and polyG) at 0.5% (*w*/*v*) for 30 min at 15 °C, followed by a boiling water bath for 10 min to terminate the reaction. One unit of enzymatic activity was defined as the amounts of enzyme required to increase absorbance at 235 nm (extinction coefficient: 6150 $M^{-1}\cdot cm^{-1}$) by 0.01 per min. Substrate specificity was determined by the activity of TAPL7A in response to three different substrates (0.5% *w*/*v* sodium alginate, 0.5% *w*/*v* polyM and 0.5% *w*/*v* polyG). The kinetic parameters of the TAPL7A towards sodium alginate, polyM, and polyG were evaluated by measuring the enzyme activity with substrate at different concentrations as described previously [49]. The Lineweaver–Burk plots were used to calculate the kinetic parameters K_m and V_{max} based on the reaction rates of the enzymes with different concentrations of the three substrates (0.2–10.0 mg/mL) at 235 nm. The ratio of V_{max} versus enzyme concentration ([E]) was used to calculate the turnover number (k_{cat}) of the enzyme. All experiments were performed with three replicates.

4.5. Effect of Temperature and pH on TAPL7A

The reactions were performed at 5–50 °C to investigate the optimal temperature for TAPL7A. TAPL7A was incubated at 5–50 °C for 1 h and then reacted with alginate at 15 °C for 30 min to evaluate its temperature stability. Purified TAPL7A and substrate were mixed in a 1:3 ratio in buffers of different pH values (4.0–12.0) and reacted at 15 °C for 30 min, and the activity was measured under the following standard conditions. In detail, the purified enzyme was mixed with the substrate in buffers with different pHs, which were 50 mM phosphate-citrate (pH 4.0–5.0), 50 mM NaH_2PO_4-Na_2HPO_4 (pH 6.0–8.0), 50 mM Tris-HCl (pH 7.0–9.0), 50 mM glycine-NaOH (pH 9.0–10.0), and 50 mM Na_2HPO_4-NaOH at 15 °C for 30 min. After incubation of TAPL7A in buffers of different pH values (4.0–12.0) for 24 h (4 °C), the residual activity of TAPL7A was assayed after 30 min of reaction with the substrate at the optimal temperature to assess the pH stability.

4.6. Effect of Metal Ions on TAPL7A

TAPL7A was incubated with various metal compounds and EDTA at a final concentration of 1 mM (50 mM Tris-HCl buffer, pH 8.0) at 4 °C for 24 h. The effect of metal ions was evaluated by detecting the participation of the enzyme after 30 min of reaction at 15 °C. In addition, the activity of the reaction mixture without any metal ion was regarded as control (100% relative activity). In order to improve the credibility of the experimental data, all experiments were performed with three replicates.

4.7. Effect of NaCl on TAPL7A

The salt tolerance of TAPL7A was observed at NaCl concentrations of 0–1.0 M. The reactions were performed at 15 °C. In addition, the activity of the reaction mixture without any NaCl was regarded as control (100% relative activity). In order to improve the credibility of the experimental data, all experiments were performed with three replicates.

4.8. Products Distribution and Action Pattern of TAPL7A

FPLC with Superdex peptide 10/300 GE Colum (GE Health) at 235 nm was used to separate and monitor the products. The reaction mixtures (400 μL) containing 100 μL of purified TAPL7A, 300 μL of substrates (0.5% *w*/*v* sodium alginate, 0.5% *w*/*v* polyM, and 0.5% *w*/*v* polyG, respectively) were incubated at 15 °C for 0–48 h. The samples were taken after reaction for 0 min, 5 min, 15 min, 30 min, 1 h, 2 h, 6 h, 24 h, and 48 h, respectively. The mixture was eluted with 0.2 M NH_4HCO_3 at flow rate of 0.8 mL/min. In addition, the final degradation products were identified by ESI-MS in negative ion mode, and the specific conditions of ESI-MS were as follows: ion source voltage, 4.5 kV; capillary temperature, 275–300 °C; tube lens, 250 V; sheath gas, 30 arbitrary units (AU); and the scanning mass range, 150–2000 m/z.

4.9. Molecular Modeling

The structure of alginate lyase AlyA5 (PDB ID: 4B3E) from *Zobellia galactanivorans* was used as the homology template, and the online software PHYRE 2.0 (http://www.sbg.bio.ic.ac.uk/phyre/html/page.cgi?id=index, accessed on 10 November 2021) was used to successfully construct the structural model of TAPL7A with 100% confidence.

Author Contributions: S.C. conducted the main experiments, analyzed the data, and wrote the manuscript; L.L. helped with the experimental procedures; B.Z. was the supervisor for this work and revised the manuscript; Z.Y. revised the manuscript. All authors have read and agreed to the published version of the manuscript.

Funding: This work was funded by the National Natural Science Foundation of China (No. 31601410), the Graduate Research and Innovation Projects of Jiangsu Province (No. KYCX22_1348) in Jiangsu Province, China.

Institutional Review Board Statement: Not applicable.

Informed Consent Statement: Not applicable.

Data Availability Statement: Not applicable.

Acknowledgments: Authors gratefully acknowledges the financially support of Jiangsu Overseas Visiting Scholar Program for University Prominent Young and Middle-aged Teachers and Presidents.

Conflicts of Interest: The authors declare no conflict of interest.

References

1. Lee, K.Y.; Mooney, D.J. Alginate: Properties and Biomedical Applications. *Prog. Polym. Sci.* **2012**, *37*, 106–126. [CrossRef]
2. Turquois, T.; Gloria, H. Determination of the Absolute Molecular Weight Averages and Molecular Weight Distributions of Alginates Used as Ice Cream Stabilizers by Using Multiangle Laser Light Scattering Measurements. *J. Agric. Food Chem.* **2000**, *48*, 5455–5458. [CrossRef]
3. Wang, Y.; Han, F.; Hu, B.; Li, J.; Yu, W. In vivo Prebiotic Properties of Alginate Oligosaccharides Prepared Through Enzymatic Hydrolysis of Alginate. *Nutr. Res.* **2006**, *26*, 597–603. [CrossRef]
4. Xu, Y.I.; Yoshie, K.; Tatsuya, O.; Tsuyoshi, M. Root Growth-promoting Activity of Unsaturated Oligomeric Uronates from Alginate on Carrot and Rice Plants. *Biosci. Biotechnol. Biochem.* **2003**, *67*, 2022–2025. [CrossRef]
5. Peng, C.; Wang, Q.; Lu, D.; Han, W.; Li, F. A Novel Bifunctional Endolytic Alginate Lyase with Variable Alginate-Degrading Modes and Versatile Monosaccharide-Producing Properties. *Front. Microbiol.* **2018**, *9*, 167. [CrossRef]
6. Li, Q.; Zheng, L.; Guo, Z.; Tang, T.; Zhu, B. Alginate Degrading Enzymes: An Updated Comprehensive Review of the Structure, Catalytic mechanism, Modification Method and Applications of Alginate Lyases. *Crit. Rev. Biotechnol.* **2021**, *41*, 953–968. [CrossRef]
7. Yang, J.; Cui, D.; Ma, S.; Chen, W.; Chen, D.; Shen, H. Characterization of a Novel PL 17 Family Alginate Lyase with Exolytic and Endolytic Cleavage Activity from Marine Bacterium *Microbulbifer* sp. SH-1. *Int. J. Biol. Macromol.* **2021**, *169*, 551–563. [CrossRef]
8. Zhu, B.; Hu, F.; Yuan, H.; Sun, Y.; Yao, Z. Biochemical Characterization and Degradation Pattern of a Unique pH-Stable PolyM-Specific Alginate Lyase from Newly Isolated *Serratia marcescens* NJ-07. *Mar. Drugs* **2018**, *16*, 129. [CrossRef]
9. Cavicchioli, R.; Charlton, T.; Ertan, H.; Mohd Omar, S.; Siddiqui, K.S.; Williams, T.J. Biotechnological Uses of Enzymes from Psychrophiles. *Microb. Biotechnol.* **2011**, *4*, 449–460. [CrossRef]
10. Li, S.Y.; Wang, Z.P.; Wang, L.N.; Peng, J.X.; Wang, Y.N.; Han, Y.T.; Zhao, S.F. Combined Enzymatic Hydrolysis and Selective Fermentation for Green Production of Alginate Oligosaccharides from *Laminaria japonica*. *Bioresour. Technol.* **2019**, *281*, 84–89. [CrossRef]
11. Siddiqui, K.S.; Cavicchioli, R. Cold-adapted Enzymes. *Annu. Rev. Biochem.* **2006**, *75*, 403–433. [CrossRef]
12. Xu, F.; Dong, F.; Wang, P.; Cao, H.Y.; Li, C.Y.; Li, P.Y.; Pang, X.H.; Zhang, Y.Z.; Chen, X.L. Novel Molecular Insights into the Catalytic Mechanism of Marine Bacterial Alginate Lyase AlyGC from Polysaccharide Lyase Family 6. *J. Biol. Chem.* **2017**, *292*, 4457–4468. [CrossRef]
13. Xu, F.; Chen, X.L.; Sun, X.H.; Dong, F.; Li, C.Y.; Li, P.Y.; Ding, H.; Chen, Y.; Zhang, Y.Z.; Wang, P. Structural and Molecular Basis for the Substrate Positioning Mechanism of a New PL7 Subfamily Alginate Lyase from the Arctic. *J. Biol. Chem.* **2020**, *295*, 16380–16392. [CrossRef]
14. He, M.; Guo, M.; Zhang, X.; Chen, K.; Yan, J.; Irbis, C. Purification and Characterization of Alginate Lyase from *Sphingomonas* sp. ZH0. *J. Biosci. Bioeng.* **2018**, *126*, 310–316. [CrossRef]
15. Thomas, F.; Lundqvist, L.C.; Jam, M.; Jeudy, A.; Barbeyron, T.; Sandstrom, C.; Michel, G.; Czjzek, M. Comparative Characterization of Two Marine Alginate Lyases from *Zobellia galactanivorans* Reveals Distinct Modes of Action and Exquisite Adaptation to Their Natural Substrate. *J. Biol. Chem.* **2013**, *288*, 23021–23037. [CrossRef]
16. Tang, L.; Wang, Y.; Gao, S.; Wu, H.; Wang, D.; Yu, W.; Han, F. Biochemical characteristics and molecular mechanism of an exo-type alginate lyase VxAly7D and its use for the preparation of unsaturated monosaccharides. *Biotechnol. Biofuels* **2020**, *13*, 99. [CrossRef]
17. Li, S.; Yang, X.; Zhang, L.; Yu, W.; Han, F. Cloning, Expression, and Characterization of a Cold-Adapted and Surfactant-Stable Alginate Lyase from Marine Bacterium *Agarivorans* sp. L11. *J. Microbiol. Biotechnol.* **2015**, *25*, 681–686. [CrossRef]
18. Hicks, S.J.; Gacesa, P. Heterologous Expression of Full-length and Truncated Forms of the Recombinant Guluronate-specific Alginate Lyase of *Klebsiella pneumoniae*. *Enzyme Microb. Technol.* **1996**, *19*, 68–73. [CrossRef]
19. Kim, H.T.; Ko, H.J.; Kim, N.; Kim, D.; Lee, D.; Choi, I.G.; Woo, H.C.; Kim, M.D.; Kim, K.H. Characterization of a Recombinant Endo-type Alginate Lyase (Alg7D) from *Saccharophagus degradans*. *Biotechnol. Lett.* **2012**, *34*, 1087–1092. [CrossRef]
20. Singh, S.M.; Panda, A.K. Solubilization and Refolding of Bacterial Inclusion Body Proteins. *J. Biosci. Bioeng.* **2005**, *99*, 303–310. [CrossRef]
21. Hu, F.; Li, Q.; Zhu, B.; Ni, F.; Sun, Y.; Yao, Z. Effects of Module Truncation on Biochemical Characteristics and Products Distribution of a New Alginate Lyase with Two Catalytic Modules. *Glycobiology* **2019**, *29*, 876–884. [CrossRef]
22. Zhang, Z.; Tang, L.; Bao, M.; Liu, Z.; Yu, W.; Han, F. Functional Characterization of Carbohydrate-Binding Modules in a New Alginate Lyase, TsAly7B, from *Thalassomonas* sp. LD5. *Mar. Drugs* **2019**, *18*, 25. [CrossRef]
23. Wang, Z.P.; Cao, M.; Li, B.; Ji, X.F.; Zhang, X.Y.; Zhang, Y.Q.; Wang, H.Y. Cloning, Secretory Expression and Characterization of a Unique pH-Stable and Cold-Adapted Alginate Lyase. *Mar. Drugs* **2020**, *18*, 189. [CrossRef]
24. Gao, S.; Zhang, Z.; Li, S.; Su, H.; Tang, L.; Tan, Y.; Yu, W.; Han, F. Characterization of a New Endo-type Polysaccharide Lyase (PL) Family 6 Alginate Lyase with Cold-adapted and Metal Ions-resisted Property. *Int. J. Biol. Macromol.* **2018**, *120*, 729–735. [CrossRef]
25. Akira Inoue, C.M.; Toshiki, U.; Naotsune, S.; Koji, M.; Takao, O. Characterization of an Eukaryotic PL-7 Alginate Lyase in the Marine Red Alga *Pyropia yezoensis*. *Curr. Biotechnol.* **2015**, *4*, 240–248. [CrossRef]

26. Chen, X.L.; Dong, S.; Xu, F.; Dong, F.; Li, P.Y.; Zhang, X.Y.; Zhou, B.C.; Zhang, Y.Z.; Xie, B.B. Characterization of a New Cold-Adapted and Salt-Activated Polysaccharide Lyase Family 7 Alginate Lyase from *Pseudoalteromonas* sp. SM0524. *Front. Microbiol.* **2016**, *7*, 1120. [CrossRef]
27. Cheng, D.; Jiang, C.; Xu, J.; Liu, Z.; Mao, X. Characteristics and Applications of Alginate Lyases: A review. *Int. J. Biol. Macromol.* **2020**, *164*, 1304–1320. [CrossRef]
28. Li, S.; Yang, X.; Bao, M.; Wu, Y.; Yu, W.; Han, F. Family 13 Carbohydrate-binding Module of Alginate Lyase from *Agarivorans* sp. L11 Enhances Its Catalytic Efficiency and Thermostability, and Alters Its Substrate Preference and Product Distribution. *FEMS Microbiol. Lett.* **2015**, *362*, fnv054. [CrossRef]
29. Yang, M.; Yang, S.X.; Liu, Z.M.; Li, N.N.; Li, L.; Mou, H.J. Rational Design of Alginate Lyase from *Microbulbifer* sp. Q7 to Improve Thermal Stability. *Mar. Drugs* **2019**, *17*, 378. [CrossRef]
30. Zhu, B.; Ni, F.; Ning, L.; Sun, Y.; Yao, Z. Cloning and Characterization of a New pH-stable Alginate Lyase with High Salt Tolerance from Marine *Vibrio* sp. NJ-04. *Int. J. Biol. Macromol.* **2018**, *115*, 1063–1070. [CrossRef]
31. Huang, H.; Li, S.; Bao, S.; Mo, K.; Sun, D.; Hu, Y. Expression and Characterization of a Cold-Adapted Alginate Lyase with Exo/Endo-Type Activity from a Novel Marine Bacterium *Alteromonas portus* HB161718(T). *Mar. Drugs* **2021**, *19*, 155. [CrossRef]
32. Zhu, B.; Tan, H.; Qin, Y.; Xu, Q.; Du, Y.; Yin, H. Characterization of a New Endo-type Alginate Lyase from *Vibrio* sp. W13. *Int. J. Biol. Macromol.* **2015**, *75*, 330–337. [CrossRef]
33. Uchimura, K.; Miyazaki, M.; Nogi, Y.; Kobayashi, T.; Horikoshi, K. Cloning and Sequencing of Alginate Lyase Genes from Deep-sea Strains of *Vibrio* and *Agarivorans* and Characterization of a New *Vibrio* Enzyme. *Mar. Biotechnol.* **2010**, *12*, 526–533. [CrossRef]
34. Huang, G.; Wang, Q.; Lu, M.; Xu, C.; Li, F.; Zhang, R.; Liao, W.; Huang, S. AlgM4: A New Salt-Activated Alginate Lyase of the PL7 Family with Endolytic Activity. *Mar. Drugs* **2018**, *16*, 120. [CrossRef]
35. Lian, F.B.; Jiang, S.; Ren, T.Y.; Zhou, B.J.; Du, Z.J. *Thalassotalea algicola* sp. nov., an Alginate-utilizing Bacterium Isolated from a Red Alga. *Antonie Van Leeuwenhoek* **2021**, *114*, 835–844. [CrossRef]
36. Enquist-Newman, M.; Faust, A.M.E.; Bravo, D.D.; Santos, C.N.S.; Raisner, R.M.; Hanel, A.; Sarvabhowman, P.; Le, C.; Regitsky, D.D.; Cooper, S.R.; et al. Efficient Ethanol Production from Brown Macroalgae Sugars by a Synthetic Yeast Platform. *Nature* **2014**, *505*, 239–243. [CrossRef]
37. Yamasaki, M.; Moriwaki, S.; Miyake, O.; Hashimoto, W.; Murata, K.; Mikami, B. Structure and Function of a Hypothetical *Pseudomonas aeruginosa* Protein PA1167 Classified into Family PL-7: A Novel Alginate Lyase with a β-sandwich Fold. *J. Biol. Chem.* **2004**, *279*, 31863–31872. [CrossRef]
38. Qin, H.M.; Miyakawa, T.; Inoue, A.; Nishiyama, R.; Nakamura, A.; Asano, A.; Ojima, T.; Tanokura, M. Structural Basis for Controlling the Enzymatic Properties of Polymannuronate Preferred Alginate Lyase FlAlyA from the PL-7 Family. *Chem. Commun.* **2018**, *54*, 555–558. [CrossRef]
39. Zeinali, F.; Homaei, A.; Kamrani, E.; Patel, S. Use of Cu/Zn-superoxide dismutase tool for biomonitoring marine environment pollution in the Persian Gulf and the Gulf of Oman. *Ecotoxicol. Environ. Saf.* **2018**, *151*, 236–241. [CrossRef]
40. Zeinali, F.; Homaei, A.; Kamrani, E. Identification and kinetic characterization of a novel superoxide dismutase from *Avicennia marina*: An antioxidant enzyme with unique features. *Int. J. Biol. Macromol.* **2017**, *105*, 1556–1562. [CrossRef]
41. Sharifian, S.; Homaei, A.; Kim, S.-K.; Satari, M. Production of newfound alkaline phosphatases from marine organisms with potential functions and industrial applications. *Process Biochem.* **2018**, *64*, 103–115. [CrossRef]
42. Beygmoradi, A.; Homaei, A.; Hemmati, R.; Arco, J.D.; Fernandez-Lucas, J. Identification of a novel tailor-made chitinase from white shrimp *Fenneropenaeus merguiensis*. *Colloids Surf. B Biointerfaces* **2021**, *203*, 111747. [CrossRef]
43. Shojaei, F.; Homaei, A.; Taherizadeh, M.R.; Kamrani, E. Characterization of biosynthesized chitosan nanoparticles from *Penaeus vannamei* for the immobilization of *P. vannameiprotease*: An eco-friendly nanobiocatalyst. *Int. J. Food Prop.* **2017**, *20*, 1413–1423.
44. Qeshmi, F.I.; Homaei, A.; Fernandes, P.; Hemmati, R.; Dijkstra, B.W.; Khajeh, K. Xylanases from marine microorganisms: A brief overview on scope, sources, features and potential applications. *Biochim. Biophys. Acta Proteins Proteom.* **2020**, *1868*, 140312. [CrossRef]
45. Izadpanah Qeshmi, F.; Homaei, A.; Khajeh, K.; Kamrani, E.; Fernandes, P. Production of a Novel Marine *Pseudomonas aeruginosa* Recombinant L-Asparaginase: Insight on the Structure and Biochemical Characterization. *Mar. Biotechnol.* **2022**, *24*, 599–613. [CrossRef]
46. Dadshahi, Z.; Homaei, A.; Zeinali, F.; Sajedi, R.H.; Khajeh, K. Extraction and purification of a highly thermostable alkaline caseinolytic protease from wastes *Penaeus vannamei* suitable for food and detergent industries. *Food Chem.* **2016**, *202*, 110–115. [CrossRef]
47. Federico Abascal, A.V. Abascal—Automatic Annotation of Protein Function Based on Family Identification. *Proteins* **2003**, *53*, 683–692. [CrossRef]
48. Fischer, B.; Summner, I.; Goodenough, P. Isolation, Renaturation, and Formation of Disulfide Bonds of Eukaryotic Proteins Expressed in *Escherichia coli* as Inclusion Bodies. *Biotechnol. Bioeng.* **1993**, *41*, 3–13. [CrossRef]
49. Zhu, B.; Ni, F.; Ning, L.; Yao, Z.; Du, Y. Cloning and Biochemical Characterization of a Novel κ-carrageenase from Newly Isolated Marine Bacterium *Pedobacter hainanensis* NJ-02. *Int. J. Biol. Macromol.* **2018**, *108*, 1331–1338. [CrossRef]

marine drugs

MDPI

Article

Anti-Inflammatory Effect of Sulfated Polysaccharides Isolated from *Codium fragile* In Vitro in RAW 264.7 Macrophages and In Vivo in Zebrafish

Lei Wang [1], Jun-Geon Je [2], Caoxing Huang [3], Jae-Young Oh [4], Xiaoting Fu [1], Kaiqiang Wang [1,5], Ginnae Ahn [6], Jiachao Xu [1], Xin Gao [1] and You-Jin Jeon [2,7,*]

1 College of Food Science and Engineering, Ocean University of China, Qingdao 266003, China; leiwang2021@ouc.edu.cn (L.W.); xiaotingfu@ouc.edu.cn (X.F.); wkq@ouc.edu.cn (K.W.); xujia@ouc.edu.cn (J.X.); xingao@ouc.edu.cn (X.G.)
2 Department of Marine Life Sciences, Jeju National University, Jeju 63243, Korea; wpwnsrjs@naver.com
3 Co-Innovation Center for Efficient Processing and Utilization of Forest Products, College of Chemical Engineering, Nanjing Forestry University, Nanjing 210037, China; hcx@njfu.edu.cn
4 Food Safety and Processing Research Division, National Institute of Fisheries Science, Busan 46083, Korea; ojy0724@naver.com
5 Fujian Provincial Key Laboratory of Breeding Lateolabrax Japonicus, Fujian 355299, China
6 Department of Marine Bio Food Science, Chonnam National University, Yeosu 59626, Korea; gnahn@chonnam.ac.kr
7 Marine Science Institute, Jeju National University, Jeju 63333, Korea
* Correspondence: youjinj@jejunu.ac.kr; Tel.: +82-64-754-3475; Fax: +82-64-756-3493

Citation: Wang, L.; Je, J.-G.; Huang, C.; Oh, J.-Y.; Fu, X.; Wang, K.; Ahn, G.; Xu, J.; Gao, X.; Jeon, Y.-J. Anti-Inflammatory Effect of Sulfated Polysaccharides Isolated from *Codium fragile* In Vitro in RAW 264.7 Macrophages and In Vivo in Zebrafish. *Mar. Drugs* **2022**, *20*, 391. https://doi.org/10.3390/md20060391

Academic Editor: Bill J. Baker

Received: 23 March 2022
Accepted: 11 June 2022
Published: 13 June 2022

Abstract: In this study, the anti-inflammatory activity of sulfated polysaccharides isolated from the green seaweed *Codium fragile* (CFCE-PS) was investigated in lipopolysaccharide (LPS)-stimulated RAW 264.7 macrophages and zebrafish. The results demonstrated that CFCE-PS significantly increased the viability of LPS-induced RAW 264.7 cells in a concentration-dependent manner. CFCE-PS remarkably and concentration-dependently reduced the levels of inflammatory molecules including prostaglandin E_2, nitric oxide (NO), interleukin-1 beta, tumor necrosis factor-alpha, and interleukin-6 in LPS-stimulated RAW 264.7 cells. In addition, in vivo test results indicated that CFCE-PS effectively reduced reactive oxygen species, cell death, and NO levels in LPS-stimulated zebrafish. Thus, these results indicate that CFCE-PS possesses in vitro and in vivo anti-inflammatory activities and suggest it is a potential ingredient in the functional food and pharmaceutical industries.

Keywords: *Codium fragile*; sulfated polysaccharides; anti-inflammatory activity; RAW 264.7 cells; zebrafish

1. Introduction

Inflammatory responses are immune responses that protect the organs from infection and tissue injury. Inflammatory responses are also associated with the pathogenesis of various diseases such as diabetes, cardiovascular diseases, obesity, arthritis, stroke, and cancer [1]. Inflammatory responses are associated with the release of inflammatory molecules such as histamine, prostaglandins, nitric oxide (NO), bradykinin, and pro-inflammatory cytokines [2]. The over-generation of these inflammatory molecules can cause uncontrolled inflammation, which leads to chronic inflammation and promotes the development of chronic inflammation-related diseases [3–5]. Thus, the inhibition of the production of inflammatory molecules is thought as a way to control the development of inflammation.

Seaweeds are rich in bioactive compounds. Seaweed-derived compounds possess several health benefits such as antiviral, anti-aging, antioxidant, anti-cancer, anti-obesity, anti-inflammatory, and anti-hypertensive effects [6,7]. Sulfated polysaccharides isolated from seaweeds possess strong anti-inflammatory activities [8,9]. Lipopolysaccharide (LPS), a component of the cell wall in Gram-negative bacteria, stimulates inflammatory responses. Thus, LPS-stimulated in vitro and in vivo models were used to investigate the anti-inflammatory activities of natural products. Sanjeewa et al. isolated a sulfated polysaccharide from the brown seaweed *Sargassum horneri*, which could inhibit lipopolysaccharide (LPS)-stimulated inflammation in RAW 264.7 cells and zebrafish [10]. Cui et al. purified a sulfated polysaccharide from *Gelidium pacificum* Okamura, which could suppress LPS-stimulated inflammation in human monocytic cells [8]. Rodrigues et al. investigated the anti-inflammation effect of the sulfated polysaccharide isolated from *Caulerpa cupressoides* (Cc-SP2). The results suggested that Cc-SP2 effectively suppressed acute inflammation in mice [9].

Codium fragile is a popular edible green seaweed. *C. fragile* contains various bioactive compounds such as fatty acids, carbohydrates, pigments, phenolic compounds, and proteins [11,12]. The anti-coagulation, antioxidant, anti-angiogenesis, anti-obesity, and immunoregulatory activities of *C. fragile* have been reported [13–15]. In previous studies, we evaluated the antioxidant activity of sulfated polysaccharides isolated from an enzymatic digest of *C. fragile* (CFCE-PS). The results demonstrated that CFCE-PS significantly suppressed hydrogen peroxide-induced oxidative damage in in vitro and in vivo models [16]. To further investigate the bioactivities of CFCE-PS, we evaluated the anti-inflammatory activity of CFCE-PS in LPS-stimulated RAW 264.7 cells and zebrafish.

2. Results and Discussion

2.1. CFCE-PS Suppressed Cytotoxicity and Inflammatory Molecules Production in LPS-Induced RAW 264.7 Cells

Sulfated polysaccharides isolated from seaweeds possess strong anti-inflammatory and immunostimulatory effects [17,18]. The anti-inflammatory activities of sulfated polysaccharides isolated from seaweeds, such as *Saccharina japonica*, *Sargassum horneri*, *Padina commersonii*, and *Chnoospora minima* have been investigated in our previous studies [19–22]. The results further confirm the potential of seaweed-derived sulfated polysaccharides in anti-inflammatory effects. Thus, in the present study, we evaluated the anti-inflammatory activity of CFCE-PS in in vitro and in vivo models.

In the present study, the effects of CFCE-PS on LPS-induced cytotoxicity and inflammatory molecule production were evaluated. As shown in Figure 1A, the viability of LPS-stimulated RAW 264.7 cells was decreased to 78.84% compared to the cells non-treated with sample and LPS (control group, 100%), whereas the viabilities of the LPS-treated RAW 264.7 cells were increased to 84.36, 85.55, and 89.90% by CFCE-PS at concentrations of 25, 50, and 100 μg/mL, respectively (Figure 1A). In addition, LPS significantly stimulated the production of NO and prostaglandin E_2 (PGE_2) in RAW 264.7 cells (Figure 1B,C). However, the production of NO and PGE_2 in LPS-treated RAW 264.7 cells was significantly reduced by CFCE-PS treatment in a concentration-dependent manner (Figure 1B,C). As shown in Figure 2, LPS significantly stimulated the production of pro-inflammatory cytokines including interleukin-1 beta (IL-1β), tumor necrosis factor-alpha (TNF-α), and interleukin-6 (IL-6) in RAW 264.7 cells. However, the production of these pro-inflammatory cytokines in RAW 264.7 cells was effectively suppressed by CFCE-PS treatment in a concentration-dependent manner (Figure 2). These results indicate that CFCE-PS protected RAW 264.7 cells against LPS-stimulated cell death by inhibiting inflammatory molecule production.

Anti-inflammatory effects of the algal sulfated polysaccharides were related to their sulfated content and proportion of monosaccharides. Previous reports suggested that the polysaccharides contain high amounts of the sulfate group, fucose, and galactose, which could inhibit the LPS-induced inflammatory response in RAW 264.7 cells [23–27]. CFCE-PS contains 21.06% sulfate and 70.19% galactose, and significantly inhibited the production of the inflammatory molecules in LPS-stimulated RAW 264.7 cells. According to the previous and present results, CFCE-PS suppressed LPS-stimulated cytotoxicity and the production of inflammatory molecules in RAW 264.7 cells. This action may be due to it containing a high amount of the sulfate group and galactose.

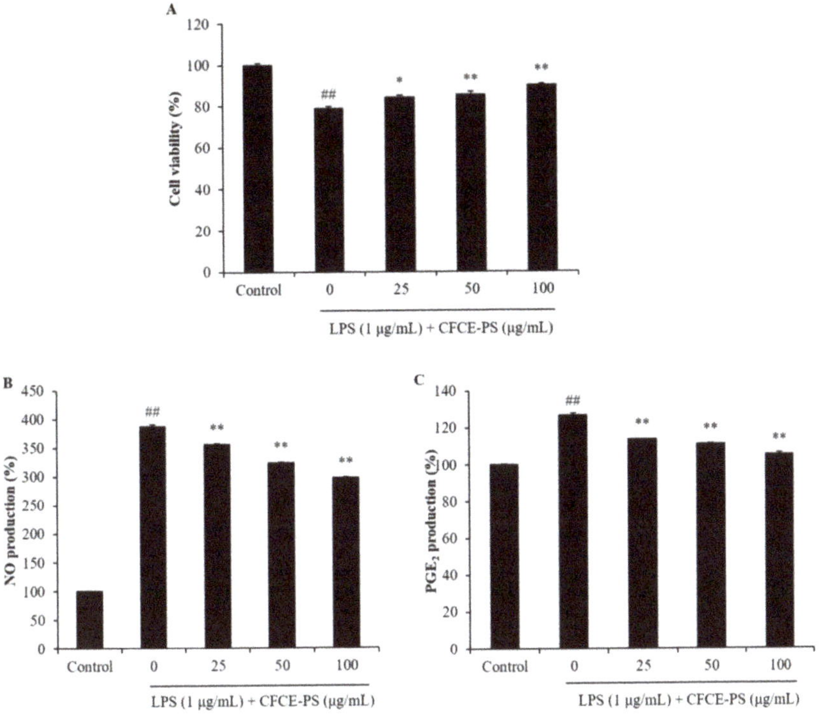

Figure 1. Effect of CFCE-PS on LPS-induced cytotoxicity in RAW 264.7 cells. (**A**) The viability of LPS-stimulated RAW 264.7 cells; the production levels of NO (**B**) and PGE_2 (**C**) in LPS-stimulated RAW 264.7 cells. The cells non-treated with CFCE-PS and LPS are referred to as the control group. The experiments were conducted in triplicate and the data are expressed as mean ± SE. * $p < 0.05$, ** $p < 0.01$ as compared to the LPS-stimulated group and ## $p < 0.01$ as compared to control group.

2.2. *Protective Effect of CFCE-PS against LPS-Stimulated Inflammatory Response in Zebrafish*

LPS-stimulated zebrafish embryo has been successfully used to investigate the in vivo anti-inflammatory effects of sulfated polysaccharides in our previous studies [21]. Therefore, in this study, the LPS-stimulated zebrafish embryo was used as the in vivo model to investigate the anti-inflammatory effect of CFCE-PS. As shown in Figure 3, the survival rate of LPS-stimulated zebrafish decreased to 56.67% compared to the control group (100%), whereas the survival rates of zebrafish treated with 50 and 100 μg/mL CFCE-PS were remarkably increased to 63.33 and 73.33%, respectively (Figure 3). In addition, the ROS level of LPS-treated zebrafish was increased to 172.65% compared to the control group (100%). However, the levels of ROS in CFCE-PS-treated zebrafish were significantly decreased in a dose-dependent manner (Figure 4A). As shown in Figure 4B, LPS significantly stimulated cell death in zebrafish, whereas the cell death levels of zebrafish treated with 25, 50, and 100 μg/mL CFCE-PS were decreased from 295.22% to 277.72, 217.68, and 185.58%, respectively (Figure 4B). Furthermore, the NO production level of zebrafish stimulated with LPS was increased to 220.45% compared to the control group (100%). However, the NO level of LPS-stimulated zebrafish was reduced to 172.99, 154.53, and 133.51% by the treatment of 25, 50, and 100 μg/mL CFCE-PS, respectively (Figure 4C). These results demonstrate that CFCE-PS remarkably protected zebrafish against LPS-stimulated inflammation.

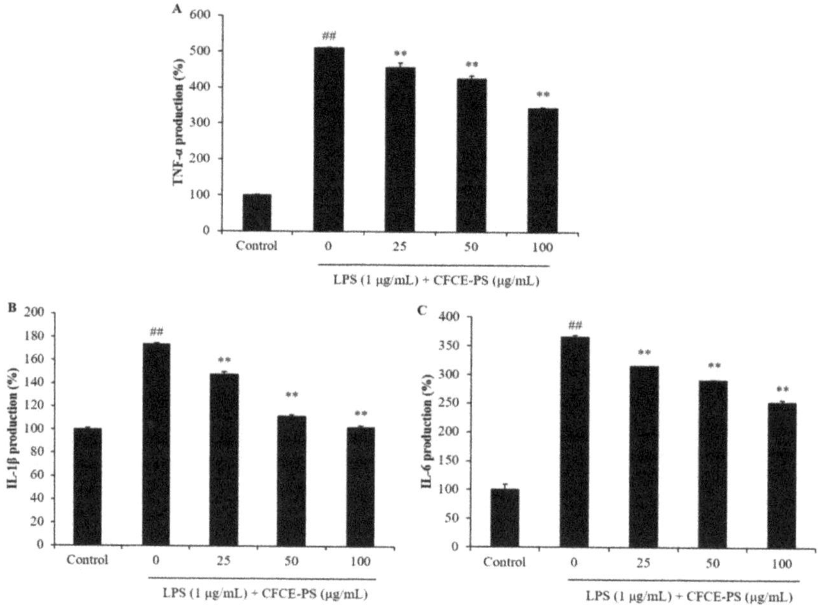

Figure 2. Effect of CFCE-PS on the production of pro-inflammatory cytokines in LPS-stimulated RAW 264.7 cells. (**A**) Production of TNF-α; (**B**) production of IL-1β; and (**C**) production of IL-6. The cells non-treated with CFCE-PS and LPS are referred to as the control group. The experiments were conducted in triplicate and the data are expressed as mean ± SE. ** $p < 0.01$ as compared to LPS-stimulated group and ## $p < 0.01$ as compared to control group.

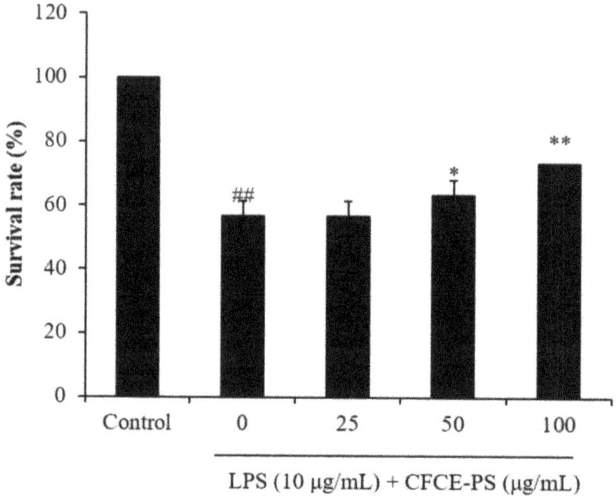

Figure 3. Survival rate of zebrafish after being treated with CFCE-PS or/and with LPS. The zebrafish non-treated with CFCE-PS and LPS are referred to as the control group. The experiments were conducted in triplicate and the data are expressed as the mean ± SE. * $p < 0.05$, ** $p < 0.01$ as compared to the LPS-stimulated group and ## $p < 0.01$ as compared to the control group.

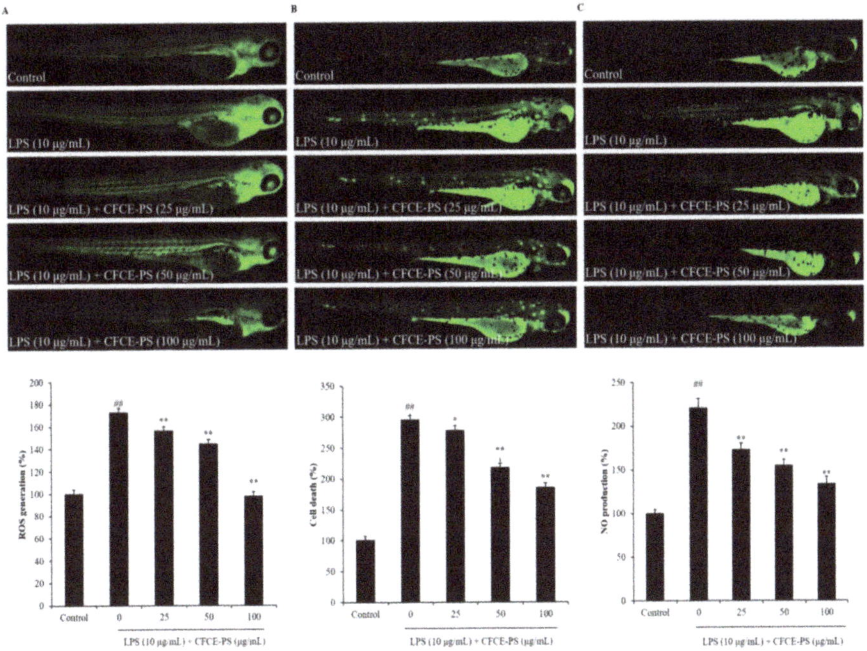

Figure 4. Effect of CFCE-PS on inflammatory responses in LPS-induced zebrafish. (**A**) ROS level of LPS-stimulated zebrafish; (**B**) cell death of LPS-stimulated zebrafish; and (**C**) NO production in LPS-stimulated zebrafish. The zebrafish non-treated with CFCE-PS and LPS are referred to as the control group. The relative amounts of ROS, cell death, and NO of zebrafish were measured using ImageJ software. The experiments were conducted in triplicate and the data are expressed as the mean ± SE. * $p < 0.05$, ** $p < 0.01$ as compared to the LPS-treated group and ## $p < 0.01$ as compared to control group.

In summary, in this study, the in vitro and in vivo anti-inflammatory effects of CFCE-PS were evaluated in LPS-stimulated RAW 264.7 cells and zebrafish. The results indicate that CFCE-PS inhibited LPS-induced inflammatory response by inhibiting the production of NO and PGE_2, and decreasing the levels of pro-inflammatory cytokines in RAW 264.7 cells. In addition, the in vivo test showed that CFCE-PS remarkably suppressed the survival rate and reduced the levels of ROS, cell death, and NO in LPS-stimulated zebrafish. These results indicate that CFCE-PS possesses in vitro and in vivo anti-inflammatory effects. It could be used as a functional material in food and pharmaceutical industries.

3. Materials and Methods

3.1. Reagents and Chemicals

LPS, MTT, and DMSO were purchased from Sigma-Aldrich (St. Louis, MO, USA). Enzyme-linked immunosorbent assay (ELISA) kits used for measurement of IL-1β, TNF-α, PGE_2, and IL-6 were purchased from R&D Systems Inc. (Minneapolis, MN, USA).

3.2. Preparation of CFCE-PS

C. fragile was collected in June 2019 from the coastal area of Jeju Island, South Korea. CFCE-PS was prepared based on the protocol described in the previous study [16]. CFCE-PS contained 76.84% sulfated polysaccharides, including 21.06% sulfate and 55.78% carbohydrates, which were composed of galactose (70.19%), arabinose (18.71%), glucose (9.10%), and xylose (1.99%).

3.3. Measurement of NO Level and Cell Viability

RAW 264.7 macrophages (RAW 264.7 cells, TIB-71^{TM}) were purchased from ATCC (Manassas, WV, USA). Cells were seeded in a 24-well plate (1×10^5 cells/mL) for 24 h. The cells were treated with 25, 50, and 100 μg/mL CFCE-PS. The cells non-treated with CFCE-PS and LPS are referred to as the control group. CFCE-PS-treated cells were incubated for 1 h and the plate was replaced with the media containing 1 μg/mL LPS. After 24 h incubation, the viability of LPS-treated RAW264.7 cells was measured using an MTT assay, and the production of NO was determined using a Griess assay [28].

3.4. ELISA

RAW 264.7 cells were seeded in a 24-well plate (1×10^5 cells/mL) for 24 h. The cells were treated with 25, 50, and 100 μg/mL CFCE-PS. CFCE-PS-treated cells were incubated for 1 h and stimulated with 1 μg/mL LPS. After 24 h, the cell culture media was collected. The levels of pro-inflammatory cytokines and PGE_2 were evaluated using ELISA kits [28].

3.5. Application of CFCE-PS and LPS to Zebrafish

The adult zebrafish were purchased from a commercial market (Seoul Aquarium, Korea) and maintained according to the condition described in our previous study [29]. After approximately 7–9 h of post-fertilization (hpf), the embryos were treated with 25, 50, and 100 μg/mL CFCE-PS. After 1 h of incubation, the embryos were incubated with the media containing 10 μg/mL LPS until 24 hpf. The zebrafish non-treated with CFCE-PS and LPS are referred to as the control group. The survival rate of zebrafish was measured at 3 days post-fertilization. The levels of cell death, ROS, and NO in LPS-induced zebrafish were measured in live zebrafish larvae by acridine orange, DCFH2-DA, and DAF-FM-DA staining, respectively [30].

3.6. Statistical Analysis

The experiments were conducted in triplicate and the data are expressed as the mean ± standard error (SE). One-way analysis of variance used to compare the mean values of each treatment using SPSS 20.0. Significant differences between the means were estimated using Tukey's test.

4. Conclusions

In this study, the in vitro and in vivo anti-inflammatory activities of sulfated polysaccharides of the edible seaweed *C. fragile* (CFCE-PS) were investigated. The results demonstrated that CFCE-PS effectively inhibited LPS-stimulated inflammation in vitro in RAW 264.7 cells and in vivo in zebrafish. These results suggest that CFCE-PS is a potential anti-inflammatory ingredient in functional food and the pharmaceutical industry. However, to develop CFCE-PS as a therapeutic agent to treat inflammatory-related diseases, the clinical study is vital in further research.

Author Contributions: L.W., G.A. and Y.-J.J. designed this study. L.W., X.F. and Y.-J.J. wrote the manuscript. L.W., J.-Y.O., K.W. and J.-G.J. performed the experiments. L.W., C.H., J.X. and X.G. analyzed the data. All authors have read and agreed to the published version of the manuscript.

Funding: This research was supported by the Start-up Fund for Young-talent Program (Grant No.: 862101013159) funded by the Ocean University of China, the Qingdao Postdoctoral Applied Research Project (Grant No.: 862105040061), and the Basic Science Research Program through the National Research Foundation of Korea (NRF) funded by the Ministry of Education (Grant No.:2019R1A6A1A03033553).

Institutional Review Board Statement: Not applicable.

Informed Consent Statement: Not applicable.

Data Availability Statement: Not applicable.

Conflicts of Interest: The authors declare no conflict of interest.

References

1. Sanjeewa, K.K.A.; Herath, K.H.I.N.M.; Yang, H.-W.; Choi, C.S.; Jeon, Y.-J. Anti-Inflammatory Mechanisms of Fucoidans to Treat Inflammatory Diseases: A Review. *Mar. Drugs* **2021**, *19*, 678. [CrossRef]
2. Li, Z.; Wang, K.; Ji, X.; Wang, H.; Zhang, Y. ACE2 suppresses the inflammatory response in LPS-induced porcine intestinal epithelial cells via regulating the NF-κB and MAPK pathways. *Peptides* **2022**, *149*, 170717. [CrossRef]
3. Lima Correa, B.; El Harane, N.; Gomez, I.; Rachid Hocine, H.; Vilar, J.; Desgres, M.; Bellamy, V.; Keirththana, K.; Guillas, C.; Perotto, M.; et al. Extracellular vesicles from human cardiovascular progenitors trigger a reparative immune response in infarcted hearts. *Cardiovasc. Res.* **2021**, *117*, 292–307. [CrossRef]
4. Ryu, D.H.; Cho, J.Y.; Sadiq, N.B.; Kim, J.-C.; Lee, B.; Hamayun, M.; Lee, T.S.; Kim, H.S.; Park, S.H.; Nho, C.W.; et al. Optimization of antioxidant, anti-diabetic, and anti-inflammatory activities and ganoderic acid content of differentially dried *Ganoderma lucidum* using response surface methodology. *Food Chem.* **2020**, *335*, 127645. [CrossRef]
5. Hirano, T. IL-6 in inflammation, autoimmunity and cancer. *Int. Immunol.* **2021**, *33*, 127–148. [CrossRef]
6. Rajauria, G.; Ravindran, R.; Garcia-Vaquero, M.; Rai, D.K.; Sweeney, T.; O'Doherty, J. Molecular characteristics and antioxidant activity of laminarin extracted from the seaweed species *Laminaria hyperborea*, using hydrothermal-assisted extraction and a multi-step purification procedure. *Food Hydrocoll.* **2020**, *112*, 106332. [CrossRef]
7. Zhong, Q.-W.; Zhou, T.-S.; Qiu, W.-H.; Wang, Y.-K.; Xu, Q.-L.; Ke, S.-Z.; Wang, S.-J.; Jin, W.-H.; Chen, J.-W.; Zhang, H.-W.; et al. Characterization and hypoglycemic effects of sulfated polysaccharides derived from brown seaweed *Undaria pinnatifida*. *Food Chem.* **2020**, *341*, 128148. [CrossRef]
8. Cui, M.; Wu, J.; Wang, S.; Shu, H.; Zhang, M.; Liu, K.; Liu, K. Characterization and anti-inflammatory effects of sulfated polysaccharide from the red seaweed *Gelidium pacificum* Okamura. *Int. J. Biol. Macromol.* **2019**, *129*, 377–385. [CrossRef]
9. Rodrigues, J.A.G.; Vanderlei, E.D.S.; Silva, L.M.; De Araújo, I.W.; De Queiroz, I.N.; De Paula, G.A.; Abreu, T.M.; Ribeiro, N.A.; Bezerra, M.M.; Chaves, H.V.; et al. Antinociceptive and anti-inflammatory activities of a sulfated polysaccharide isolated from the green seaweed Caulerpa cupressoides. *Pharmacol. Rep.* **2012**, *64*, 282–292. [CrossRef]
10. Sanjeewa, K.K.A.; Jayawardena, T.U.; Kim, S.-Y.; Kim, H.-S.; Ahn, G.; Kim, J.; Jeon, Y.-J. Fucoidan isolated from invasive *Sargassum horneri* inhibit LPS-induced inflammation via blocking NF-κB and MAPK pathways. *Algal Res.* **2019**, *41*, 101561. [CrossRef]
11. Ahn, J.; Kim, M.J.; Yoo, A.; Ahn, J.; Ha, T.Y.; Jung, C.H.; Seo, H.D.; Jang, Y.J. Identifying Codium fragile extract components and their effects on muscle weight and exercise endurance. *Food Chem.* **2021**, *353*, 129463. [CrossRef]
12. Kim, J.; Choi, J.H.; Oh, T.; Ahn, B.; Unno, T. Codium fragile Ameliorates High-Fat Diet-Induced Metabolism by Modulating the Gut Microbiota in Mice. *Nutrients* **2020**, *12*, 1848. [CrossRef]
13. Li, P.; Yan, Z.; Chen, Y.; He, P.; Yang, W. Analysis of monosaccharide composition of water-soluble polysaccharides from *Codium fragile* by ultra-performance liquid chromatography-tandem mass spectrometry. *J. Sep. Sci.* **2021**, *44*, 1452–1460. [CrossRef]
14. Kim, T.I.; Kim, Y.-J.; Kim, K. Extract of Seaweed *Codium fragile* Inhibits Integrin αIIbβ3-Induced Outside-in Signaling and Arterial Thrombosis. *Front. Pharmacol.* **2021**, *12*, 685948. [CrossRef]
15. Park, H.-B.; Hwang, J.; Zhang, W.; Go, S.; Kim, J.; Choi, I.; You, S.; Jin, J.-O. Polysaccharide from *Codium fragile* Induces Anti-Cancer Immunity by Activating Natural Killer Cells. *Mar. Drugs* **2020**, *18*, 626. [CrossRef]
16. Wang, L.; Oh, J.Y.; Je, J.G.; Jayawardena, T.U.; Kim, Y.-S.; Fu, X.; Jeon, Y.-J. Protective effects of sulfated polysaccharides isolated from the enzymatic digest of Codium fragile against hydrogen peroxide-induced oxidative stress in in vitro and in vivo models. *Algal Res.* **2020**, *48*, 101891. [CrossRef]
17. Jiang, P.; Zheng, W.; Sun, X.; Jiang, G.; Wu, S.; Xu, Y.; Song, S.; Ai, C. Sulfated polysaccharides from *Undaria pinnatifida* improved high fat diet-induced metabolic syndrome, gut microbiota dysbiosis and inflammation in BALB/c mice. *Int. J. Biol. Macromol.* **2020**, *167*, 1587–1597. [CrossRef]
18. Chen, C.-Y.; Wang, S.-H.; Huang, C.-Y.; Dong, C.-D.; Huang, C.-Y.; Chang, C.-C.; Chang, J.-S. Effect of molecular mass and sulfate content of fucoidan from *Sargassum siliquosum* on antioxidant, anti-lipogenesis, and anti-inflammatory activity. *J. Biosci. Bioeng.* **2021**, *132*, 359–364. [CrossRef]
19. Fernando, I.P.S.; Sanjeewa, K.K.A.; Samarakoon, K.W.; Lee, W.W.; Kim, H.-S.; Kang, N.; Ranasinghe, P.; Lee, H.-S.; Jeon, Y.-J. A fucoidan fraction purified from *Chnoospora minima*; a potential inhibitor of LPS-induced inflammatory responses. *Int. J. Biol. Macromol.* **2017**, *104*, 1185–1193. [CrossRef]
20. Sanjeewa, K.K.A.; Fernando, I.P.S.; Kim, E.-A.; Ahn, G.; Jee, Y.; Jeon, Y.-J. Anti-inflammatory activity of a sulfated polysaccharide isolated from an enzymatic digest of brown seaweed *Sargassum horneri* in RAW 264.7 cells. *Nutr. Res. Pract.* **2017**, *11*, 3–10. [CrossRef]
21. Ni, L.; Wang, L.; Fu, X.; Duan, D.; Jeon, Y.-J.; Xu, J.; Gao, X. In vitro and in vivo anti-inflammatory activities of a fucose-rich fucoidan isolated from *Saccharina japonica*. *Int. J. Biol. Macromol.* **2020**, *156*, 717–729. [CrossRef] [PubMed]
22. Asanka Sanjeewa, K.K.; Jayawardena, T.U.; Kim, H.-S.; Kim, S.-Y.; Shanura Fernando, I.P.; Wang, L.; Abetunga, D.T.U.; Kim, W.-S.; Lee, D.-S.; Jeon, Y.-J. Fucoidan isolated from *Padina commersonii* inhibit LPS-induced inflammation in macrophages blocking TLR/NF-κB signal pathway. *Carbohydr. Polym.* **2019**, *224*, 115195. [CrossRef] [PubMed]

23. Rukshala, D.; de Silva, E.D.; Ranaweera, B.L.R.; Fernando, N.; Handunnetti, S.M. Anti-inflammatory effect of leaves of Vernonia zeylanica in lipopolysaccharide-stimulated RAW 264.7 macrophages and carrageenan-induced rat paw-edema model. *J. Ethnopharmacol.* **2021**, *274*, 114030. [CrossRef] [PubMed]
24. Kim, J.-H.; Kim, M.; Hong, S.; Kwon, B.; Song, M.W.; Song, K.; Kim, E.-Y.; Jung, H.-S.; Sohn, Y. Anti-inflammatory effects of *Fritillaria thunbergii* Miquel extracts in LPS-stimulated murine macrophage RAW 264.7 cells. *Exp. Ther. Med.* **2021**, *21*, 429. [CrossRef] [PubMed]
25. Kumar, S.; Singh, P.; Kumar, A. Targeted therapy of irritable bowel syndrome with anti-inflammatory cytokines. *Clin. J. Gastroenterol.* **2021**, *15*, 1–10. [CrossRef]
26. Xu, Z.; Ke, T.; Zhang, Y.; Guo, L.; Chen, F.; He, W. Danshensu inhibits the IL-1β-induced inflammatory response in chondrocytes and osteoarthritis possibly via suppressing NF-κB signaling pathway. *Mol. Med.* **2021**, *27*, 80. [CrossRef] [PubMed]
27. Liu, X.; Su, J.; Wang, G.; Zheng, L.; Wang, G.; Sun, Y.; Bao, Y.; Wang, S.; Huang, Y. Discovery of Phenolic Glycoside from *Hyssopus cuspidatus* Attenuates LPS-Induced Inflammatory Responses by Inhibition of iNOS and COX-2 Expression through Suppression of NF-κB Activation. *Int. J. Mol. Sci.* **2021**, *22*, 12128. [CrossRef]
28. Wang, L.; Oh, J.Y.; Jayawardena, T.U.; Jeon, Y.-J.; Ryu, B. Anti-inflammatory and anti-melanogenesis activities of sulfated polysaccharides isolated from *Hizikia fusiforme*: Short communication. *Int. J. Biol. Macromol.* **2019**, *142*, 545–550. [CrossRef]
29. Wang, L.; Oh, J.Y.; Hwang, J.; Ko, J.Y.; Jeon, Y.-J.; Ryu, B. In Vitro and In Vivo Antioxidant Activities of Polysaccharides Isolated from Celluclast-Assisted Extract of an Edible Brown Seaweed, *Sargassum fulvellum*. *Antioxidants* **2019**, *8*, 493. [CrossRef]
30. Ko, E.-Y.; Cho, S.-H.; Kwon, S.-H.; Eom, C.-Y.; Jeong, M.S.; Lee, W.; Kim, S.-Y.; Heo, S.-J.; Ahn, G.; Lee, K.P.; et al. The roles of NF-κB and ROS in regulation of pro-inflammatory mediators of inflammation induction in LPS-stimulated zebrafish embryos. *Fish Shellfish Immunol.* **2017**, *68*, 525–529. [CrossRef]

marine drugs

MDPI

Article

Multi-Step Enzymatic Production and Purification of 2-Keto-3-Deoxy-Galactonate from Red-Macroalgae-Derived Agarose

Sora Yu [1], So Young Park [1], Dong Hyun Kim [2], Eun Ju Yun [3,*] and Kyoung Heon Kim [1,4,*]

1 Department of Biotechnology, Graduate School, Korea University, Seoul 02841, Korea; sora90715@korea.ac.kr (S.Y.); thdud2502@naver.com (S.Y.P.)
2 Department of Marine Food Science and Technology, Gangneung-Wonju National University, Gangneung 25457, Gangwon, Korea; dhkim85@gwnu.ac.kr
3 Division of Biotechnology, Jeonbuk National University, Iksan 54596, Korea
4 Department of Food Bioscience and Technology, College of Life Sciences and Biotechnology, Korea University, Seoul 02841, Korea
* Correspondence: ejyun@jbnu.ac.kr (E.J.Y.); khekim@korea.ac.kr (K.H.K.)

Abstract: 2-keto-3-deoxy sugar acids, which have potential as precursors in medicinal compound production, have gained attention in various fields. Among these acids, 2-keto-3-deoxy-L-galactonate (KDGal) has been biologically produced from D-galacturonate originating from plant-derived pectin. KDGal is also found in the catabolic pathway of 3,6-anhydro-L-galactose (AHG), the main component of red-algae-derived agarose. AHG is converted to 3,6-anhydrogalactonate by AHG dehydrogenase and subsequently isomerized to KDGal by 3,6-anhydrogalactonate cycloisomerase. Therefore, we used the above-described pathway to produce KDGal from agarose. Agarose was depolymerized to AHG and to agarotriose (AgaDP3) and agaropentaose (AgaDP5), both of which have significantly higher molecular weights than AHG. When only AHG was converted to KDGal, AgaDP3 and AgaDP5 remained unreacted. Finally, KDGal was effectively purified from the enzymatic products by size-exclusion chromatography based on the differences in molecular weights. These results show that KDGal can be enzymatically produced and purified from agarose for use as a precursor to high-value products.

Keywords: keto-deoxy-sugar; 2-keto-3-deoxy sugar acid; 2-keto-3-deoxy-L-galactonate; agarose; red algae; 3,6-anhydro-L-galactose

Citation: Yu, S.; Park, S.Y.; Kim, D.H.; Yun, E.J.; Kim, K.H. Multi-Step Enzymatic Production and Purification of 2-Keto-3-Deoxy-Galactonate from Red-Macroalgae-Derived Agarose. *Mar. Drugs* **2022**, *20*, 288. https://doi.org/10.3390/md20050288

Academic Editors: Yuya Kumagai, Hideki Kishimura and Benwei Zhu

Received: 11 March 2022
Accepted: 22 April 2022
Published: 25 April 2022

1. Introduction

Keto-deoxy sugars are known to possess potential as precursors for producing medicinal compounds [1]. In particular, the demand for 2-keto-3-deoxy sugar acids, which are key intermediates of the central metabolic pathways of hexose and pentose and integral constituents of bacterial polysaccharides, have been continuously increasing in use in various fields to elucidate the mechanisms involved in microbial metabolic processes and to produce biochemicals using metabolic engineering [2]. However, there have been few attempts to produce 2-keto-3-deoxy-sugar acids such as 2-keto-3-deoxy-D-gluconate, 2-keto-3-deoxy-L-gaclatonate (KDGal), 2-keto-3-deoxy-D-xylonate, and 2-keto-3-deoxy-L-arabinonate [2–4]. These sugar acids can be produced using either chemical or biological methods. Biological methods are known to be advantageous over chemical methods because the latter often require many reaction steps and involve non-stereoselective reactions, which result in racemic product mixtures and lower yields [2]. On the contrary, biological processes involve fewer reaction steps, high specificity, and enantioselectivity and are therefore preferred over chemical processes for the synthesis of 2-keto-3-deoxy-sugar acids.

KDGal has been biologically synthesized from galacturonate derived from pectin present in plant biomass [4]. Pectin is a group of galacturonate-rich polysaccharides [5]. However, galacturonate residues, the main backbone of pectin, are known to be highly methyl-esterified [6]. In addition, pectin is considered to be the most complex polysaccharide, which complicates the saccharification process with additional steps, such as de-methyl-esterification in order to obtain galacturonate [7,8]. However, KDGal, an intermediate in the galacturonate catabolic pathway in fungi [9], has also been discovered in the metabolic pathway of 3,6-anhydro-L-galactose (AHG) of a marine bacterium recently [10]. AHG, a major monomer comprising agarose, which is a linear polysaccharide in marine biomass [11], is oxidized to 3,6-anhydrogalactonate (AHGA) and subsequently isomerized into KDGal [10]. Thus, AHG derived from agarose in marine biomass can be used as a substrate for producing KDGal. However, even though agarose has a simpler structure than that of plant biomass pectin, marine biomass agarose, unlike plant biomass, has not been utilized for producing KDGal yet [4]. In this study, we attempted to produce KDGal using agarose from marine biomass via a biocatalytic enzyme-mediated process.

In this study, we designed a three-step method for the production of KDGal from agarose: (1) enzymatic production of AHG and neoagarooligosaccharides (NAOSs) from agarose, (2) enzymatic production of KDGal from AHG, and (3) purification of KDGal from the reaction product mixture (Figure 1). Agarose is the most abundant polymer in red macroalgal biomass and has gained much attention as a sustainable source owing to its higher carbohydrate and lower lignin content compared to that of plant biomass [12,13]. AHG and D-galactose form agarose via alternative α-1,3- and β-1,4-glycosidic bonds [11]. Thus, monomeric sugars such as AHG and D-galactose can be produced by the enzymatic hydrolysis of agarose using β-agarase and α-neoagarooligosaccharide hydrolase (NAOH) (Figure 1). Accordingly, agarose can be hydrolyzed into NAOSs, including neoagarotetraose (NeoDP4) and neoagarohexaose (NeoDP6), by endo-type β-agarase. NAOH can then act on NeoDP4 and NeoDP6, leading to the production of AHG and agarotriose (AgaDP3) and AHG and agaropentaose (AgaDP5), respectively [14]. AHG can be subsequently converted to KDGal using the enzymes AHG dehydrogenase (AHGD) and AHGA cycloisomerase (ACI), which, respectively oxidize AHG into AHGA and isomerize AHGA into KDGal, found in the AHG catabolic pathway of *Vibrio* sp. strain EJY3 (Figure 1) [10]. Finally, high-purity KDGal can be obtained through a purification step using size-exclusion chromatography owing to the large differences in molecular weights between KDGal and the by-products, AgaDP3 and AgaDP5 (Figure 1). In addition, agarooligosaccharides (AOSs), including AgaDP3 and AgaDP5, which remain after KDGal separation, are known to have prebiotic, antioxidant, and anti-inflammatory activities [15–19]. Thus, even byproducts produced along with KDGal can be utilized as high-value-added products in this process. Overall, this study showed that agarose-containing red macroalgal biomass can potentially be used in the production of high-value chemicals, including KDGal.

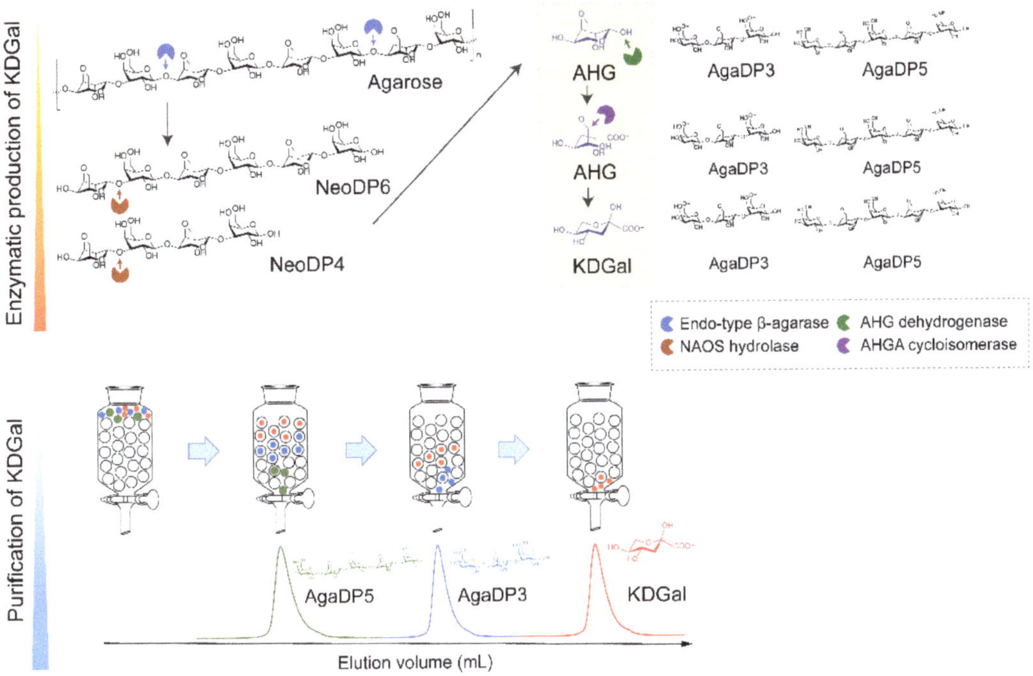

Figure 1. Scheme of KDGal production from agarose. Agarose can be degraded into AHG by two-step enzymatic hydrolysis using endo-type β-agarase and NAOS hydrolase. Subsequently, AHG is converted into KDGal by a two-step enzymatic reaction using AHG dehydrogenase and AHGA cycloisomerase. KDGal can be purified by size-exclusion chromatography using water as an eluent. Abbreviations: AHG, 3,6-anhydro-L-galactose; AHGA, 3,6-anhy-drogalactonate; KDGal, 2-keto-3-deoxy-L-gaclatonate; NAOS; neoagarooligosaccharide.

2. Results

2.1. Enzymatic Depolymerization of Agarose into AHG and AOSs

To obtain AHG as the substrate for producing KDGal from agarose saccharification, recombinant endo-type β-agarase, Aga16B, and NAOH, *Sd*NABH were purified. The purified Aga16B and *Sd*NABH were identified by SDS-PAGE based on their theoretical molecular weights of 63.7 kDa and 41.5 kDa, respectively (Figure 2A). Agarose was initially hydrolyzed mainly into NAOSs, specifically NeoDP4 and NeoDP6, via enzymatic reaction using Aga16B, as described previously [20] (Figure 2B,C). The subsequent enzymatic reaction of *Sd*NABH using Aga16B reaction products containing NeoDP4 and NeoDP6 produced AHG, AgaDP3, and AgaDP5 as reaction products, as previously described (Figure 2B,C) [21]. These results were also confirmed by HPLC analysis. In the analysis of products formed by Aga16B, two peaks corresponding to NeoDP4 and NeoDP6 were detected, and in the analysis of *Sd*NABH reaction products, three peaks corresponding to AHG, AgaDP3, and AgaDP5 were detected, which is consistent with results obtained upon TLC analysis (Figure 2B,C).

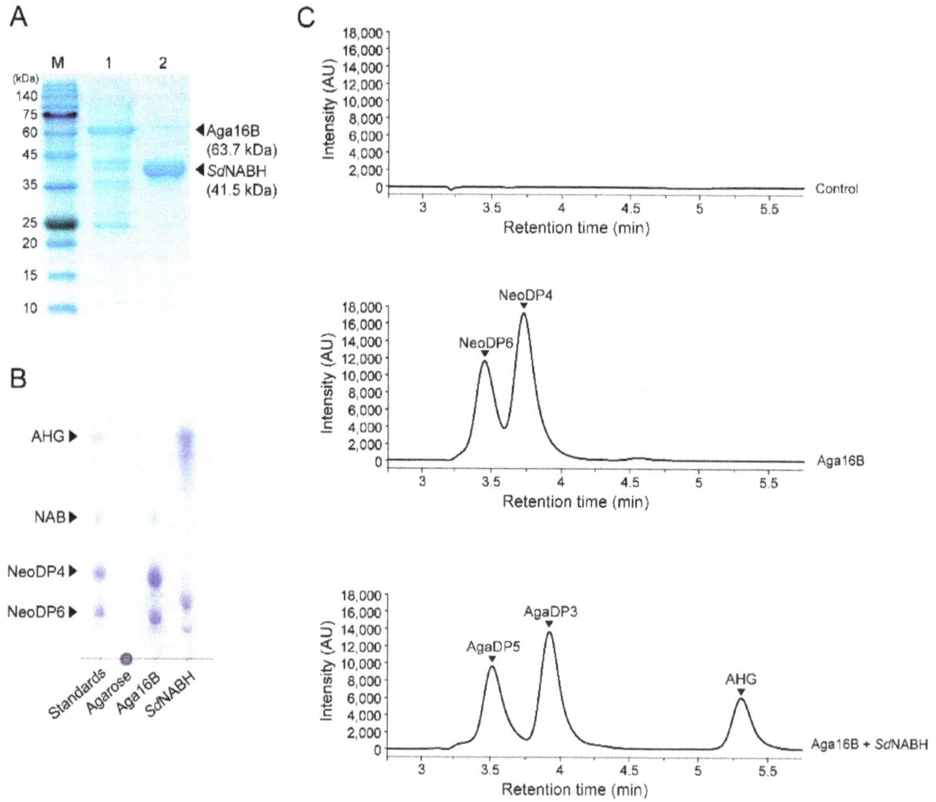

Figure 2. Enzymatic production of AHG from agarose. (**A**) SDS-PAGE analysis of the purified recombinant Aga16B and *Sd*NABH. Lanes: M, protein markers; 1, Aga16B; 2, *Sd*NABH purified by affinity chromatography. (**B**) TLC analysis of serial enzymatic reaction products of Aga16B and *Sd*NABH with agarose for producing AHG. (**C**) HPLC analysis of serial enzymatic reaction products with agarose for producing AHG. Abbreviations: AHG, 3,6-anhydro-L-galactose; AgaDP3, agarotriose; AgaDP5, agaropentaose; NAB, neoagarobiose; NeoDP4, neoagarotetraose; NeoDP6, neoagarohexaose; TLC, thin-layer chromatography; SDS-PAGE, sodium dodecyl sulfate-polyacrylamide gel electrophoresis.

2.2. Enzymatic Production of KDGal from AHG

Because we prepared *Sd*NABH products containing AHG, two-step enzymatic reactions were performed to convert AHG to KDGal. *Vej*AHGD and *Vej*ACI, originating from *Vibrio* sp. EJY3, which has been reported to metabolize AHG as the sole carbon source, were overexpressed in *E. coli*, purified, and identified by SDS-PAGE based on their theoretical molecular weights of 53.3 kDa and 40.4 kDa, respectively (Figure 3A). We confirmed that AHG was converted to AHGA, an intermediate of the AHG metabolic pathway in *Vibrio* sp. EJY3 by *Vej*AHGD (Figure 3C). Subsequently, we also observed that a peak corresponding to KDGal appeared, whereas a peak corresponding to AHGA disappeared after incubation with *Vej*ACI using GC-MS. In addition, the production of AHGA and KDGal was verified by comparing the mass fragmentation patterns of AHG, AHGA, and KDGal that were produced in this study with those observed in a previous study [10] (Figure 4). In particular, the generation of unique daughter ions at 247 and 290 m/z for AHGA and KDGal, respectively, was observed in the GC-MS analysis (Figure 4B,C).

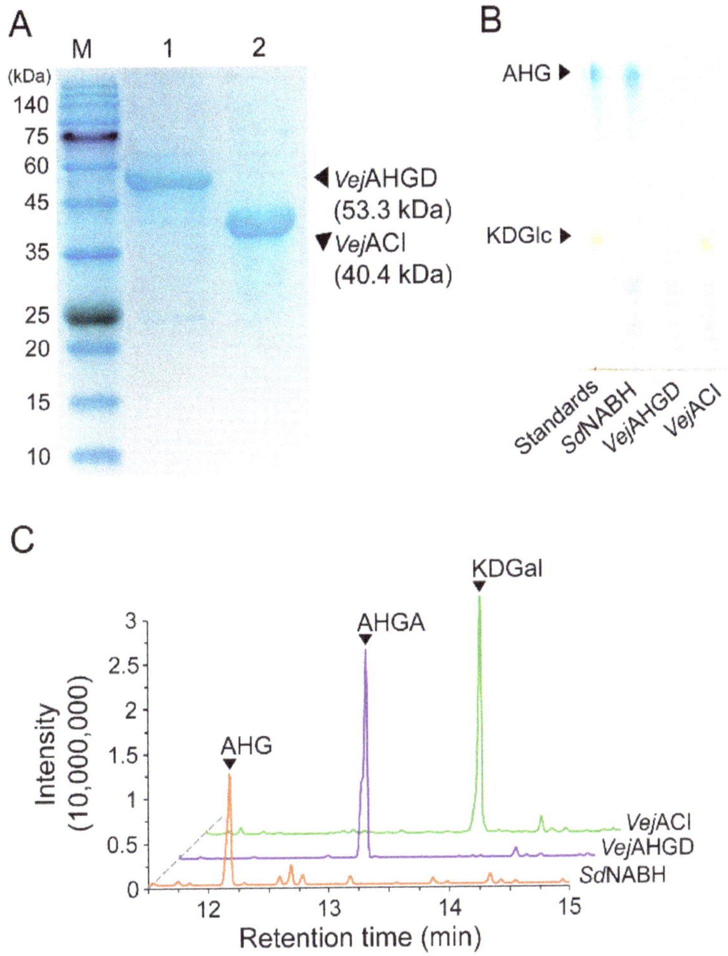

Figure 3. Enzymatic production of KDGal from AHG. (**A**) SDS-PAGE analysis of the purified recombinant *Vej*AHGD and *Vej*ACI. (**B**) TLC analysis of serial enzymatic reaction products of *Vej*AHGD and *Vej*ACI with *Sd*NABH reaction products for producing KDGal. (**C**) GC-MS total ion chromatograms of serial enzymatic reaction products of *Vej*AHGD and *Vej*ACI with *Sd*NABH reaction products. Abbreviations: AHG, 3,6-anhydro-L-galactose; AHGA, 3,6-anhydrogalactonate; KDGal, 2-keto-3-deoxy-L-gaclatonate; KDGlc, 2-keto-3-deoxy-D-gluconate; GC-MS, gas chromatography–mass spectrometry; TLC, thin-layer chromatography; SDS-PAGE, sodium dodecyl sulfate-polyacrylamide gel electrophoresis.

While the peak corresponding to AHG disappeared, the peaks corresponding to AgaDP3 and AgaDP5 were observed in TLC analysis (Figure 3B).

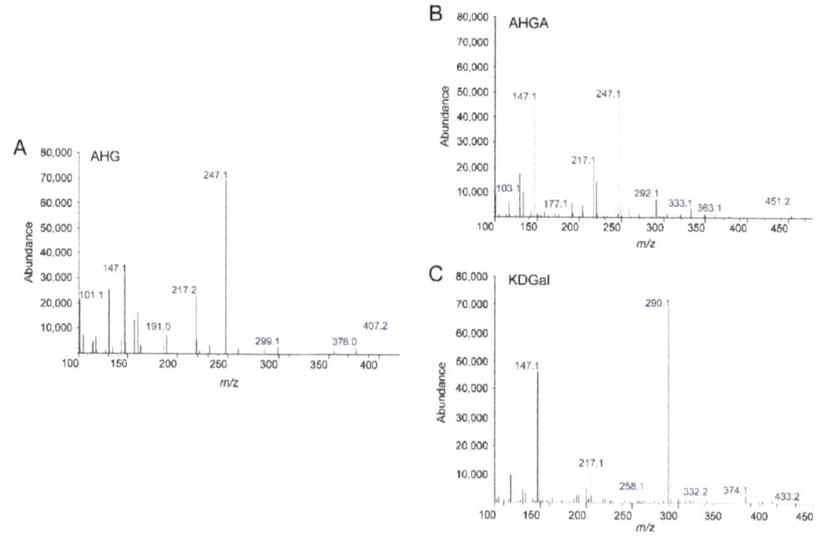

Figure 4. Analysis of the enzymatic reaction products of *Vej*AHGD and *Vej*ACI with AHG by GC-MS. The mass spectra of (**A**) AHG, (**B**) AHGA, and (**C**) KDGal. Abbreviations: AHG, 3,6-anhydro-L-galactose; AHGA, 3,6-anhydrogalactonate; KDGal, 2-keto-3-deoxy-L-gaclatonate; GC-MS, gas chromatography–mass spectrometry.

2.3. Purification of KDGal from the Enzymatic Reaction Product Mixture

The purification process is essential for obtaining high-purity KDGal. After the enzymatic reaction with *Vej*ACI, the reaction product mixture contained KDGal along with AgaDP3 and AgaDP5, which are the products of the NABH reaction with NeoDP4 and NeoDP6, respectively (Figure 3B). Molecules with different molecular weights can be separated based on their size as they pass through a size-exclusion chromatography column. Because there is a large difference between KDGal, with a molecular weight of 178.14 g/mol, and AgaDP3 and AgaDP5, with molecular weights of 486.4 and 792.7 g/mol, respectively, KDGal was able to be easily separated from the mixture containing AgaDP3 and AgaDP5 using size-exclusion chromatography (Figure 5).

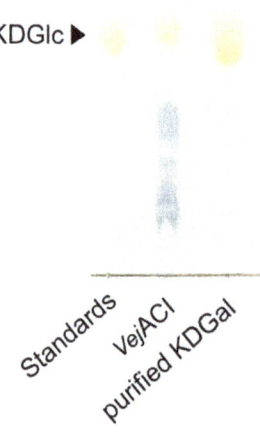

Figure 5. TLC analysis of purified KDGal from reaction products of *Vej*ACI. Abbreviations: KDGal, 2-keto-3-deoxy-L-gaclatonate; KDGlc, 2-keto-3-deoxy-D-gluconate; TLC, thin-layer chromatography.

3. Discussion

KDGal, a keto-deoxy sugar that has the potential to be used as a precursor in pharmaceutical production, is found in the catabolic pathway of AHG, which is one of the major monomeric sugars in red macroalgal agarose. As a proof of concept, we have demonstrated that KDGal, produced from plant-derived D-galacturonate so far, can also be produced from marine macroalgal agarose in this study.

Prior to KDGal production, AHG was produced with AgaDP3 and AgaDP5 from agarose by enzymatic hydrolysis. For depolymerization of agarose, the unique properties of agarose should be considered. Agarose can exist in either the sol or the gel state. Agarose in the gel state has lower accessibility to enzymes than agarose in the sol state. Thus, it is important to maintain agarose in the sol state to saccharify it efficiently, which means that agarose saccharification should be performed above the sol–gel transition temperature of agarose [20]. In addition, the near-insolubility of agarose hinders its enzymatic depolymerization. Therefore, initial pretreatment is necessary to increase the solubility of agarose in water. Chemical pretreatment of agarose has been reported to have several drawbacks, including the formation of salts and the necessary use of additional enzymes for complete depolymerization of agarose into monomeric sugars [22–24]. Moreover, it has been reported that AHG residues seem to be unstable under the mild acid conditions, leading to overdegradation of AHG to 5-hydroxymethylfurfural, ultimately leading to a lower yield of KDGal [25]. Thus, to overcome these drawbacks, enzymatic liquefaction, which can replace chemical pretreatment, has been suggested [20]. Therefore, the importance of thermostable ento-type β-agarases in the depolymerization of agarose has been highlighted previously [20].

Thus far, β-agarase has been the most reported and characterized agar-degrading enzyme. Aga16B is an enzyme with an optimal temperature of 60 °C, the highest temperature among those β-agarases that produce NeoDP4 or NeoDP6 as the major end products [26]. In addition, we selected Aga16B for agarose hydrolysis because Aga16B produces NeoDP4 and NeoDP6 as the main products and rarely produces neoagarobiose (NeoDP2). In the NAOH reaction, NeoDP2 is degraded into AHG and D-galactose, which have a small difference in size, making the final KDGal purification step using size-exclusion chromatography difficult. Therefore, considering the final purification process, Aga16B, an endo-type β-agarase that does not produce NeoDP2, is an appropriate choice for saccharifying agarose.

KDGal production was finally achieved using a two-step enzymatic reaction carried out by *Vej*AHGD and *Vej*ACI. Regarding KDGal production from *Sd*NABH enzymatic reaction products containing mainly AHG, AgaDP3, and AgaDP5, AgaDP3 and AgaDP5 remained after two-step enzymatic reactions of *Vej*AHGD and *Vej*ACI, while AHG was converted to KDGal (Figure 3). *Vej*AHGD has been revealed to display very high substrate specificity toward AHG [27]. While most aldehyde dehydrogenases are known to have broad substrate specificities toward various aldehyde substrates, *Vej*AHGD showed almost no activity toward other aldehyde sugars, including D-galactose, which has been associated with the unique structure of its substrate, AHG, comprising a bridged bicyclic structure [27]. Although the purification process for separating AHG from AgaDP5 and AgaDP3 in KDGal production was omitted, owing to the high substrate specificity of *Vej*AHGD, only the desired reaction, that is, oxidation of AHG without additional byproducts, was achieved. This is advantageous in reducing the number of overall processing steps by omitting the purification step prior to *Vej*AHGD reaction.

The purification process was essential since the reaction product mixture contained KDGal along with AgaDP3 and AgaDP5 after the enzymatic reaction with *Vej*ACI. We separated KDGal from the remaining AgaDP3 and AgaDP5 using size-exclusion chromatography with distilled water as the eluent. To simplify the purification step, agarose was intentionally hydrolyzed into NeoDP4 and NeoDP6 using Aga16B. If agarose had been hydrolyzed into NeoDP2, it would have been degraded into AHG and D-galactose by *Sd*NABH. The final enzymatic reaction mixture then would have contained KDGal and D-galactose, which have similar molecular weights, thereby making it much more difficult to purify KDGal from the enzymatic reaction mixture containing D-galactose using size-exclusion chromatography. Therefore, in this case, although the hydrolysis of agarose into NeoDP4 and NeoDP6 would result in a lower yield of KDGal than that obtained by decomposing agarose into NeoDP2, it has the advantage of being a simpler purification process. Another advantage is the AOSs, including AgaDP3 and AgaDP5 obtained as byproducts; they are known to have prebiotic, antioxidant, and anti-inflammatory activities and can therefore be utilized as high value-added products [15–19].

In addition to these advantages, the use of water, a non-toxic solvent as an eluent also provides an advantage in the purification step of this KDGal production process, whereas toxic solvents, such as methanol and chloroform, have been used as eluents for adsorption chromatography for the purification of AHG, which is the substrate for KDGal production [28]. This makes the purification of KDGal simpler and safer.

This study shows that agarose, one of the major carbohydrate components of red macroaglae, can also be used for the production of KDGal via enzymatic reactions and a simple purification process.

4. Materials and Methods

4.1. Overexpression and Purification of Recombinant Proteins

To produce KDGal from agarose, four recombinant enzymes were used: endo-type β-agarase (Aga16B originating from *Saccharophagus degradans* 2-40^T) [20], NAOH (*Sd*NABH originating from *S. degradans* 2-40^T) [21], AHGD (*Vej*AHGD originating from *Vibrio* sp. EJY3) [10,27], and AHGA cycloisomerase (*Vej*ACI originating from *Vibrio* sp. EJY3) [10]. To produce the recombinant enzymes, each plasmid encoding each protein was transformed into *Escherichia coli* BL21(DE3) by using the heat-shock method, and transformants were selected on agar plates containing 100 µg/mL ampicillin (Sigma-Aldrich, St. Louis, MO, USA). *E. coli* BL21(DE3) harboring genes encoding each of the proteins was grown at 37 °C in Luria-Bertani (LB; BD, San Jose, CA, USA) medium containing 100 µg/mL ampicillin until the mid-exponential phase of growth. Protein overexpression was induced by adding 0.5 mM IPTG (Sigma-Aldrich, St. Louis, MO, USA) for Aga16B, *Sd*NABH, and *Vej*ACI or 0.2% L-(+)-arabinose (Sigma-Aldrich, St. Louis, MO, USA) for *Vej*AHGD at 16 °C for 16 h. The cell pellet was collected by centrifugation at 6000 rpm for 30 min at 4 °C and resuspended in ice-cold Tris-HCl buffer (pH 7.4). Cell disruption was then performed using a sonicator (Branson Korea, Gunpo, Korea). The supernatant was collected by centrifugation at 16,000 rpm for 30 min at 4 °C to purify the soluble recombinant protein. The overexpressed recombinant protein was further purified via affinity chromatography using a HisTrap column (GE Healthcare Life Sciences, Piscataway, NJ, USA), followed by desalting and concentration using an Amicon ultrafiltration membrane (Millipore, Burlington, MA, USA). The protein concentration was determined using a BCA protein assay kit (Thermo Fisher Scientific, Waltham, MA, USA). The purified recombinant enzymes were identified using sodium dodecyl sulfate-polyacrylamide gel electrophoresis (SDS-PAGE) based on their theoretical molar mass.

4.2. Enzymatic Production of AHG from Agarose

To produce AHG as a substrate for KDGal production, we performed enzymatic depolymerization of agarose using the recombinant enzymes Aga16B and *Sd*NABH. To produce NAOSs from agarose, including NeoDP4 and NeoDP6, 4 mg of Aga16B was added to 100 mL of 2% (*w*/*v*) agarose (agarose, for molecular biology, Sigma-Aldrich, St. Louis, MO, USA) in 20 mM Tris-HCl (pH 7.4), and the reaction mixture was incubated at 50 °C overnight. To produce AHG from Aga16B reaction products, NeoDP4 and NeoDP6, 2 mg of *Sd*NABH was then added to the Aga16B reaction mixture, followed by incubation at 30 °C for 5 h.

4.3. HPLC and TLC Analyses

The enzymatic reaction products of Aga16B and *Sd*NABH were analyzed using high-performance liquid chromatography (HPLC; Agilent Technologies, Santa Clara, CA, USA) equipped with a Rezex ROA-Organic Acid H^+ (8%) column (Phenomenex, Torrance, CA, USA) and a refractive index (RI) detector (Agilent Technologies, Santa Clara, CA, USA). The temperature of the column and RI detector was set to 50 °C. The column was eluted using 0.005 N H_2SO_4 as the mobile phase at a flow rate of 0.6 mL/min.

The enzymatic reaction products of Aga16B and *Sd*NABH were also identified using thin-layer chromatography (TLC). Each enzymatic reaction product (1 µL) was loaded onto silica gel 60 TLC plates (Merck, Darmstadt, Germany), which were developed with a mobile phase consisting of n-butanol, ethanol, and water (3:1:1, *v*/*v*/*v*). The plate was visualized using 10% (*v*/*v*) H_2SO_4 and 0.2% (*w*/*v*) 1,3-dihydroxynaphthalene in ethanol, as previously described [28].

4.4. Enzymatic Production of KDGal from AHG

Two recombinant enzymes, *Vej*AHGD and *Vej*ACI, were used to convert AHG to KDGal. First, to oxidize AHG into AHGA using AHGD, *Vej*AHGD was added to the NABH reaction products containing mainly AHG, AgaDP3, and AgaDP5. The AHGD reaction mixture containing 2 mM AHG, 3 mM NAD^+ as a cofactor, and 0.05 mg/mL of *Vej*AHGD was incubated at 30 °C and 100 rpm. After 12 h, 0.05 mg/mL of *Vej*ACI was finally added to the reaction product of *Vej*AHGD to isomerize AHGA into KDGal. Subsequently, the reaction mixture was incubated at 30 °C and 100 rpm for 12 h.

4.5. GC-MS Analysis of KDGal

To confirm the production of KDGal, the enzymatic reaction products of *Vej*AHGD and *Vej*ACI were analyzed using gas chromatography–mass spectrometry (GC-MS). For GC-MS analysis, the reaction products of *Vej*AHGD and *Vej*ACI were derivatized as previously described [10]. Before the derivatization step, the enzymatic reaction mixtures of *Vej*AHGD and *Vej*ACI were centrifuged at 4 °C and 16,000 rpm for 5 min. Then, 20 µL of the supernatant was dried for 1 h using a speed vacuum evaporator, and methoxyamination and trimethylsilylation were subsequently performed for derivatization. Briefly, 10 µL of 40 mg/mL methoxyamine hydrochloride in pyridine (Sigma-Aldrich, St. Louis, MO, USA) was added to the dried sample and incubated at 30 °C. After 90 min, the sample was treated with 45 µL of N-methyl-N-(trimethylsilyl)trifluoroacetamide (Sigma-Aldrich, St. Louis, MO, USA) for 30 min at 37 °C. The chemically derivatized samples were analyzed using an Agilent 7890A GC/5975C MSD system (Agilent Technologies, Santa Clara, CA, USA) equipped with a DB5-MS column (30 m length, 0.25 mm diameter, and 0.25 µm film thickness, Agilent Technologies). The derivatized sample, 1 µL in volume, was injected into the GC column in the splitless mode. The oven was programmed to maintain an initial temperature of 100 °C for 3.5 min and then for the temperature to be increased to 160 °C at 15 °C/min and held for 20 min, increased to 200 °C at 20 °C/min and held for 20 min, and finally to 280 °C at 20 °C/min and held for 5 min. Electron ionization was performed at 70 eV, and the temperature of the ion source was 230 °C. The mass range was 85–700 *m*/*z*. The reaction products of *Vej*AHGD and *Vej*ACI were also analyzed using TLC, as described above.

4.6. Purification of KDGal from the Enzymatic Reaction Mixture

For the purification of KDGal from the enzymatic reaction mixtures, size-exclusion chromatography using Bio-Gel P-2 Gel (Bio-Rad, Hercules, CA, USA) was performed. Distilled water was used for elution at a flow rate of 0.3 mL/min. To obtain high-purity KDGal, the fractions containing only KDGal were collected and freeze-dried. The purified KDGal was finally analyzed using TLC.

Author Contributions: S.Y., D.H.K., E.J.Y. and K.H.K. designed the experiments; S.Y. and S.Y.P. performed the experiments and analyzed the data; K.H.K. conceived the project and analyzed the data; S.Y., D.H.K., E.J.Y., S.Y.P. and K.H.K. wrote the manuscript. All authors have read and agreed to the published version of the manuscript.

Funding: This work was supported by the Mid-career Researcher Program through the National Research Foundation of Korea (2020R1A2B5B02002631) and by the Korea Institute of Planning and Evaluation for Technology in Food, Agriculture, Forestry, and Fisheries, funded by the Ministry of Agriculture, Food, and Rural Affairs (32136-05-1-SB010). This work was also supported by the Korea University Food Safety Hall for the Institute of Biomedical Science and Food Safety and by a Korea University Grant. The article processing charge was supported by an LG Chem grant.

Informed Consent Statement: Not applicable.

Conflicts of Interest: The authors declare that they have no competing interest.

References

1. Hiroshi, I.; Takashi, Y. Production of 2-keto-3-deoxyaldonic Acid Derivative and Production Thereof. Japanese Patent JP62258342, 1987.
2. Matsubara, K.; Köhling, R.; Schönenberger, B.; Kouril, T.; Esser, D.; Bräsen, C.; Siebers, B.; Wohlgemuth, R. One-step synthesis of 2-keto-3-deoxy-D-gluconate by biocatalytic dehydration of D-gluconate. *J. Biotechnol.* **2014**, *191*, 69–77. [CrossRef] [PubMed]
3. Archer, R.M.; Royer, S.F.; Mahy, W.; Winn, C.L.; Danson, M.J.; Bull, S.D. Syntheses of 2-keto-3-deoxy-D-xylonate and 2-keto-3-deoxy-L-arabinonate as stereochemical probes for demonstrating the metabolic promiscuity of sulfolobus solfataricus towards D-xylose and L-arabinose. *Chem. Eur. J.* **2013**, *19*, 2895–2902. [CrossRef]
4. Wiebe, M.G.; Mojzita, D.; Hilditch, S.; Ruohonen, L.; Penttilä, M. Bioconversion of D-galacturonate to keto-deoxy-L-galactonate (3-deoxy-L-threo-hex-2-ulosonate) using filamentous fungi. *BMC Biotechnol.* **2010**, *10*, 1–8. [CrossRef]
5. Willats, W.G.; McCartney, L.; Mackie, W.; Knox, J.P. Pectin: Cell biology and prospects for functional analysis. *Plant Mol. Biol.* **2001**, *47*, 9–27. [CrossRef] [PubMed]
6. O'Neill, M.; Albersheim, P.; Darvill, A. The pectic polysaccharides of primary cell walls. In *Methods in Plant Biochemistry*; Elsevier: Amsterdam, The Netherlands, 1990; Volume 2, pp. 415–441.
7. Mohnen, D. Pectin structure and biosynthesis. *Curr. Opin. Plant Biol.* **2008**, *11*, 266–277. [CrossRef] [PubMed]
8. Lionetti, V.; Francocci, F.; Ferrari, S.; Volpi, C.; Bellincampi, D.; Galletti, R.; D'Ovidio, R.; De Lorenzo, G.; Cervone, F. Engineering the cell wall by reducing de-methyl-esterified homogalacturonan improves saccharification of plant tissues for bioconversion. *Proc. Natl. Acad. Sci. USA* **2010**, *107*, 616–621. [CrossRef]
9. Richard, P.; Hilditch, S. D-galacturonic acid catabolism in microorganisms and its biotechnological relevance. *Appl. Microbiol. Biotechnol.* **2009**, *82*, 597–604. [CrossRef]
10. Yun, E.J.; Lee, S.; Kim, H.T.; Pelton, J.G.; Kim, S.; Ko, H.J.; Choi, I.-G.; Kim, K.H. The novel catabolic pathway of 3,6-anhydro-L-galactose, the main component of red macroalgae, in a marine bacterium. *Environ. Microbiol.* **2015**, *17*, 1677–1688. [CrossRef]
11. Araki, C. Structure of the agarose constituent of agar-agar. *Bull. Chem. Soc. Jpn.* **1956**, *29*, 543–544. [CrossRef]
12. Wei, N.; Quarterman, J.; Jin, Y.-S. Marine macroalgae: An untapped resource for producing fuels and chemicals. *Trends Biotechnol.* **2013**, *31*, 70–77. [CrossRef]
13. Yun, E.J.; Choi, I.-G.; Kim, K.H. Red macroalgae as a sustainable resource for bio-based products. *Trends Biotechnol.* **2015**, *33*, 247–249. [CrossRef] [PubMed]
14. Yu, S.; Yun, E.J.; Kim, D.H.; Park, S.Y.; Kim, K.H. Dual agarolytic pathways in a marine bacterium, *Vibrio* sp. strain EJY3: Molecular and enzymatic verification. *Appl. Environ. Microbiol.* **2020**, *86*, e02724-19. [CrossRef] [PubMed]
15. Chen, H.; Yan, X.; Zhu, P.; Lin, J. Antioxidant activity and hepatoprotective potential of agaro-oligosaccharides in vitro and in vivo. *Nutr. J.* **2006**, *5*, 31. [CrossRef] [PubMed]
16. Li, M.; Li, G.; Zhu, L.; Yin, Y.; Zhao, X.; Xiang, C.; Yu, G.; Wang, X. Isolation and characterization of an agaro-oligosaccharide (AO)-hydrolyzing bacterium from the gut microflora of Chinese individuals. *PLoS ONE* **2014**, *9*, e91106. [CrossRef]
17. Higashimura, Y.; Naito, Y.; Takagi, T.; Mizushima, K.; Hirai, Y.; Harusato, A.; Ohnogi, H.; Yamaji, R.; Inui, H.; Nakano, Y. Oligosaccharides from agar inhibit murine intestinal inflammation through the induction of heme oxygenase-1 expression. *J. Gastroenterol.* **2013**, *48*, 897–909. [CrossRef]
18. Enoki, T.; Okuda, S.; Kudo, Y.; Takashima, F.; Sagawa, H.; Kato, I. Oligosaccharides from agar inhibit pro-inflammatory mediator release by inducing heme oxygenase 1. *Biosci. Biotechnol. Biochem.* **2010**, *74*, 766–770. [CrossRef]
19. Higashimura, Y.; Naito, Y.; Takagi, T.; Uchiyama, K.; Mizushima, K.; Ushiroda, C.; Ohnogi, H.; Kudo, Y.; Yasui, M.; Inui, S. Protective effect of agaro-oligosaccharides on gut dysbiosis and colon tumorigenesis in high-fat diet-fed mice. *Am. J. Physiol. Gastrointest. Liver Physiol.* **2016**, *310*, G367–G375. [CrossRef]
20. Kim, J.H.; Yun, E.J.; Seo, N.; Yu, S.; Kim, D.H.; Cho, K.M.; An, H.J.; Kim, J.-H.; Choi, I.-G.; Kim, K.H. Enzymatic liquefaction of agarose above the sol–gel transition temperature using a thermostable endo-type β-agarase, Aga16B. *Appl. Microbiol. Biotechnol.* **2017**, *101*, 1111–1120. [CrossRef]

21. Ha, S.C.; Lee, S.; Lee, J.; Kim, H.T.; Ko, H.-J.; Kim, K.H.; Choi, I.-G. Crystal structure of a key enzyme in the agarolytic pathway, α-neoagarobiose hydrolase from *Saccharophagus degradans* 2–40. *Biochem. Biophys. Res. Commun.* **2011**, *412*, 238–244. [CrossRef]
22. Kim, H.T.; Lee, S.; Kim, K.H.; Choi, I.-G. The complete enzymatic saccharification of agarose and its application to simultaneous saccharification and fermentation of agarose for ethanol production. *Bioresour. Technol.* **2012**, *107*, 301–306. [CrossRef]
23. Lee, C.H.; Kim, H.T.; Yun, E.J.; Lee, A.R.; Kim, S.R.; Kim, J.-H.; Choi, I.-G.; Kim, K.H. A novel agarolytic β-galactosidase acts on agarooligosaccharides for complete hydrolysis of agarose into monomers. *Appl. Environ. Microbiol.* **2014**, *80*, 5965–5973. [CrossRef] [PubMed]
24. Lee, C.H.; Yun, E.J.; Kim, H.T.; Choi, I.-G.; Kim, K.H. Saccharification of agar using hydrothermal pretreatment and enzymes supplemented with agarolytic β-galactosidase. *Process Biochem.* **2015**, *50*, 1629–1633. [CrossRef]
25. Yang, B.; Yu, G.; Zhao, X.; Jiao, G.; Ren, S.; Chai, W. Mechanism of mild acid hydrolysis of galactan polysaccharides with highly ordered disaccharide repeats leading to a complete series of exclusively odd-numbered oligosaccharides. *FEBS J.* **2009**, *276*, 2125–2137. [CrossRef] [PubMed]
26. Park, S.H.; Lee, C.-R.; Hong, S.-K. Implications of agar and agarase in industrial applications of sustainable marine biomass. *Appl. Microbiol. Biotechnol.* **2020**, *104*, 2815–2832. [CrossRef]
27. Yu, S.; Choi, I.-G.; Yun, E.J.; Kim, K.H. High substrate specificity of 3, 6-anhydro-L-galactose dehydrogenase indicates its essentiality in the agar catabolism of a marine bacterium. *Process Biochem.* **2018**, *64*, 130–135. [CrossRef]
28. Yun, E.J.; Lee, S.; Kim, J.H.; Kim, B.B.; Kim, H.T.; Lee, S.H.; Pelton, J.G.; Kang, N.J.; Choi, I.-G.; Kim, K.H. Enzymatic production of 3, 6-anhydro-L-galactose from agarose and its purification and in vitro skin whitening and anti-inflammatory activities. *Appl. Microbiol. Biotechnol.* **2013**, *97*, 2961–2970. [CrossRef]

marine drugs

Article

Characterization of an Unknown Region Linked to the Glycoside Hydrolase Family 17 β-1,3-Glucanase of *Vibrio vulnificus* Reveals a Novel Glucan-Binding Domain

Yuya Kumagai [1,*], Hideki Kishimura [1], Weeranuch Lang [2], Takayoshi Tagami [2], Masayuki Okuyama [2] and Atsuo Kimura [2,*]

1 Faculty of Fisheries Sciences, Hokkaido University, Hakodate 041-8611, Japan; i-dulse@fish.hokudai.ac.jp
2 Research Faculty of Agriculture, Hokkaido University, Sapporo 060-8589, Japan; weranuch@abs.agr.hokudai.ac.jp (W.L.); tagami@abs.agr.hokudai.ac.jp (T.T.); okuyama@abs.agr.hokudai.ac.jp (M.O.)
* Correspondence: yuyakumagai@fish.hokudai.ac.jp (Y.K.); kimura@abs.agr.hokudai.ac.jp (A.K.)

Abstract: The glycoside hydrolase family 17 β-1,3-glucanase of *Vibrio vulnificus* (VvGH17) has two unknown regions in the N- and C-termini. Here, we characterized these domains by preparing mutant enzymes. VvGH17 demonstrated hydrolytic activity of β-(1→3)-glucan, mainly producing laminaribiose, but not of β-(1→3)/β-(1→4)-glucan. The C-terminal-truncated mutants (ΔC466 and ΔC441) showed decreased activity, approximately one-third of that of the WT, and ΔC415 lost almost all activity. An analysis using affinity gel containing laminarin or barley β-glucan revealed a shift in the mobility of the ΔC466, ΔC441, and ΔC415 mutants compared to the WT. Tryptophan residues showed a strong affinity for carbohydrates. Three of four point-mutations of the tryptophan in the C-terminus (W472A, W499A, and W542A) showed a reduction in binding ability to laminarin and barley β-glucan. The C-terminus was predicted to have a β-sandwich structure, and three tryptophan residues (Trp472, Trp499, and Trp542) constituted a putative substrate-binding cave. Linker and substrate-binding functions were assigned to the C-terminus. The N-terminal-truncated mutants also showed decreased activity. The WT formed a trimer, while the N-terminal truncations formed monomers, indicating that the N-terminus contributed to the multimeric form of VvGH17. The results of this study are useful for understanding the structure and the function of GH17 β-1,3-glucanases.

Keywords: glucanase; *Vibrio*; carbohydrate-binding domain; glycoside hydrolase family 17

Citation: Kumagai, Y.; Kishimura, H.; Lang, W.; Tagami, T.; Okuyama, M.; Kimura, A. Characterization of an Unknown Region Linked to the Glycoside Hydrolase Family 17 β-1,3-Glucanase of *Vibrio vulnificus* Reveals a Novel Glucan-Binding Domain. *Mar. Drugs* **2022**, *20*, 250. https://doi.org/10.3390/md20040250

Academic Editor: Hitoshi Sashiwa

Received: 25 February 2022
Accepted: 29 March 2022
Published: 31 March 2022

1. Introduction

Marine algae convert marine carbon into algal polysaccharides by photosynthesis. Algal polysaccharides are made up of a variety of glycans. The recycling of algal polysaccharides into carbon dioxide gives us a better understanding of the global marine carbon cycle [1]. Recently, the involvement of marine bacteria in this cycle has been gradually revealed [2]. Laminarin is a major glucose polymer found in marine environments [3]. Therefore, an understanding of the mechanisms underlying the degradation of large algal polysaccharides by enzymes and their modules is useful in order to produce sustainable and renewable raw materials for use in valuable compounds, feeds, and fuels [4].

Endo-β-1,3-glucanases catalyze the hydrolysis of internal β-(1→3)-glucosidic linkages. Endo-β-1,3-glucanases mainly belong to the enzyme families GH16, GH17, and GH3 [5]. The GH16 family is mainly composed of bacterial enzymes that catalyze β-(1→3)-glucan and β-(1→3)/β-(1→4)-glucan [6]. Laminarin is a natural β-(1→3)-glucan with occasional β-(1→6)-glucosyl branches found in marine micro- and macroalgae. Bacteria degrade and metabolize laminarin as a source of glucose [7–12]. The successive hydrolysis of laminarin by GH16 enzymes and GH3 enzymes, a family containing various kinds of glycosidases, has been reported [13–18]. On the other hand, the GH17 family is mainly composed of plant and fungal enzymes. They are classified as pathogen-related proteins [19–21] that contribute to the degradation and biosynthesis of the cell wall. Recently, many GH17 bacterial enzymes have been discovered due to the progress made in sequencing technology; however, the biological functions of bacterial enzymes are still unclear. Studies have shown that proteobacterial species produce an antibiotic biofilm via GH17 glucosyltransferase activity [22,23]. Another study reported that glucosyltransferase activity was modulated to a glucanase activity by a single mutation [24].

The CAZy database provides the taxonomic distribution of the GH17 family (cazy.org/IMG/krona/GH17_krona.html, accessed on 23 February 2022), revealing that a large number of bacterial enzymes are found within the phylum Proteobacteria (recently renamed Pseudomonadota). Within Proteobacteria, GH17 enzymes are commonly found within the genus *Pseudomonas*, with its diverse members and metabolism. While many *Vibrio* species, which belong to the class Gammaproteobacteria, have GH16 enzymes, a limited number possess enzymes of the GH17 family. The genome of *V. vulnificus* has been sequenced and annotated, and sequence analysis has revealed that one GH16 enzyme (VvGH16) and one GH17 enzyme (VvGH17) exist adjacently in the genome. One GH3 enzyme is located close to the other two enzymes. On the other hand, three GH16 (VbGH16A, VbGH16B, and VbGH16C) and one GH17 (VbGH17A) enzyme of *Vibrio breoganii* 1C10 have been characterized [25].

Several CAZymes have various domains in addition to the catalytic domain, including carbohydrate-binding modules (CBMs) [26–28]. These domains are involved in carbohydrate binding. Tryptophan is an important amino acid residue in carbohydrate binding [26]. The VvGH17 C-terminus has several tryptophan residues. Therefore, we predicted that this region may have functions, such as carbohydrate binding, that can increase the catalytic efficiency or specificity. In this study, we characterized GH17 β-1,3-glucanase of *V. vulnificus* to clarify the unknown region of the protein and found that the N- and C- terminal regions were affiliated with the assembly of monomeric subunits into the multimeric form and the affinity for the substrate, respectively.

2. Results

2.1. Bioinformatic Analysis of VvGH17

VvGH17 is composed of 615 amino acids (AAs) comprising 1–22 AAs as signal peptides, 23–86 AAs as an unknown N-terminal region (Uk-N), 87–415 AAs as the GH17 domain, and 416–615 AAs as an unknown C-terminal region (Uk-C) (Figure 1a). Secondary structure prediction showed that Uk-N had a random coil structure, while Uk-C was composed of a β-sheet structure. The structure of VvGH17 was predicted using AlphaFold2 [29] (Figure 1b). The GH17 domain and C-terminus of Uk-C were predicted to have a $(\beta/\alpha)_8$ barrel structure and a β-sandwich structure, respectively. It was expected that the Uk-C structure possessed some function. Therefore, we attempted to characterize the impact of Uk-N and Uk-C on the catabolic properties of the enzymes.

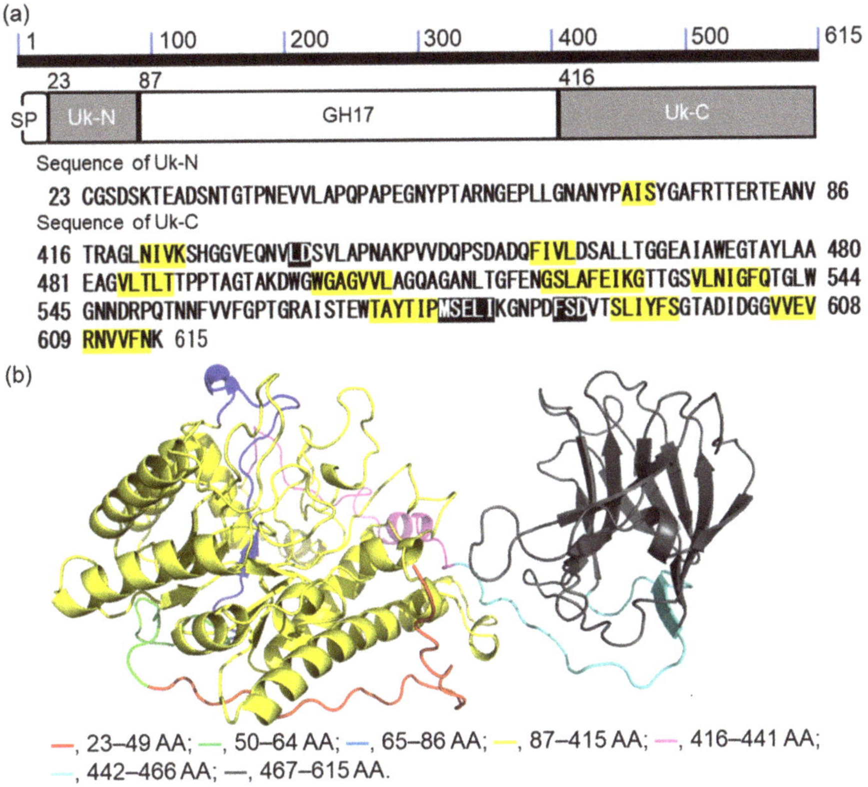

Figure 1. Sequence and predicted structure of VvGH17. (**a**) The scheme of VvGH17. SP—signal peptide; Uk-N—unknown N-terminal region; GH17—catalytic domain of GH17; Uk-C—unknown C-terminal region. Characters highlighted in yellow and those highlighted in black in the sequences are predicted α-fold and β-sheet structures, respectively. (**b**) Predicted three-dimensional structure. Colors are related to the truncated mutation region in this study.

2.2. Biochemical Properties of VvGH17

VvGH17 was produced in an *Escherichia coli* expression system and isolated using a TALON affinity resin (Takara Bio, Otsu, Japan). The purified enzyme (20 mg) was obtained from one liter of medium and showed a single band of approximately 63 kDa on SDS-PAGE. The optimal temperature and pH were 50 °C and 5.0–6.5, respectively (Figure 2a,b). The temperature required for the half inactivation of the hydrolysis activity of VvGH17 at 30 min was 47 °C (Figure 2c). The activity of VvGH17 decreased by approximately 80% in the presence of 0.5 M NaCl and retained the activity up to 4.0 M (Figure 2d). The specific activity of VvGH17 in optimal conditions was 65.5 U/mg. VvGH17 hydrolyzed curdlan (insoluble β-(1→3)-glucan) and laminarin, mainly producing laminaribiose, glucose, and laminaritriose; it did not hydrolyze barley β-glucan, which as β-(1→3)- and β-(1→4)-linkages (Figure 2e). The products of laminarin hydrolysis by VvGH17 were monitored from 0 to 60 min using gel filtration; the results revealed that VvGH17 hydrolyzed laminarin via an endolytic mechanism (Figure 2f).

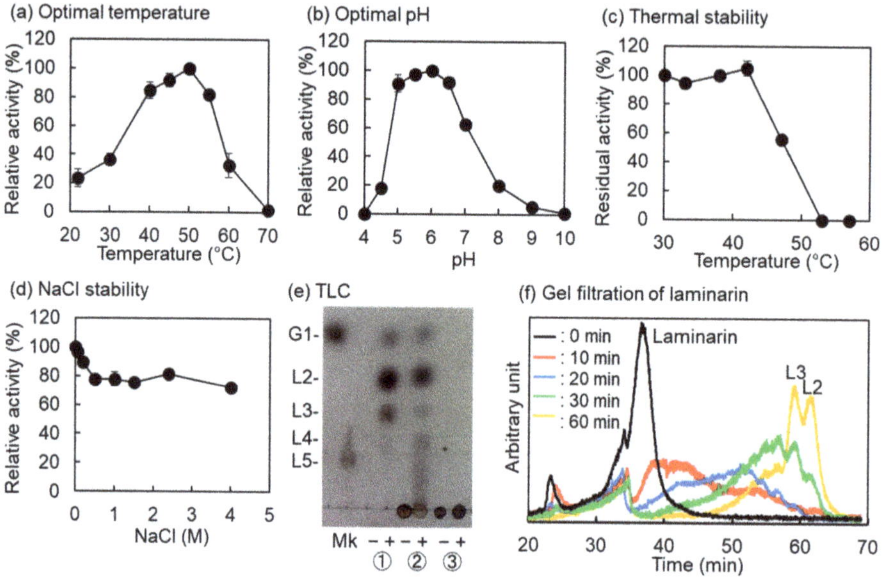

Figure 2. Characterization of VvGH17. (**a**) The effect of temperature on VvGH17 activity. The enzyme reaction was conducted in a mixture containing 50 mM MES buffer (pH 6.0), 1% (*w/v*) laminarin, and 0.02 mg/mL VvGH17 at 20–70 °C for 10 min. (**b**) The effect of pH on VvGH17 activity. The enzyme reaction was conducted in a mixture containing 1% (*w/v*) laminarin, 0.02 mg/mL VvGH17, and 100 mM Britton–Robinson buffer (pH 4.0–10.0) at 45 °C for 10 min. (**c**) The effect of temperature on VvGH17 stability. A mixture containing 50 mM MES buffer (pH 6.0) and 0.2 mg/mL VvGH17 was incubated at the indicated temperature for 30 min and placed on ice for 10 min. Then, the enzyme activity was assayed in a mixture containing 50 mM MES buffer (pH 6.0), 1% (*w/v*) laminarin, and 0.02 mg/mL VvGH17 at 45 °C for 10 min. (**d**) The effect of NaCl on VvGH17 activity. The enzyme reaction was conducted in a mixture containing 50 mM MES buffer (pH 6.0), 1% (*w/v*) laminarin, 0.02 mg/mL VvGH17, and 0–4.0 M NaCl at 45 °C for 10 min. (**e**) Thin layer chromatography (TLC) analyses of the hydrolysis products obtained using VvGH17. One microliter of each reaction mixture was applied for TLC analysis. Mk—marker of glucose and laminaripentaose; '–'—without VvGH17; '+'—with VvGH17. ①—curdlan; ②—laminarin; ③—β-glucan. (**f**) Gel filtration chromatography analysis for the hydrolysis of laminarin by VvGH17.

2.3. *C-terminal-Truncated Mutant*

C-terminal-truncated mutants of VvGH17 were constructed for the characterization of Uk-C. The position from 87–415 AA was demonstrated as the conserved domain of GH17. Therefore, Uk-C was defined as the position from 416–615 AA in VvGH17, and the three C-terminal-truncated mutants (ΔC466, ΔC441, and ΔC415) were constructed (Figure 3a). Recombinant proteins of the three mutants were successfully expressed, and we evaluated the enzyme kinetics (Figure 3b, Table 1). The enzyme kinetics k_{cat}/K_m of the WT toward laminarin was 93.0 mM^{-1} s^{-1}, and 32.8 and 30.5 mM^{-1} s^{-1} for ΔC466 and ΔC441, respectively, which are approximately one-third of the k_{cat}/K_m values in the WT. The k_{cat}/K_m values of ΔC415 were less than 2% of those in the WT. To confirm whether the loss of activity in ΔC415 was derived from folding, the secondary structure was compared using circular dichroism (CD) spectroscopy (Figure 3c). The difference in the CD spectrum (deg cm^2 $dmol^{-1}$) between 210 and 230 nm may be a result of the deletion of the C-terminus in VvGH17. From these results, the truncation of the C-terminus in Uk-C (AA 442–615) resulted in a decrease in the catalytic efficiency of VvGH17, and the truncation of the whole Uk-C (416–615 AA) caused the loss of the majority of its activity, suggesting that this is an essential region.

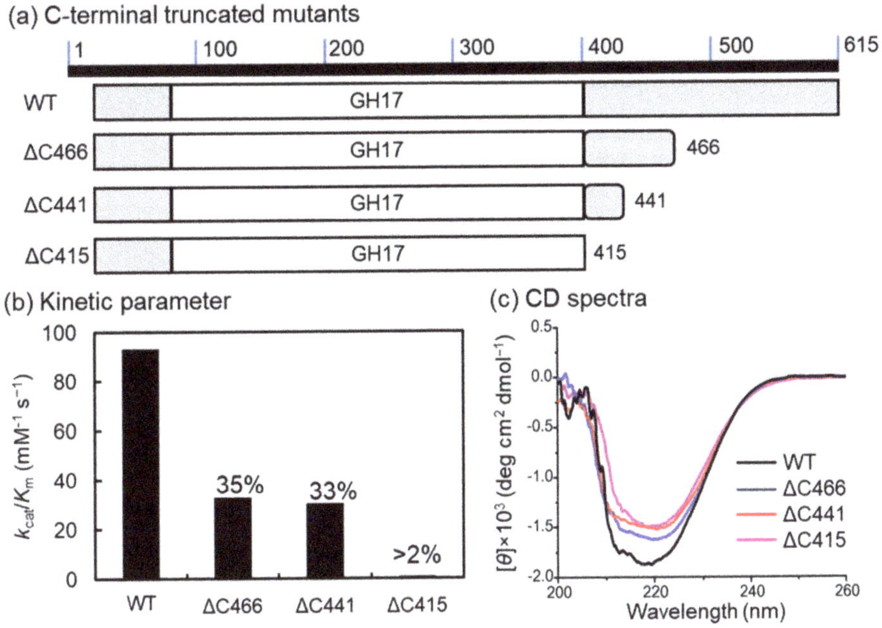

Figure 3. C-terminal-truncated mutants of VvGH17. (**a**) Scheme of C-terminal-truncated mutants. (**b**) Enzyme kinetics using laminarin as a substrate. The k_{cat}/K_m value of the WT (93.0 mM^{-1} s^{-1}) was set at 100%, and the relative values of the other mutants are indicated in the figure. (**c**) CD spectra of the WT and mutants. WT—black line; ΔC466—blue line; ΔC441—red line; ΔC415—pink line.

Table 1. Enzyme kinetics of VvGH17 and mutants using laminarin as a substrate.

	k_{cat}/K_m (mM^{-1} s^{-1})	k_{cat} (s^{-1})	K_m (mM^{-1})
VvGH17	93.0	148	1.60
ΔC466	35.3	81.7	2.49
ΔC441	32.7	87.6	2.87
ΔC415	0.2	1.4	9.39
ΔN50	67.5	143.3	2.12
ΔN65	24.7	86.8	3.52

2.4. Affinity Gel Analysis of C-Terminal-Truncated Mutants of VvGH17

The truncation of the VvGH17 C-terminus revealed that this region affects the enzyme kinetics (k_{cat} and K_m). This indicates that Uk-C has the potential for carbohydrate binding. To investigate the Uk-C function further, affinity gel analysis was performed (Figure 4). The WT and three C-terminal-truncated mutants showed two bands with and without substrates. The two bands were confirmed as monomers and oligomers (trimer) of the enzyme, as discussed in Section 2.7. Bovine serum albumin (BSA) was used as a marker protein for the mobility shift assay. No affinity toward curdlan was found in the tested enzymes, compared to the gel without substrate. The mobility of the WT monomer was clearly shifted from below the BSA band (without substrate) to upper the BSA band in the gels, confirming its affinity toward laminarin and β-glucan.

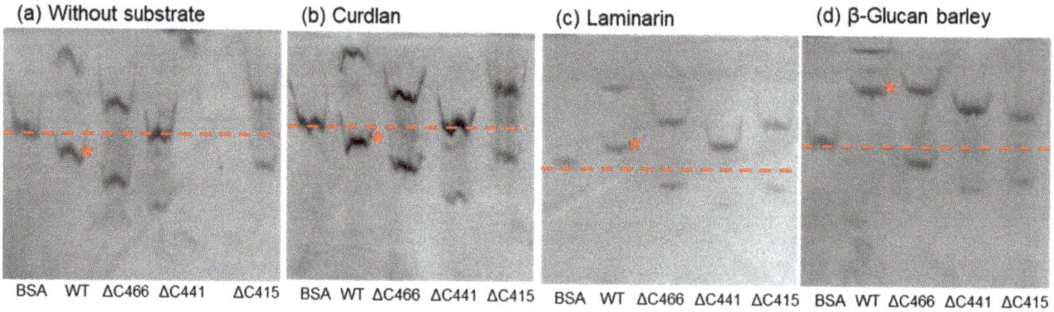

Figure 4. Affinity gel analysis of the WT and C-terminal-truncated mutants of VvGH17. (**a**) Affinity gel without substrate; (**b**) gel containing curdlan; (**c**) gel containing laminarin; (**d**) gel containing barley β-glucan. Asterisks show the WT monomer bands. The dashed lines show the mobility of BSA.

2.5. Affinity Gel Analysis of Uk-C and Point Mutants of VvGH17

The affinity of Uk-C and the C-terminus of VvGH17 toward laminarin and β-glucan was revealed. To confirm the important amino acids for substrate binding, point mutants of Uk-C and VvGH17 were constructed. Affinity toward substrates was also evaluated by the mobility as compared with BSA (Figure 5). The mobility of Uk-C in the gel containing laminarin and β-glucan was decreased compared to the gel without substrate. This indicated that Uk-C had a binding ability for laminarin and β-glucan. Tryptophan is an important amino acid for carbohydrate binding [26]. Therefore, we mutated four tryptophans in Uk-C to alanines (W472A, W499A, W542A, and W567A), and the affinity was evaluated by mobility shift assays. The WT and four mutants showed the same mobilities without a substrate. The mobilities of W472A, W499A, and W542A in the gel containing laminarin and β-glucan differed from those of the WT and W567A. The decreased mobility of W472A, W499A, and W542A indicated reduced binding ability, suggesting that the three tryptophans are essential amino acids for substrate binding.

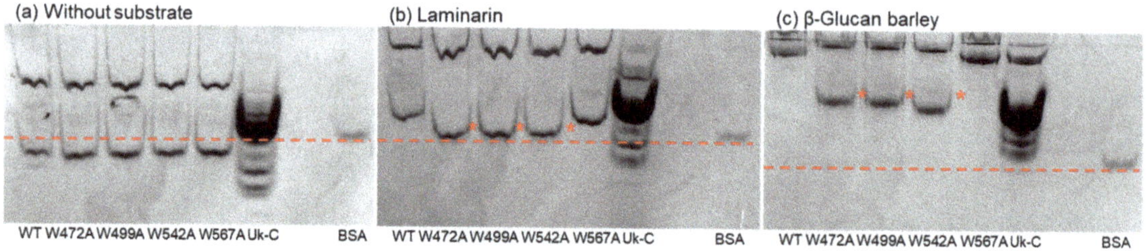

Figure 5. Affinity gel analysis of the WT, point mutants of VvGH17, and Uk-C. (**a**) Affinity gel without substrate; (**b**) gel containing laminarin; (**c**) gel containing barley β-glucan. Asterisks indicate the monomer bands showing different mobility. The dashed lines show the mobility of BSA.

2.6. Prediction of Uk-C Structure and Function

We attempted to clarify the relationship between the predicted three-dimensional structure of Uk-C (AA 441–615 of VvGH17) and the binding ability of the mutants. The predicted Uk-C had two domains: the N-terminus of Uk-C (AA 416–462 of VvGH17) was predicted to be a linker between GH17 and the binding region, and the C-terminus of Uk-C (AA 463–615 of VvGH17) was predicted to be a β-sandwich structure with a possible carbohydrate-binding ability (Figure 1b). Three tryptophan residues (Trp472, Trp499, and Trp542) were located in the putative substrate binding region in the β-sandwich structure (Figure 6). On the other hand, the predicted structure suggested that Trp567 was located outside of the putative substrate binding region. The results of the mutation experiments agreed with the predicted structure.

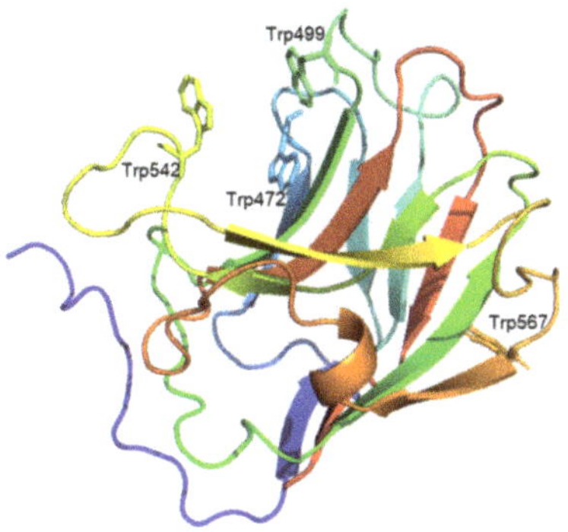

Figure 6. Structural prediction of the C-terminus of VvGH17. AA 441-615 of VvGH17 as predicted by AlphaFold2. Colors from blue to red show the sequence from AA 441 to 615. The locations of the four tryptophans (Trp472, Trp499, Trp542, and Trp567) are indicated.

2.7. *N-Terminal-Truncated Mutants of VvGH17*

The catalytic domain of VvGH17 was mapped from AA 87 to 415, and AA 1–22 of VvGH17 were predicted as a signal peptide. The function of the N-terminus in VvGH17 (AA 23–86) was unclear. Therefore, we constructed two N-terminal-truncated mutants (ΔN50 and ΔN65) and evaluated their activity (Figure 7). The k_{cat}/K_m values of ΔN50 and ΔN65 toward laminarin were 67.5 and 24.7 mM^{-1} s^{-1}, respectively. The predicted three-dimensional structure of VvGH17 showed that the region of AA 51–65 was composed of the bottom of the $(\beta/\alpha)_8$ barrel structure (Figure 1b). Consequently, the loss of this region in the ΔN65 mutant led to structural instability, resulting in decreased catalytic efficiency (K_{cat}/k_m) (Table 1).

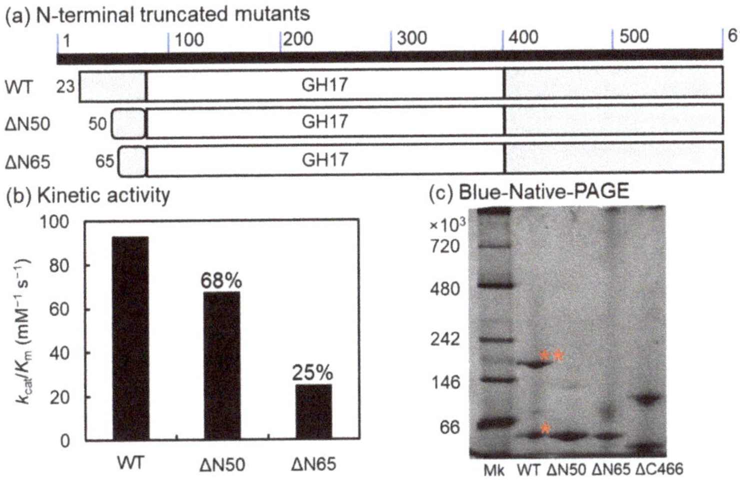

Figure 7. N-terminal-truncated mutants of VvGH17. (**a**) Scheme of N-terminal-truncated mutants. (**b**) Enzyme kinetics using laminarin as substrate. The k_{cat}/K_m value of the WT (93.0 mM^{-1} s^{-1}) was set at 100% and the relative values of the other mutants are indicated in the figure. (**c**) Blue native PAGE of the WT and N- and C-terminal-truncated mutants. *—WT monomer; **—putative WT trimer from molecular weight.

Two bands from the WT and C-terminal-truncated mutants were observed in native PAGE, as shown in Section 2.4. To confirm the assembly of monomeric subunits into the multimeric form, blue native PAGE was performed for the WT and N- and C-terminal-truncated mutants (Figure 7c). The WT and ΔC466 mutant clearly showed two bands (monomers and putative trimers from the molecular mass), while ΔN50 and ΔN65 showed a single band corresponding to the monomer.

3. Discussion

In this study, we characterized the GH17 enzymes of *V. vulnificus* using an *E. coli* expression system. Functionally, GH17 enzymes have been reported to be β-(1→3)-glucan hydrolases and transglycosylases. In particular, endo-type β-(1→3)-glucanases are classified into the enzyme commission (EC) number EC 3.2.1.6 endo-1,3(4)-β-glucanase; EC 3.2.1.39 represents glucan endo-1,3-β-D-glucosidase; and EC 3.2.1.73 indicates licheninase. Our results showed that VvGH17 was classified into EC 3.2.1.39 due to its endolytic mechanism and specificity for β-(1→3)-glucan.

VvGH17 produced laminaribiose as the main product regardless of soluble and insoluble β-(1→3)-glucans, showing its potential for oligosaccharide production. The amino acid identity between VvGH17 and VbGH17A from *V. breoganii* 1C10 was low (42% identity). VbGH17A contains a signal peptide, the GH17 catalytic domain, and an unknown region of the C-terminus from amino acid (AA) 411 to 634 [18]. The catalytic domains of VvGH17 and VbGH17A shared 56% identity; however, the identity between the C-termini was low (21%). The hydrolysis products of VbGH17A were oligosaccharides, which were larger than a degree of polymerization (DP) of 4. *V. breoganii* 1C10 has four endo-type β-(1→3)-glucanases, which presumably show synergic activity during the hydrolysis of β-(1→3)-glucans. On the other hand, *V. vulnificus* has two endo-type β-(1→3)-glucanases. We expected several enzymes; however, there was only GH16, which had 57% identity with VbGH16A and produced mainly DP 3 and 4. The GH3 enzymes of *Vibrio* sp. have been shown to have activity toward laminaribiose [30]. Therefore, *V. vulnificus* may metabolize β-(1→3)-glucan by producing small DP oligosaccharides using two endo-type enzymes and then hydrolyzing them using the GH3 enzyme.

In this study, we identified the Uk-C as a carbohydrate binding-domain. VvGH17 formed a trimer, and the complex structure also showed carbohydrate binding activity. It can be concluded that the N-terminal region is affiliated with the trimerization of VvGH17. A more detailed structure-function analysis is needed. Uk-C showed binding activity with β-(1→3)-glucan and β-(1→3)/β-(1→4)-glucan and no binding activity with curdlan, an insoluble triple helix β-(1→3)-glucan. The TLC results indicated that VvGH17 hydrolyzed curdlan as well as laminarin without the assistance of Uk-C (Figure 2e). This study investigated the affinity of Uk-C for insoluble curdlan, but not the affinity for curdlan gel. Therefore, the binding specificity of Uk-C for a linear β-(1→3)-glucan should be further investigated. Curdlan is produced by the soil bacterium *Agrobacterium* sp., and *V. vulnificus* is a marine bacterium. Therefore, Uk-C might be specific for the marine polysaccharide laminarin. Laminarin is a soluble β-(1→3)-glucan with a β-(1→6)-glycosyl side chain. The difference in polysaccharide structure could affect the binding specificity. CBMs are classified into three types by their ligand binding sites. A-type CBMs recognize crystalline polysaccharide-like cellulose and chitin. B-type CBMs recognize a single glycan by binding a cleft or groove. C-type CBMs recognize the glycan terminus by binding pockets [26]. The Uk-C structure was predicted to be a B-type groove with three tryptophan residues. We confirmed that the mutations constituted the groove. Therefore, the mutation of tryptophan residues decreased the glucan binding ability. A BLAST search of Uk-C (416–615 AA) showed identity with CBM domains linked to other GH17 enzymes. A high AA identity of more than 95% was shared with the CBM domains of the GH17 enzymes from *Vibrio* sp., including *V. fluvialis*, *V. cholerae*, *V. metoecus*, and *V. metschnikovii*. A total of 30–70% identities were shared with enzymes from bacterial species, such as *Enterovibrio* sp., *Porticoccaceae* sp., *Bacteroidetes* sp., and *Grimontia* sp. (Table S1). The CBMs were classified into 89 families in the CAZy database (accessed on 16 February 2022). Among them, an affinity for β-(1→3)-glucan or β-(1→3)/β-(1→4)-glucan was demonstrated by 18 families: CBM4, 6, 11, 22, 28, 39, 43, 52, 54, 56, 65, 72, 76, 78, 79, 80, 81, and 85. CBM43, linked to eukaryotic GH17 enzymes, generally consists of 90-100 AAs [31]. The C-terminus of VvGH17 consisted of 150 AAs. Therefore, the sequences of CBMs belonging to nine families with around 150 AA residues were selected and aligned using ClustalW (https://www.genome.jp/tools-bin/clustalw, accessed on 23 February 2022) after removing the His-tag sequence, and we visualized the tree using iTOL [32] (Figure 8). The C-terminus of VvGH17 showed the closest relationship to the CBM79 cluster. The AA identity between Uk-C and CBM79 was 15.6-17.2% (Figure S1, Supplementary Materials). The complete genome sequence of *V. vulnificus* was determined in 2011 [33], and CBM79 family was recorded in 2016 [34]; however, Uk-C has not been included. In addition, the Uk-C sequence was not hit by a BLASTP search using CBM79 as query sequence. The distance of VvGH17 and CBM79 was similar to other CBM clusters (Figure 8), indicating that Uk-C is a novel soluble β-(1→3)-glucan and β-(1→3)/β-(1→4)-glucan-binding protein.

Figure 8. Phylogenetic tree of VvGH17 C-terminal domain and relatives. The tree was constructed based on ClustalW pairwise sequence alignment using the iTOL visualizing software. The following amino acid sequences were used: CBM4, laminarinase 16A from *Thermotoga maritima*, accession number (AN)—AAD35118, protein data bank (PDB) —1GUI [35]; CBM6, β-1,3-glucanase from *Alkalihalobacillus halodurans* C-125, AN—BAB03955, PDB—1W9T [36]; CBM6, endo-β-1,3-glucanase from *Zobellia galactanivorans*, AN—CAZ95067, PDB—5FUI [36]; CBM22, xylanase Xyn10B from *Acetivibrio thermocellus* YS, AN—CAA58242, PDB—1DYO [37]; CBM65, endoglucanase (EcCel5A) from *Eubacterium cellulosolvens* 5, AN—BAE46390, PDB—2YPJ [38]; CBM72, endoglucanase from uncultured microorganism, AN—EU449484 [39]; CBM76, GH44 from *Ruminococcus flavefaciens*, AN—AAA95959 [34]; CBM78, GH5 from *R. flavefaciens*, AN—WP_009983134, PDB—4V17 [34]; CBM79, GH9 from *R. flavefaciens*, AN—WP_009984389 [34]; CBM85, GH10 xylanase from metagenomic data, AN—MH727997 [27]; and VvGH17 from 451–615 AA. His-tag sequences from CBM6_5FUI, CBM65_2YPJ, and CBM78_4V17 were removed. The alignment of the tree and VvGH17 and CBM79 are shown in Figure S1 and Figure S2, respectively.

4. Materials and Methods

4.1. Materials

Curdlan was purchased from Fujifilm Wako Pure Chemicals Industries Ltd. (Osaka, Japan); laminarin (*Laminaria digitata*) was from Sigma-Aldrich Corp. (St. Louis, MO, USA); and β-glucan (barley; medium viscosity) was from Megazyme International Ireland Ltd. (Bray, Ireland). Laminaripentaose was prepared by the hydrolysis of curdlan with KfGH64 [40]. All the other reagents were purchased from Wako Pure Chemical Industries (Osaka, Japan).

4.2. Bioinformatic Analysis of VvGH17

The GH17 gene from *Vibrio vulnificus* (hypothetical protein AOT11_01225) was obtained from GenBank (accession no. ASM98089.1). The putative conserved domain was searched using BLASTP [41]. The signal peptide was predicted using the SignalP 4.1 server [42]. Secondary structure prediction was performed using the PSIPRED server [43] and the structure was predicted by AlphaFold2 [29]. Homolog proteins of the C-terminus of VvGH17 (416–615 AA) were searched by BLASTP with the standard algorithm, excluding *Vibrio vulnificus* (taxid: 672); we also removed query covers of less than 40%. A phylogenetic tree was constructed by pairwise sequence alignment.

4.3. Construction, Expression, and Purification of VvGH17

The expression plasmid of the gene putatively encoding β-(1→3)-glucanase (VvGH17) was constructed as follows: a codon-optimized mature *Vvgh17* gene was synthesized (Eurofins Genomics) for expression in *E. coli* harboring *Nde*I and *Hin*dIII sites at 5′ and 3′, respectively. Then, the *Vvgh17* gene was cloned into the *Nde*I-*Hin*dIII site of pET28a to construct an expression vector of pET28a(VvGH17). The recombinant protein was produced in *E. coli* BL21-RIL (DE3) cells (Agilent Technologies, Palo Alto, CA, USA) harboring pET28a(VvGH17) and was purified as previously described [44]. The protein concentrations were determined by absorbance at 280 nm using the molar extinction coefficients for VvGH17 [45].

4.4. Construction of VvGH17 Mutants

The C-terminal-truncated mutants (ΔC466, ΔC441, and ΔC415), N-terminal-truncated mutants (ΔN50, ΔN65, and UK-C), and point mutants (W472A, W499A, W542A, and W567A) were constructed by polymerase chain reaction using PrimeSTAR MAX DNA polymerase (Takara Bio, Otsu, Japan), primers (Table 2), and pET28a(VvGH17) as a template.

Table 2. Sequences of the primers used in this study.

Primer Name	Primer Sequence (5′-3′)	Purpose
ΔC466-S	TGATGGCAAGCTTGCGGCCGCACTC	Truncation of 149 AAs from C-terminus
ΔC466-AS	GCAAGCTTGCCATCAAACGCGCCGGC	
ΔC441-S	GACCGGCAAGCTTGCGGCCGCACTC	Truncation of 174 AAs from C-terminus
ΔC441-AS	GCAAGCTTGCCGGTCAGTAATGCACT	
ΔC415-S	TGCTCCGTGAAAGCTTGCGGCCGCACTC	Truncation of 200 AAs from C-terminus
ΔC415-AS	GCAAGCTTTCACGGAGCAAGAACGGAAT	
ΔN50-S	CCATATGGGCAACTATCCGACAGCT	Truncation of 50 AAsf rom N-terminus
ΔN50-AS	TAGTTGCCCATATGGCTGCCGCGCGG	
ΔN65-S	CCATATGGGCAACGCGAATTATCCG	Truncation of 65 AAs from N-terminus
ΔN65-AS	GCGTTGCCCATATGGCTGCCGCGCGG	
UK-C-S	CCATATGGCCGGCGCGTTTGATGGC	Truncation of 410 AAs from N-terminus
UK-C-AS	GCGCCGGCCATATGGCTGCCGCGCGG	
W472A-S	ATCGCAgcgGAAGGTACCGCCTATCTG	Mutation of Trp472 to Ala472
W472A-AS	ACCTTCcgcTGCGATCGCTTCCCCGCC	
W499A-S	TGGGGTgcgGGAGCGGGCGTCGTGCTC	Mutation of Trp499 to Ala499
W499A-AS	CGCTCCcgcACCCCAGTCTTTTGCAGT	
W542A-S	GGCCTGgcgGGCAACAACGACCGTCCG	Mutation of Trp542 to Ala542
W542A-AS	GTTGCCcgcCAGGCCGGTCTGAAATCC	
W567A-S	ACCGAAgcgACAGCCTACACGATTCCG	Mutation of Trp567 to Ala567
W567A-AS	GGCTGTcgcTTCGGTTGAAATGGCACG	

Small characters show amino acid mutations from tryptophan to alanine.

4.5. VvGH17 Standard Activity Assay

VvGH17 activity was determined at 45 °C for 10 min with an appropriate amount of enzyme, 1% (*w/v*) laminarin, and 50 mM 2-morpholinoethanesulfonic acid (MES; pH 6.0). The amount of reducing sugars was determined using the dinitrosalicylic acid method (DNS) [46]. One unit of activity was defined as the amount of enzyme that liberated reducing sugars equivalent to 1.0 μmol glucose per minute. The optimal temperature of VvGH17 was measured as follows: a reaction mixture containing 1% (*w/v*) laminarin and 50 mM MES (pH 6.0) was incubated at 22–70 °C for 10 min. The optimal pH of VvGH17 was measured as follows: a reaction mixture containing 1% (*w/v*) laminarin and 100 mM Britton–Robinson buffer (a mixture containing sodium acetate buffer, sodium phosphate buffer, and glycine–NaOH buffer; pH 4.0–10.0) was incubated at 45 °C for 10 min. Temperature stability was determined by measuring the residual activity after incubation in 50 mM MES (pH 6.0) at 30–57 °C for 30 min. The effect of NaCl was determined using a mixture containing 1% (*w/v*) laminarin, 50 mM MES (pH 6.0), and 0–4.0 M NaCl at 45 °C for 10 min. The V_{max} and K_m with laminarin (0.5–40 mg/mL) were determined by the standard Michaelis–Menten equation using nonlinear regression (Origin Software, Lightstone Corp., Tokyo, Japan). All the activity assays were performed in triplicate.

4.6. Analysis of Hydrolysis Products by TLC and Gel Filtration Chromatography

The products of VvGH17 hydrolysis were analyzed by TLC using a silica gel 60 plate (Merck). The substrates (curdlan, laminarin, and β-glucan: 10 mg/mL) were hydrolyzed with 0.01 U/mL of VvGH17 for 24 h, and the reaction was terminated by heating at 100 °C for 10 min. The hydrolysis products (1 μL) were developed in ethyl acetate, acetic acid, and water (2:2:1, *v/v/v*); sugars were detected by spraying a solution of 10% (*v/v*) sulfuric acid in ethanol and then heating at 100 °C for 10 min.

The distribution of the hydrolysis products of laminarin was analyzed using high-performance liquid chromatography (HPLC) with a Superdex Peptide 10/300 GL column (GE Healthcare UK Ltd., Little Chalfont, UK) and a Corona Charged Aerosol Detector (Thermo Scientific Inc., Chelmsford, MA, USA). Laminarin (10 mg/mL) was hydrolyzed with 0.01 U/mL of VvGH17 from 0 to 60 min, and the reaction was terminated by heating at 100 °C for 10 min. The samples were eluted using water with a flow rate of 0.3 mL/min.

4.7. CD Spectroscopy

The secondary structures of VvGH17 were determined by CD spectroscopy using a J-720WI spectrometer (Jasco Corp. Tokyo, Japan). The proteins were dissolved at a final concentration of 0.1 mg/mL in 50 mM MES buffer (pH 6.0). The spectra were acquired at 37 °C using a 0.2 cm cuvette. The molar ellipticities (per residue) were calculated using the equation $[\theta] = 100(\theta)/(lcN)$, where $[\theta]$ is the molar ellipticity per residue, (θ) is the observed ellipticity in degrees, l is the optical path length in centimeters, c is the molar concentration of the protein, and N is the number of residues in the protein.

4.8. Polyacrylamide Gel Electrophoresis (PAGE) Analysis

The assays for the binding activity of the proteins were performed by affinity gel electrophoresis, according to the procedure described by Zhang et al. [47]. A stacking gel containing 3 wt% polyacrylamide in 1.5 M Tris-HCl buffer (pH 8.3), a native gel with 12 wt% polyacrylamide containing 0.1 wt% polysaccharides (curdlan, laminarin, and barley β-glucan), and a control gel without polysaccharides were prepared. Each protein (1 μg) was loaded onto the gel, and the gels were electrophoresed at 4 °C and 100 V for 3 h. The gels were then stained with Coomassie brilliant blue G-250 for protein visualization.

Blue native PAGE was performed using a 5–10% gradient gel at 4 °C and 150 V held constant for 3.5 h using an anode buffer (50 mM tricine, 15 mM bis-Tris/HCl, pH 7) and cathode buffer (50 mM tricine, 15 mM bis-Tris/HCl, pH 7, 0.02% (*w/v*) Coomassie blue G250).

5. Conclusions

In this study, we characterized the unknown domains of the GH17 β-(1→3)-glucanase of *V. vulnificus*. The WT formed a trimer, but the N-terminal truncations formed monomers. Therefore, the N-terminus contributes to the assembly of monomeric subunits into the multimeric form of VvGH17. The C-terminal region showed an affinity for β-(1→3)-glucan and β-(1→3)/β-(1→4)-glucan. The C-terminus was predicted to have a β-sandwich structure, and three tryptophan residues (Trp472, Trp499, and Trp542) were located at the substrate binding site using mutational analysis. A BLAST search revealed that the C-terminal region of GH17 was conserved among Gammaproteobacteria. The results of this study are useful for understanding bacterial GH17 enzymes and oligosaccharide preparation.

Supplementary Materials: The following supporting information can be downloaded at: https://www.mdpi.com/article/10.3390/md20040250/s1, Table S1: BLAST search result for Uk-C; Figure S1: AA alignment of Uk-C and CBM79; Figure S2: AA alignment of Figure 8.

Author Contributions: Conceptualization, Y.K.; methodology, Y.K., H.K., W.L., T.T., M.O. and A.K.; writing—original draft preparation, Y.K.; writing—review and editing, W.L., T.T. and M.O.; supervision, H.K. and A.K.; funding acquisition, Y.K. All authors have read and agreed to the published version of the manuscript.

Funding: This research was funded by the Japan Society for the Promotion of Science KAKENHI Grant No. 16K18748.

Conflicts of Interest: The funders had no role in the design of the study; in the collection, analyses, or interpretation of data; in the writing of the manuscript; or in the decision to publish the results.

References

1. Field, C.B.; Behrenfeld, M.J.; Randerson, J.T.; Falkowski, P. Primary Production of the Biosphere: Integrating Terrestrial and Oceanic Components. *Science* **1998**, *281*, 237–240. [CrossRef] [PubMed]
2. Worden, A.Z.; Follows, M.J.; Giovannoni, S.J.; Wilken, S.; Zimmerman, A.E.; Keeling, P.J. Rethinking the marine carbon cycle: Factoring in the multifarious lifestyles of microbes. *Science* **2015**, *347*, 1257594. [CrossRef] [PubMed]
3. Stefan, B.; Jan, T.; Sarah, C.; Karen, W.; Hvitfeldt, I.M.; Tilmann, H.; Kai-Uwe, H.; Jan-Hendrik, H. Laminarin is a major molecule in the marine carbon cycle. *Proc. Natl. Acad. Sci. USA* **2020**, *117*, 6599–6607. [CrossRef]
4. Lim, H.G.; Kwak, D.H.; Park, S.; Woo, S.; Yang, J.-S.; Kang, C.W.; Kim, B.; Noh, M.H.; Seo, S.W.; Jung, G.Y. *Vibrio* sp. dhg as a platform for the biorefinery of brown macroalgae. *Nat. Commun.* **2019**, *10*, 2486. [CrossRef] [PubMed]
5. Drula, E.; Garron, M.-L.; Dogan, S.; Lombard, V.; Henrissat, B.; Terrapon, N. The carbohydrate-active enzyme database: Functions and literature. *Nucleic Acids Res.* **2022**, *50*, D571–D577. [CrossRef]
6. Viborg, A.H.; Terrapon, N.; Lombard, V.; Michel, G.; Czjzek, M.; Henrissat, B.; Brumer, H. A subfamily roadmap of the evolutionarily diverse glycoside hydrolase family 16 (GH16). *J. Biol. Chem.* **2019**, *294*, 15973–15986. [CrossRef]
7. Jian, Y.; Yuqun, X.; Takuya, M.; Lijuan, L.; Masaru, T.; Ning-Yi, Z. Molecular Basis for Substrate Recognition and Catalysis by a Marine Bacterial Laminarinase. *Appl. Environ. Microbiol.* **2022**, *86*, e01796-20. [CrossRef]
8. Burkhardt, C.; Schäfers, C.; Claren, J.; Schirrmacher, G.; Antranikian, G. Comparative Analysis and Biochemical Characterization of Two Endo-β-1,3-Glucanases from the Thermophilic Bacterium *Fervidobacterium* sp. *Catalysts* **2019**, *9*, 830. [CrossRef]
9. Liberato, M.V.; Teixeira Prates, E.; Gonçalves, T.A.; Bernardes, A.; Vilela, N.; Fattori, J.; Ematsu, G.C.; Chinaglia, M.; Machi Gomes, E.R.; Migliorini Figueira, A.C.; et al. Insights into the dual cleavage activity of the GH16 laminarinase enzyme class on β-1,3 and β-1,4 glycosidic bonds. *J. Biol. Chem.* **2021**, *296*, 100385. [CrossRef]
10. Mitsuya, D.; Sugiyama, T.; Zhang, S.; Takeuchi, Y.; Okai, M.; Urano, N.; Ishida, M. Enzymatic properties and the gene structure of a cold-adapted laminarinase from *Pseudoalteromonas* species LA. *J. Biosci. Bioeng.* **2018**, *126*, 169–175. [CrossRef]
11. Oda, M.; Inaba, S.; Kamiya, N.; Bekker, G.-J.; Mikami, B. Structural and thermodynamic characterization of endo-1,3-β-glucanase: Insights into the substrate recognition mechanism. *Biochim. Biophys. Acta-Proteins Proteom.* **2018**, *1866*, 415–425. [CrossRef]
12. Li, Z.; Liu, W.; Lyu, Q. Biochemical Characterization of a Novel Endo-1,3-β-Glucanase from the Scallop *Chlamys farreri*. *Mar. Drugs* **2020**, *18*, 466. [CrossRef] [PubMed]
13. Singh, R.P.; Thakur, R.; Kumar, G. Human gut *Bacteroides uniformis* utilizes mixed linked β-glucans via an alternative strategy. *Bioact. Carbohydr. Diet. Fibre* **2021**, *26*, 100282. [CrossRef]
14. Unfried, F.; Becker, S.; Robb, C.S.; Hehemann, J.-H.; Markert, S.; Heiden, S.E.; Hinzke, T.; Becher, D.; Reintjes, G.; Krüger, K.; et al. Adaptive mechanisms that provide competitive advantages to marine bacteroidetes during microalgal blooms. *ISME J.* **2018**, *12*, 2894–2906. [CrossRef] [PubMed]
15. Xue, C.; Xie, Z.-X.; Li, Y.-Y.; Chen, X.-H.; Sun, G.; Lin, L.; Giovannoni, S.J.; Wang, D.-Z. Polysaccharide utilization by a marine heterotrophic bacterium from the SAR92 clade. *FEMS Microbiol. Ecol.* **2021**, *97*, fiab120. [CrossRef]
16. Déjean, G.; Tamura, K.; Cabrera, A.; Jain, N.; Pudio, N.A.; Pereira, G.; Viborg, A.H.; van Petegem, F.; Martens, E.C.; Brumer, H. Synergy between Cell Surface Glycosidases and Glycan-Binding Proteins Dictates the Utilization of Specific Beta(1,3)-Glucans by Human Gut Bacteroides. *MBio* **2022**, *11*, e00095-20. [CrossRef]
17. Armstrong, Z.; Liu, F.; Kheirandish, S.; Chen, H.M.; Mewis, K.; Duo, T.; Morgan-Lang, C.; Hallam, S.J.; Withers, S.G. High-Throughput Recovery and Characterization of Metagenome-Derived Glycoside Hydrolase-Containing Clones as a Resource for Biocatalyst Development. *mSystems* **2022**, *4*, e00082-19. [CrossRef]
18. Kappelmann, L.; Krüger, K.; Hehemann, J.-H.; Harder, J.; Markert, S.; Unfried, F.; Becher, D.; Shapiro, N.; Schweder, T.; Amann, R.I.; et al. Polysaccharide utilization loci of North Sea *Flavobacteriia* as basis for using SusC/D-protein expression for predicting major phytoplankton glycans. *ISME J.* **2019**, *13*, 76–91. [CrossRef]
19. Bagnaresi, P.; Biselli, C.; Orrù, L.; Urso, S.; Crispino, L.; Abbruscato, P.; Piffanelli, P.; Lupotto, E.; Cattivelli, L.; Valè, G. Comparative Transcriptome Profiling of the Early Response to *Magnaporthe oryzae* in Durable Resistant vs Susceptible Rice (*Oryza sativa* L.) Genotypes. *PLoS ONE* **2012**, *7*, e51609. [CrossRef]

20. Wu, J.; Lee, D.Y.; Wang, Y.; Kim, S.T.; Baek, S.-B.; Kim, S.G.; Kang, K.Y. Protein profiles secreted from phylloplane of rice leaves free from cytosolic proteins: Application to study rice-Magnaporthe Oryzae interactions. *Physiol. Mol. Plant Pathol.* **2014**, *88*, 28–35. [CrossRef]
21. Marqués-Gálvez, J.E.; Miyauchi, S.; Paolocci, F.; Navarro-Ródenas, A.; Arenas, F.; Pérez-Gilabert, M.; Morin, E.; Auer, L.; Barry, K.W.; Kuo, A.; et al. Desert truffle genomes reveal their reproductive modes and new insights into plant–fungal interaction and ectendomycorrhizal lifestyle. *New Phytol.* **2021**, *229*, 2917–2932. [CrossRef] [PubMed]
22. Sadovskaya, I.; Vinogradov, E.; Li, J.; Hachani, A.; Kowalska, K.; Filloux, A. High-level antibiotic resistance in Pseudomonas aeruginosa biofilm: The ndvB gene is involved in the production of highly glycerol-phosphorylated β-(1→3)-glucans, which bind aminoglycosides. *Glycobiology* **2010**, *20*, 895–904. [CrossRef] [PubMed]
23. Hreggvidsson, G.O.; Dobruchowska, J.M.; Fridjonsson, O.H.; Jonsson, J.O.; Gerwig, G.J.; Aevarsson, A.; Kristjansson, J.K.; Curti, D.; Redgwell, R.R.; Hansen, C.-E.; et al. Exploring novel non-Leloir β-glucosyltransferases from proteobacteria for modifying linear (β1→3)-linked gluco-oligosaccharide chains. *Glycobiology* **2011**, *21*, 304–328. [CrossRef]
24. Qin, Z.; Yan, Q.; Yang, S.; Jiang, Z. Modulating the function of a β-1,3-glucanosyltransferase to that of an endo-β-1,3-glucanase by structure-based protein engineering. *Appl. Microbiol. Biotechnol.* **2016**, *100*, 1765–1776. [CrossRef]
25. Badur, A.H.; Ammar, E.M.; Yalamanchili, G.; Hehemann, J.-H.; Rao, C.V. Characterization of the GH16 and GH17 laminarinases from *Vibrio breoganii* 1C10. *Appl. Microbiol. Biotechnol.* **2020**, *104*, 161–171. [CrossRef]
26. Boraston, A.B.; Bolam, D.N.; Gilbert, H.J.; Davies, G.J. Carbohydrate-binding modules: Fine-tuning polysaccharide recognition. *Biochem. J.* **2004**, *382*, 769–781. [CrossRef] [PubMed]
27. Fredriksen, L.; Stokke, R.; Jensen, M.S.; Westereng, B.; Jameson, J.-K.; Steen, I.H.; Eijsink, V.G.H.; Stabb, E.V. Discovery of a Thermostable GH10 Xylanase with Broad Substrate Specificity from the Arctic Mid-Ocean Ridge Vent System. *Appl. Environ. Microbiol.* **2019**, *85*, e02970-18. [CrossRef]
28. Leth, M.L.; Ejby, M.; Workman, C.; Ewald, D.A.; Pedersen, S.S.; Sternberg, C.; Bahl, M.I.; Licht, T.R.; Aachmann, F.L.; Westereng, B.; et al. Differential bacterial capture and transport preferences facilitate co-growth on dietary xylan in the human gut. *Nat. Microbiol.* **2018**, *3*, 570–580. [CrossRef]
29. Jumper, J.; Evans, R.; Pritzel, A.; Green, T.; Figurnov, M.; Ronneberger, O.; Tunyasuvunakool, K.; Bates, R.; Žídek, A.; Potapenko, A.; et al. Highly accurate protein structure prediction with AlphaFold. *Nature* **2021**, *596*, 583–589. [CrossRef]
30. Wang, Z.; Robertson, K.L.; Liu, C.; Liu, J.L.; Johnson, B.J.; Leary, D.H.; Compton, J.R.; Vuddhakul, V.; Legler, P.M.; Vora, G.J. A novel *Vibrio* beta-glucosidase (LamN) that hydrolyzes the algal storage polysaccharide laminarin. *FEMS Microbiol. Ecol.* **2015**, *91*, fiv087. [CrossRef]
31. Barral, P.; Suárez, C.; Batanero, E.; Alfonso, C.; Alché, J.d.D.; Rodríguez-García, M.I.; Villalba, M.; Rivas, G.; Rodríguez, R. An olive pollen protein with allergenic activity, Ole e 10, defines a novel family of carbohydrate-binding modules and is potentially implicated in pollen germination. *Biochem. J.* **2005**, *390*, 77–84. [CrossRef] [PubMed]
32. Letunic, I.; Bork, P. Interactive Tree Of Life (iTOL) v5: An online tool for phylogenetic tree display and annotation. *Nucleic Acids Res.* **2021**, *49*, W293–W296. [CrossRef] [PubMed]
33. Park, J.H.; Cho, Y.-J.; Chun, J.; Aeok, Y.-J.; Lee, J.K.; Kim, K.-S.; Lee, K.-H.; Park, S.-J.; Choi, S.H. Complete Genome Sequence of *Vibrio vulnificus* MO6-24/O. *J. Bacteriol.* **2011**, *193*, 2062–2063. [CrossRef] [PubMed]
34. Venditto, I.; Luis, A.S.; Rydahl, M.; Schückel, J.; Fernandes, V.O.; Vidal-Melgosa, S.; Bule, P.; Goyal, A.; Pires, V.M.R.; Dourado, C.G.; et al. Complexity of the *Ruminococcus flavefaciens* cellulosome reflects an expansion in glycan recognition. *Proc. Natl. Acad. Sci. USA* **2016**, *113*, 7136–7141. [CrossRef] [PubMed]
35. Boraston, A.B.; Nurizzo, D.; Notenboom, V.; Ducros, V.; Rose, D.R.; Kilburn, D.G.; Davies, G.J. Differential Oligosaccharide Recognition by Evolutionarily-related β-1,4 and β-1,3 Glucan-binding Modules. *J. Mol. Biol.* **2002**, *319*, 1143–1156. [CrossRef]
36. Van Bueren, A.L.; Morland, C.; Gilbert, H.J.; Boraston, A.B. Family 6 Carbohydrate Binding Modules Recognize the Non-reducing End of β-1,3-Linked Glucans by Presenting a Unique Ligand Binding Surface. *J. Biol. Chem.* **2005**, *280*, 530–537. [CrossRef] [PubMed]
37. Charnock, S.J.; Bolam, D.N.; Turkenburg, J.P.; Gilbert, H.J.; Ferreira, L.M.A.; Davies, G.J.; Fontes, C.M.G.A. The X6 "Thermostabilizing" Domains of Xylanases Are Carbohydrate-Binding Modules: Structure and Biochemistry of the *Clostridium thermocellum* X6b Domain. *Biochemistry* **2000**, *39*, 5013–5021. [CrossRef]
38. Luís, A.S.; Venditto, I.; Temple, M.J.; Rogowski, A.; Baslé, A.; Xue, J.; Knox, J.P.; Prates, J.A.M.; Ferreira, L.M.A.; Fontes, C.M.G.A.; et al. Understanding How Noncatalytic Carbohydrate Binding Modules Can Display Specificity for Xyloglucan. *J. Biol. Chem.* **2013**, *288*, 4799–4809. [CrossRef]
39. Duan, C.-J.; Feng, Y.-L.; Cao, Q.-L.; Huang, M.-Y.; Feng, J.-X. Identification of a novel family of carbohydrate-binding modules with broad ligand specificity. *Sci. Rep.* **2016**, *6*, 19392. [CrossRef]
40. Kumagai, Y.; Okuyama, M.; Kimura, A. Heat treatment of curdlan enhances the enzymatic production of biologically active β-(1,3)-glucan oligosaccharides. *Carbohydr. Polym.* **2016**, *146*, 396–401. [CrossRef]
41. Marchler-Bauer, A.; Bo, Y.; Han, L.; He, J.; Lanczycki, C.J.; Lu, S.; Chitsaz, F.; Derbyshire, M.K.; Geer, R.C.; Gonzales, N.R.; et al. CDD/SPARCLE: Functional classification of proteins via subfamily domain architectures. *Nucleic Acids Res.* **2017**, *45*, D200–D203. [CrossRef] [PubMed]
42. Nielsen, H. Predicting Secretory Proteins with SignalP. In *Protein Function Prediction*, 1st ed.; Kihara, D., Ed.; Methods in Molecular Biology; Springer: Cham, Switzerland, 2017; Volume 1611, pp. 59–73. [CrossRef]

43. Buchan, D.W.A.; Jones, D.T. The PSIPRED Protein Analysis Workbench: 20 years on. *Nucleic Acids Res.* **2019**, *47*, W402–W407. [CrossRef] [PubMed]
44. Kumagai, Y.; Usuki, H.; Yamamoto, Y.; Yamasato, A.; Arima, J.; Mukaihara, T.; Hatanaka, T. Characterization of calcium ion sensitive region for β-Mannanase from *Streptomyces thermolilacinus*. *Biochim. Biophys. Acta-Proteins Proteom.* **2011**, *1814*, 1127–1133. [CrossRef] [PubMed]
45. Gill, S.C.; von Hippel, P.H. Calculation of protein extinction coefficients from amino acid sequence data. *Anal. Biochem.* **1989**, *182*, 319–326. [CrossRef]
46. Waffenschmidt, S.; Jaenicke, L. Assay of reducing sugars in the nanomole range with 2,2′-bicinchoninate. *Anal. Biochem.* **1987**, *165*, 337–340. [CrossRef]
47. Zhang, M.; Chekan, J.R.; Dodd, D.; Hong, P.-Y.; Radlinski, L.; Revindran, V.; Nair, S.K.; Mackie, R.I.; Cann, I. Xylan utilization in human gut commensal bacteria is orchestrated by unique modular organization of polysaccharide-degrading enzymes. *Proc. Natl. Acad. Sci. USA* **2014**, *111*, E3708–E3717. [CrossRef]

marine drugs

Article

Identification and Characterization of Three Chitinases with Potential in Direct Conversion of Crystalline Chitin into N,N′-diacetylchitobiose

Xue-Bing Ren [1], Yan-Ru Dang [1], Sha-Sha Liu [1], Ke-Xuan Huang [1], Qi-Long Qin [1,2], Xiu-Lan Chen [1,3], Yu-Zhong Zhang [1,2,3], Yan-Jun Wang [1,4,*] and Ping-Yi Li [1,*]

1 State Key Laboratory of Microbial Technology, Institute of Marine Science and Technology, Shandong University, Qingdao 266237, China; 201611626@mail.sdu.edu.cn (X.-B.R.); dangyanru@mail.sdu.edu.cn (Y.-R.D.); 202012644@mail.sdu.edu.cn (S.-S.L.); 202112533@mail.sdu.edu.cn (K.-X.H.); qinqilong@sdu.edu.cn (Q.-L.Q.); cxl0423@sdu.edu.cn (X.-L.C.); zhangyz@sdu.edu.cn (Y.-Z.Z.)
2 College of Marine Life Sciences, Frontiers Science Center for Deep Ocean Multispheres and Earth System, Ocean University of China, Qingdao 266003, China
3 Laboratory for Marine Biology and Biotechnology, Pilot National Laboratory for Marine Science and Technology, Qingdao 266237, China
4 Institute of Wetland Agriculture and Ecology, Shandong Academy of Agricultural Sciences, Jinan 250100, China
* Correspondence: wangyanjun1@shandong.cn (Y.-J.W.); lipingyipeace@sdu.edu.cn (P.-Y.L.)

Abstract: Chitooligosaccharides (COSs) have been widely used in agriculture, medicine, cosmetics, and foods, which are commonly prepared from chitin with chitinases. So far, while most COSs are prepared from colloidal chitin, chitinases used in preparing COSs directly from natural crystalline chitin are less reported. Here, we characterize three chitinases, which were identified from the marine bacterium *Pseudoalteromonas flavipulchra* DSM 14401^T, with an ability to degrade crystalline chitin into $(GlcNAc)_2$ (*N,N′*-diacetylchitobiose). Strain DSM 14401 can degrade the crystalline α-chitin in the medium to provide nutrients for growth. Genome and secretome analyses indicate that this strain secretes six chitinolytic enzymes, among which chitinases Chia4287, Chib0431, and Chib0434 have higher abundance than the others, suggesting their importance in crystalline α-chitin degradation. These three chitinases were heterologously expressed, purified, and characterized. They are all active on crystalline α-chitin, with temperature optima of 45–50 °C and pH optima of 7.0–7.5. They are all stable at 40 °C and in the pH range of 5.0–11.0. Moreover, they all have excellent salt tolerance, retaining more than 92% activity after incubation in 5 M NaCl for 10 h at 4 °C. When acting on crystalline α-chitin, the main products of the three chitinases are all $(GlcNAc)_2$, which suggests that chitinases Chia4287, Chib0431, and Chib0434 likely have potential in direct conversion of crystalline chitin into $(GlcNAc)_2$.

Keywords: chitinases; crystalline chitin; chitooligosaccharides; *N,N′*-diacetylchitobiose; *Pseudoalteromonas*

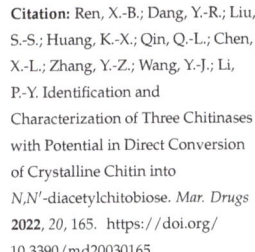

Citation: Ren, X.-B.; Dang, Y.-R.; Liu, S.-S.; Huang, K.-X.; Qin, Q.-L.; Chen, X.-L.; Zhang, Y.-Z.; Wang, Y.-J.; Li, P.-Y. Identification and Characterization of Three Chitinases with Potential in Direct Conversion of Crystalline Chitin into *N,N′*-diacetylchitobiose. *Mar. Drugs* **2022**, *20*, 165. https://doi.org/10.3390/md20030165

Academic Editors: Yuya Kumagai, Hideki Kishimura and Benwei Zhu

Received: 12 January 2022
Accepted: 23 February 2022
Published: 24 February 2022

1. Introduction

Chitin is a polymer of *N*-acetyl-D-glucosamine (GlcNAc) and is the second most abundant polysaccharide after cellulose in nature. Chitin is mainly present in arthropod exoskeletons, fungal cell walls, and insect cuticles in a crystalline form, which is intractable, highly hydrophobic, and insoluble in water [1]. Chitin has three polymorphic isomers, including α-chitin, β-chitin, and γ-chitin. Among them, α-chitin is the most common form found in fungi, insect exoskeletons, and shells of crustaceans. α-chitin is harder to degrade than β-chitin and γ-chitin as it has a higher degree of recalcitrance, which decreases the accessibility of the individual polymer chains [2]. Colloidal chitin is normally prepared by treating natural chitin with strong acids to break the crystal structure and increase the accessibility of the substrate to enzymes. Therefore, colloidal chitin is usually used as the substrate for chitinase characterization.

The annual production of chitin in the ocean exceeds billions of tons [3,4], which is a good source for the production of chitooligosaccharides (COSs) and GlcNAc. Due to their various bioactive activities, COSs and GlcNAc have been widely applied in agriculture, medicine, cosmetics, and foods. For example, COSs have protective effects against infections and enhanced antitumor properties [5,6]. GlcNAc and $(GlcNAc)_2$ (*N,N'*-diacetylchitobiose) can serve as cosmetic ingredients, dietary supplements, and osteoarthritis therapeutics [7–9].

The chitinolytic enzymes contain chitinases (EC 3.2.1.14), mainly from the GH18 and GH19 families, and β-*N*-acetylglucosaminidases (EC 3.2.1.52), mainly from the GH20 and GH3 families. While several β-*N*-acetylglucosaminidases have been reported to be active on chitin [10–12], the hydrolysis of chitin into COSs and/or GlcNAc is predominantly catalyzed by chitinases [13]. Chitinases include endochitinases and exochitinases, which are widely produced by bacteria [14], fungi [15], and plants [16], playing key roles in natural chitin degradation and recycling. Many bacteria-derived chitinases have been characterized, predominantly with colloidal chitin or chitooligosaccharides (or synthetic chitooligosaccharide analogs) as the substrate. Reported bacterial chitinases are mostly mesophilic enzymes with optimal temperatures at 40–60 °C [17–25]; only a few have been found to be cold-active enzymes, such as CHI II of *Glaciozyma antarctica* PI12 (15 °C) [26] and ChiA of *Pseudoalteromonas* sp. DL-6 (20 °C) [27]. The pH optima of bacterial chitinases are over a wide range. For example, chitinases from *Streptomyces chilikensis* RC1830 [24], *Pseudoalteromonas tunicata* CCUG 44952^T [25], and *Bacillus* sp. R2 [21] showed their highest activity at neutral pHs (7.0–7.5), those from *Micrococcus* sp. AG84 [22], *Pseudoalteromonas* sp. DC14 [23], and *Citrobacter freundii* haritD11 [28] at basic pHs (8.0–9.0), and those from *Moritella marina* ATCC 15381 [29] and *Paenicibacillus barengoltzii* CAU904 [17] at acidic pHs (3.5 and 5.0, respectively). Chitinases are good tools to prepare COSs and GlcNAc from chitin. Because the natural source of chitin is crystalline chitin, chitinases that can efficiently hydrolyze crystalline chitin have better application potential in preparing COSs and GlcNAc from natural chitin sources than those only active on colloidal chitin. However, so far, only a few crude enzymes produced by wild strains and recombinant chitinases have been reported to be used in preparing COSs and GlcNAc from crystalline chitin [27,30–33]. Thus, it is necessary to identify and characterize more chitinases that can efficiently hydrolyze crystalline chitin for preparing COSs and GlcNAc from natural chitin sources.

Bacteria of the genus *Pseudoalteromonas* are widely distributed in the ocean, accounting for 2–3% of total bacterial abundance in upper ocean waters [34,35]. Many strains in this genus contain multiple chitinase-encoding genes [36], and some have been reported to secrete chitinases [18,23,25,27,37,38]. Furthermore, some chitinases from *Pseudoalteromonas* have been characterized. The GH18 chitinase Chi23, from *Pseudoalteromonas aurantia* DSM6057, is a thermostable enzyme with activity towards crystalline chitin in acidic conditions (pH 3.0–6.0) [18]. The GH18 chitinases ChiA and ChiC from *Pseudoalteromonas* sp. DL-6 [27,37] and ChiB from *Pseudoalteromonas* sp. O-7 [38] are cold-active enzymes with temperature optima at 20–30 °C. The GH19 chitinase Ptchi19 from *Pseudoalteromonas tunicata* CCUG 44952^T was active at 20–50 °C and pH 6.0–9.5 [25]. The chitinase purified from the fermentation broth of *Pseudoalteromonas* sp. DC14 exhibited halo-alkali and thermo-stable properties [23]. Despite these studies, *Pseudoalteromonas* chitinases with potential in preparing COSs/GlcNAc from natural crystalline chitin have rarely been reported. The aim of this study is to identify and characterize chitinases with activity on crystalline chitin from marine *Pseudoalteromonas* bacteria and to evaluate their potential in preparing COSs/GlcNAc from natural crystalline chitin. In this study, the ability of 26 *Pseudoalteromonas* type strains to use crystalline chitin as a carbon source for growth was investigated, and *Pseudoalteromonas flavipulchra* DSM 14401^T (hereafter strain DSM 14401), which was isolated from surface seawater [39], was found to have the highest degradation rate on crystalline α-chitin. The extracellular chitinases secreted by strain DSM 14401 were further identified by genome and secretome analyses. Three chitinases with high abundance in the secretome were heterologously expressed in *Escherichia coli* BL21 (DE3) and biochemically characterized. The hydrolytic products released from crystalline chitin by these chitinases were further investigated. The results suggest that these chitinases likely have potential in the preparation of $(GlcNAc)_2$ from natural crystalline chitin.

2. Results and Discussion

2.1. The Ability of Strain DSM 14401 to Utilize Crystalline Chitin

To obtain *Pseudoalteromonas* strains that can secrete chitinases to efficiently degrade crystalline chitin, 26 type *Pseudoalteromonas* strains (Table S1) were cultured in a liquid medium containing chitin flakes (crystalline α-chitin) as carbon source, and their growth and the degree of degradation of chitin flakes were observed. Strain DSM 14401 showed the greatest degradation rate of chitin flakes. This strain was able to degrade most of the chitin flakes in the medium in 5 days (Figure 1A). The growth curve and the extracellular chitinase activity of strain DSM 14401 during cultivation were also investigated (Figure 1B). The strain was cultured in a medium containing 0.05% peptone, 0.01% yeast powder, and 3% chitin flakes; the same medium without chitin flakes was used as a control. Strain DSM 14401 grew rapidly in the first 10 h in both media, with or without chitin flakes. After 10 h, the growth stagnated in both media, likely due to the depletion of the absorbable nutrients, such as peptone and yeast powder. After 40 h, while the cell number in the control medium began to decrease slowly and no extracellular chitinase activity was detected during the cultivation, both the cell number and the extracellular chitinase activity in the medium containing chitin flakes began to continuously increase until 68 h (Figure 1B). Based on this result, it can be speculated that, after absorbable nutrients were depleted, strain DSM 14401 began to secrete chitinases to degrade the chitin flakes in the medium into COSs/GlcNAc, which were absorbed by the strain to support its growth.

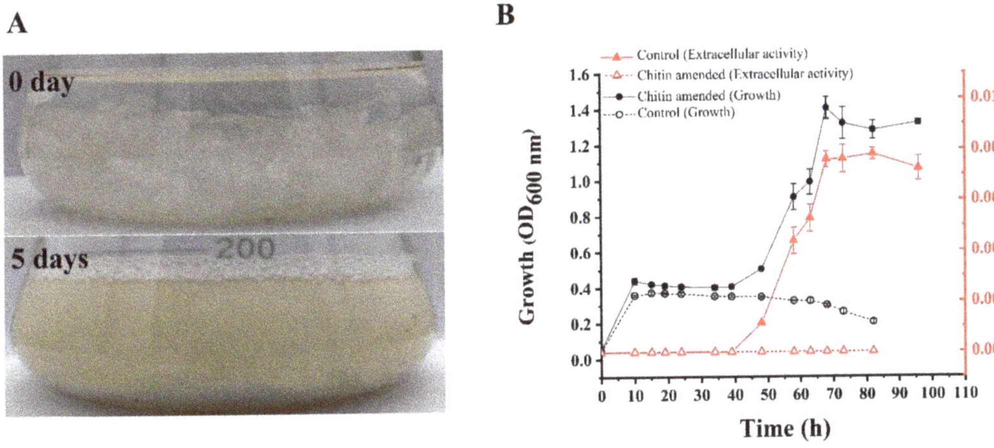

Figure 1. Growth and extracellular chitinase activity of *P. flavipulchra* DSM 14401^T cultured on crystalline chitin. (**A**) Cultures of strain DSM 14401 at 25 °C for 0 and 5 days. (**B**) The growth curve (black line) and the extracellular chitinase activity (red line) of strain DSM 14401. Strain DSM 14401 was cultured in a minimal medium containing 0.05% peptone, 0.01% yeast powder, and 3% (*w*/*v*) chitin flakes at 25 °C and 180 rpm. The extracellular chitinase activity was measured with chitin powder as the substrate at 50 °C. Strain DSM 14401 cultured in the same medium without chitin flakes and under the same conditions was used as the control.

Paulsen et al. reported that 27 *Pseudoalteromonas* strains have the ability to degrade crystalline chitin [36]. Strain *Pseudoalteromonas* sp. DC14 was also reported to be able to degrade crystalline chitin [23]. In addition, 5 chitinases from *Pseudoalteromonas* strains have been expressed and characterized, including ChiA and ChiC from *Pseudoalteromonas* sp. DL-6 [27,37], ChiB from *Pseudoalteromonas* sp. O-7 [38], PtChi19p from *P. tunicata* CCUG 44952^T [25] and Chi23 from *P. aurantia* DSM6057 [18]. Among them, chitinases ChiA, PtChi19p, and Chi23 have activity on crystalline chitin based on substrate specificity analysis [18,25,27]. These reports indicate that many *Pseudoalteromonas* strains can produce chitinases with activity on crystalline chitin. Consistently, strain DSM 14401 was most likely to secrete chitinases with activity on crystalline chitin due to its high degradation rate on crystalline α-chitin.

2.2. Identification of the Chitinases Secreted by Strain DSM 14401

To ascertain the chitinolytic enzymes secreted by strain DSM 14401, genomic analysis was carried out to find putative chitinolytic enzyme-encoding genes in strain DSM 14401. There are 11 genes encoding putative chitinolytic enzymes in strain DSM 14401, which were named Chia2822, Chib0431, Chib0434, Chia4287, Chib0889, Chib0721, Chia2290, Chia3704, Chib0633, Chib0719 and Chib0710. Chia2822, Chib0431, Chib0434, and Chia4287 are potential chitinases belonging to the GH18 family (Figure 2). Of these, Chib0431, Chib0434, and Chia4287 belong to the GH18A subfamily that mainly contains processive exochitinases [40–42], and Chia2822 belongs to the GH18B subfamily that mainly contains non-processive endochitinases [43,44]. Multiple sequence alignments suggest that all these GH18 chitinases of strain DSM 14401 contain a DxDxE catalytic motif (Figure S1), which is conserved in the GH18 chitinases [45]. Chitinase Chib0889 belongs to the GH19 family that mainly contains chitinases found in plants [46]. Two GH19 chitinases, LYS177 and LYS188, from *Pseudomonas* Ef1 have been reported to have lysozyme activity and they are clustered with phage/prophage endolysins based on the phylogenetic analysis [47]. However, the GH19 chitinase, Chib0889, of strain DSM 14401 was nested in the cluster of chitinases from Proteobacteria (Figure S2), implying that Chib0889 may function as a chitinase rather than a lysozyme. Chib0721, Chia2290, Chia3704, Chib0633, and Chib0719 from the GH20 family, and Chib0710 from the GH3 family are potential β-*N*-acetylglucosaminidases. The predicted domain architectures of these chitinolytic enzymes are shown in Figure 3. Except for Chib0710, the other chitinolytic enzymes all have a signal peptide predicted by SignalP 5.0, implying that they are likely secreted enzymes. Among these enzymes, Chib0633 and Chib0710 are single-domain enzymes, while the others are all multi-domain enzymes containing one or more carbohydrate-binding domains (Big_7, CBM_5_12, and CHB_HEX) in addition to their catalytic domains. The CBMs (carbohydrate-binding modules) in chitinases were reported to facilitate enzyme movement along a chitin chain during processive action and to stimulate the substrate to decrystallize [48–51].

Secretome analysis was further performed to identify the chitinolytic enzymes secreted by strain DSM 14401 cultured in the medium containing 3% chitin flakes as the sole carbon source. The extracellular proteins tightly absorbed on the chitin flakes were collected for secretome analysis when approximately half of the chitin flakes in the medium were degraded after 85 h. Finally, 6 of the putative chitinolytic enzymes were detected in the secretome. Of these, the 4 GH18 chitinases accounted for 97.50% of the abundance, and the GH19 and GH20 chitinolytic enzymes each accounted for 1.25% (Table 1), which suggests the importance of the GH18 chitinases in the degradation of crystalline chitin. Of the GH18 chitinases, Chia4287 was the most abundant (48.75%), followed by Chib0431 (25.00%), Chib0434 (15.00%) and Chia2822 (8.75%). The five putative β-*N*-acetylglucosaminidases with a predicted signal peptide were not found in the secretome, which may be secreted to the periplasm.

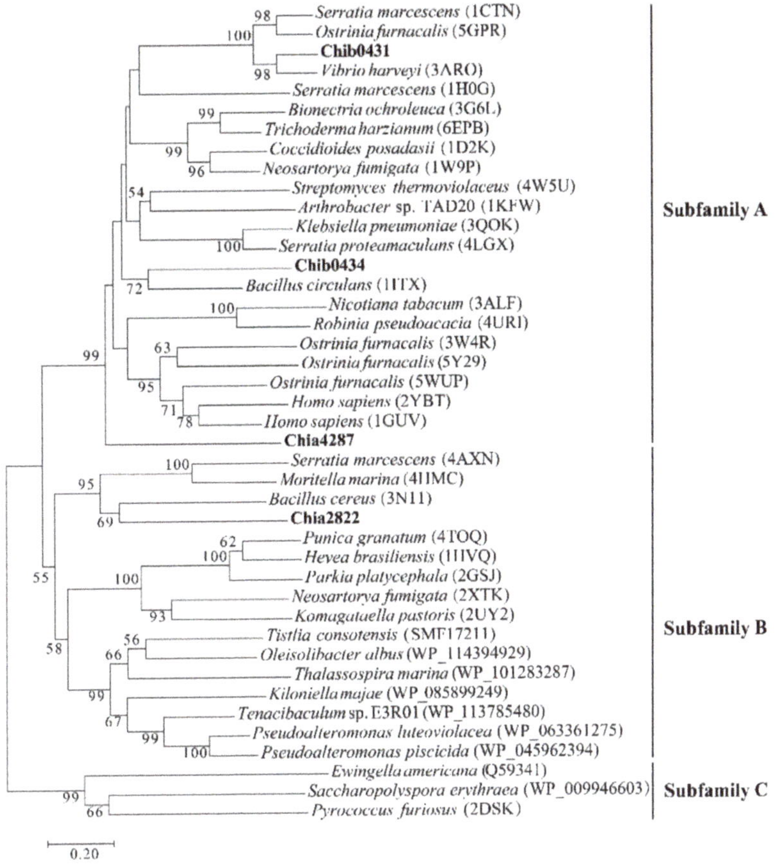

Figure 2. Phylogenetic analysis of chitinases Chib0431, Chib0434, Chia4287, and Chia2822 with other GH18 chitinases. The phylogenetic tree was constructed by the Neighbor-Joining method. Bootstrap analysis of 1000 replicates was conducted.

Table 1. The extracellular chitinolytic enzymes secreted by strain DSM 14401 identified by secretome analysis.

Chitinolytic Enzyme	Accession Number	Family	Length (aa)	Molecular Weight (kDa)	PSMs [a]	Abundance [b]
Chia4287	WP_039494805	GH18	479	50.86	39	48.75%
Chib0431	WP_039495329	GH18	822	87.51	20	25.00%
Chib0434	WP_039495331	GH18	1037	112.17	12	15.00%
Chia2822	WP_039492151	GH18	850	90.42	7	8.75%
Chib0889	WP_084204324	GH19	470	53.05	1	1.25%
Chib0721	WP_039496328	GH20	915	101.45	1	1.25%

[a] Peptide-Spectrum Matches. [b] Abundance was calculated based on the proportion of the PSMs of a chitinolytic enzyme in the sum of PSMs of all chitinolytic enzymes in the secretome.

It has been reported that chitinolytic strains belonging to the genus *Pseudoalteromonas* usually have two GH18 chitinase genes in their chitin degradation clusters [36]. In addition, many *Pseudoalteromonas* species also contain one or more GH19 chitinase genes [36]. However, the removal of the GH19 chitinase gene from strain *Pseudoalteromonas rubra* S4059 had no significant influence on the growth of the strain on crystalline α-chitin [52], suggesting that the GH19 chitinase is likely unimportant in the utilization of crystalline chitin. In contrast, the removal of the GH18 chitinase gene *chiD* from strain *Cellvibrio japonicus* Ueda107 made it unable to grow on crystalline α-chitin [53], indicating that the GH18 chitinase plays an important role in the crystalline chitin degradation of this strain. Moreover, it has been reported that $(GlcNAc)_2$ and larger chitooligosaccharides can induce the expression of chitinases in *Vibrio furnissii* 7225 and *Vibrio cholerae* O1 [54]. For strain DSM 14401, although its genome contains a GH19 chitinase gene, a GH3 β-*N*-acetylglucosaminidase gene, and 5 GH20 β-*N*-acetylglucosaminidase genes in addition to 4 GH18 chitinase genes, secretome analysis showed that it mainly secreted the GH18 chitinases when crystalline α-chitin was present, which suggests that the GH18 chitinases likely play a main role in the degradation of crystalline α-chitin in this strain.

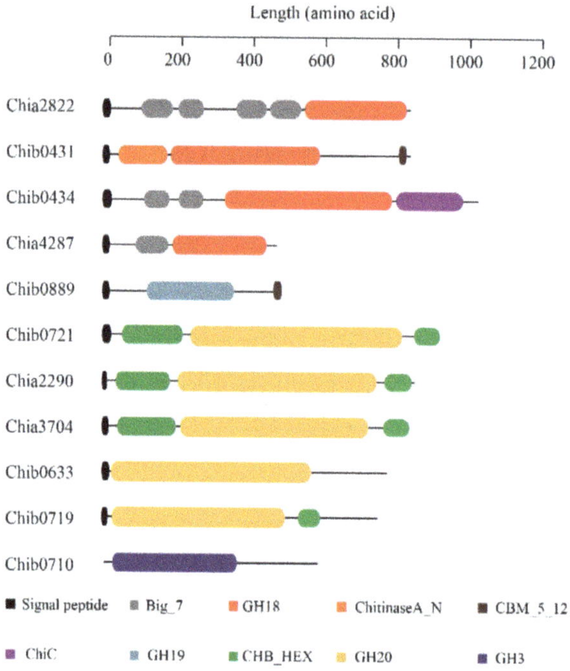

Figure 3. Domain architecture of the 11 chitinolytic enzymes of *P. flavipulchra* DSM 14401^T. Protein sequences were analyzed on the HMMER website, and domains were illustrated by different colors based on their functional annotations. The Pfam IDs corresponding to the function annotations are as follows: Big_7, bacterial Ig domain (PF17957); GH18, glycosyl hydrolases family 18 (PF00704); ChitinaseA_N, ChitinaseA_N-terminal domain (PF08329); CBM_5_12, carbohydrate-binding module (PF02839), ChiC, Chitinase C (PF06483); GH19, glycoside hydrolase family 19 (PF00182), CHB_HEX, putative carbohydrate-binding domain (PF03173); GH20, glycosyl hydrolase family 20 (PF00728); GH3, glycosyl hydrolase family 3 (PF00933).

2.3. *Characterization of the GH18 Chitinases with Activity on Crystalline Chitin*

The high abundance of the GH18 chitinases in the secretome of strain DSM 14401 implies that they are likely to be the chitinases with activity on crystalline chitin. Thus, 3 GH18 chitinases, Chia4287, Chib0431, and Chib0434, with high abundance in the secretome, were selected to be expressed and characterized. Genes encoding Chia4287, Chib0431, and Chib0434 were heterologously expressed in *E. coli* BL21 (DE3), and the recombinant proteins were purified by NTA-Ni Sepharose affinity chromatography (Figure 4). The purification folds for Chib0431, Chib0434 and Chia4287 were 6.75, 5.33, and 7.30, respectively (Table S2). As shown in Figure 4, the 3 purified recombinant proteins have apparent molecular weights of approximately 88 kDa (Chib0431), 112 kDa (Chib0434), and 51 kDa (Chia4287), consistent with their theoretical molecular weights (Table 1).

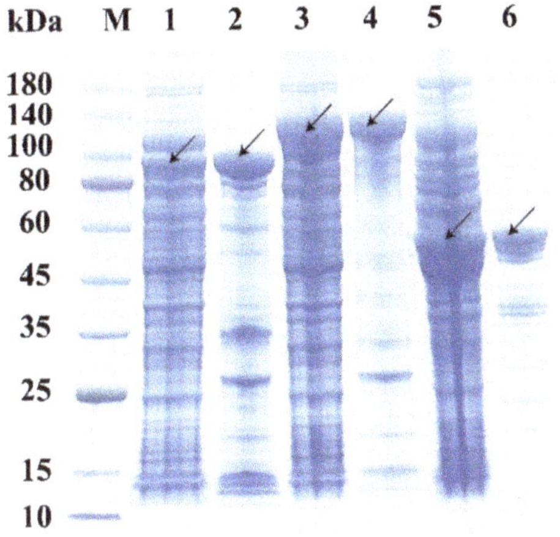

Figure 4. The SDS-PAGE analysis of recombinant proteins Chib0431, Chib0434, and Chia4287. Lane M, protein molecular mass marker; Lane 1, the cell lysate of *E. coli* containing recombinant protein Chib0431; Lane 2, the purified recombinant protein Chib0431; Lane 3, the cell lysate of *E. coli* containing recombinant protein Chib0434; Lane 4, the purified recombinant protein Chib0434; Lane 5, the cell lysate of *E. coli* containing recombinant protein Chia4287; Lane 6, the purified recombinant protein Chia4287. The enzyme bands are indicated by arrows.

To investigate the substrate specificity of these 3 chitinases, the enzyme activities of Chib0431, Chib0434, and Chia4287 toward colloidal chitin, chitin powder, chitosan, microcrystalline cellulose, 4-Methylumbelliferyl *N*-acetyl-β-D-glucosaminide (MUF-GlcNAc) [55], 4-Methylumbelliferyl-β-D-*N*,*N*′-diacetylchitobioside hydrate (MUF-$(GlcNAc)_2$) [56], and 4-Methylumbelliferyl-β-D-*N*,*N*′,*N*″-triacetylchitotrioside (MUF-$(GlcNAc)_3$) [57] were determined. As shown in Table 2, all the three chitinases had activity toward colloidal chitin, crystalline chitin, MUF-$(GlcNAc)_2$, and MUF-$(GlcNAc)_3$, but neither had activity toward chitosan, microcrystalline cellulose, or MUF-GlcNAc. Among them, Chia4287 had the highest activity towards chitin powder, followed by Chib0431 and Chib0434, which is consistent with their amount in the secretome. Chitinases Chia4287 and Chib0431 exhibited higher activities toward MUF-$(GlcNAc)_3$ than MUF-$(GlcNAc)_2$, suggesting that both enzymes likely function as endochitinases. In contrast, Chib0434 showed approximately 10-fold higher activity toward MUF-$(GlcNAc)_2$ than MUF-$(GlcNAc)_3$, suggesting that Chib0434 tends to act as an exochitinase.

With chitin powder as the substrate, the three chitinases were biochemically characterized. Both chitinases Chib0431 and Chia4287 showed optimum temperatures at 50 °C, and Chib0434 at 45 °C (Figure 5A). For their thermal stability, Chib0431 retained approximately 100% activity at 40 °C and more than 61% at 50 °C after 120 min incubation but lost all its activity at 60 °C in 15 min (Figure 5B). Chib0434 retained 100% activity at 40 °C after 120 min incubation but lost all its activity at 50 °C in 90 min and at 60 °C in 30 min (Figure 5C). Chitinase Chia4287 retained high activity (≥89%) when incubated at 40 °C for 120 min (Figure 5D). Chitinases Chib0434 and Chia4287 both showed highest activity at pH 7.5 and Chib0431 at pH 7.0 (Figure 6A). For their pH stability, the 3 chitinases all exhibited high stability (retaining ≥80% activity) from pH 5.0 to 11.0 in the Britton–Robinson buffer after 10 h incubation at 4 °C (Figure 6B). They all showed highest activity at 0 M NaCl (Figure 6C) but maintained high activity (≥92%) in 1–5 M NaCl after 10 h incubation at 4 °C (Figure 6D). Therefore, the 3 chitinases have temperature optima of 45–50 °C and pH optima of 7.0–7.5, indicating that they are all neutral and mesophilic enzymes. They are all stable at 40 °C and in the pH range of 5.0–11.0, and all have excellent salt tolerance.

Table 2. The substrate specificity of the three chitinases of strain DSM 14401 [a].

Substrate	Specific Activity (U/mg)		
	Chia4287	Chib0431	Chib0434
Colloidal chitin	0.53 ± 0.05	0.15 ± 0.04	0.09 ± 0.02
Chitin powder	0.17 ± 0.005	0.04 ± 0.002	0.01 ± 0.001
Chitosan	ND [b]	ND	ND
Microcrystalline cellulose	ND	ND	ND
MUF-GlcNAc	ND	ND	ND
MUF-(GlcNAc)$_2$	130.32 ± 3.29	19.69 ± 1.30	221.68 ± 12.15
MUF-(GlcNAc)$_3$	139.33 ± 26.96	423.12 ± 9.82	23.47 ± 3.57

[a] The data in the table are from three experiment repeats (mean ± SD). [b] ND means that the enzyme activity was not detectable.

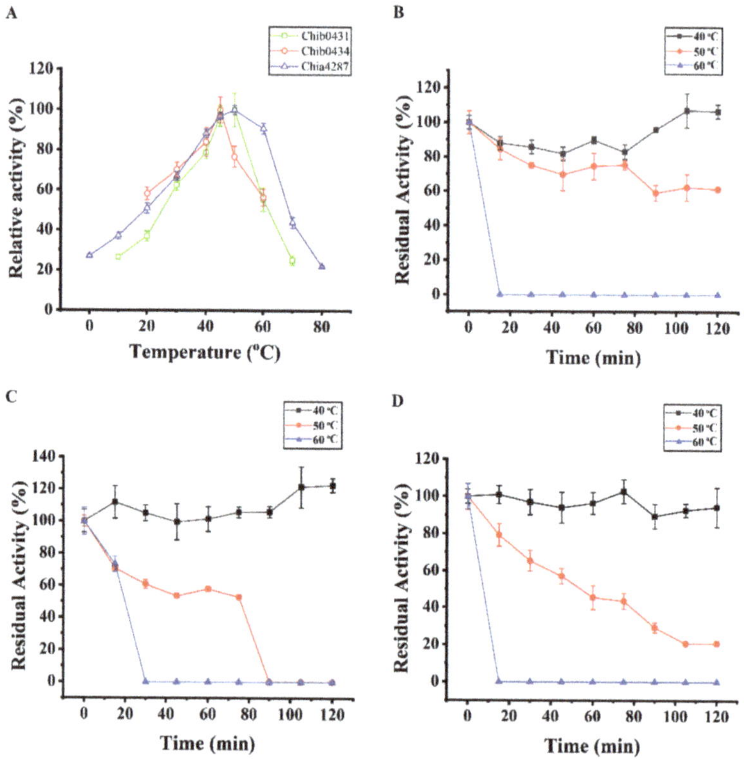

Figure 5. Effect of temperature on the activities and stabilities of chitinases Chib0431, Chib0434, and Chia4287. (**A**) Effect of temperature on the activities of Chib0431, Chib0434, and Chia4287. The activities of each enzyme were measured at its optimal pH with chitin powder as the substrate. The highest activity of each enzyme was defined as 100%. (**B**) Effect of temperature on the stability of Chib0431. (**C**) Effect of temperature on the stability of Chib0434. (**D**) Effect of temperature on the stability of Chia4287. In B, C, and D, the residual activities of each enzyme were measured at its optimal temperature and pH with chitin powder as the substrate, and the activity of each enzyme without incubation was defined as 100%. The graphs show data from triplicate experiments (mean ± SD).

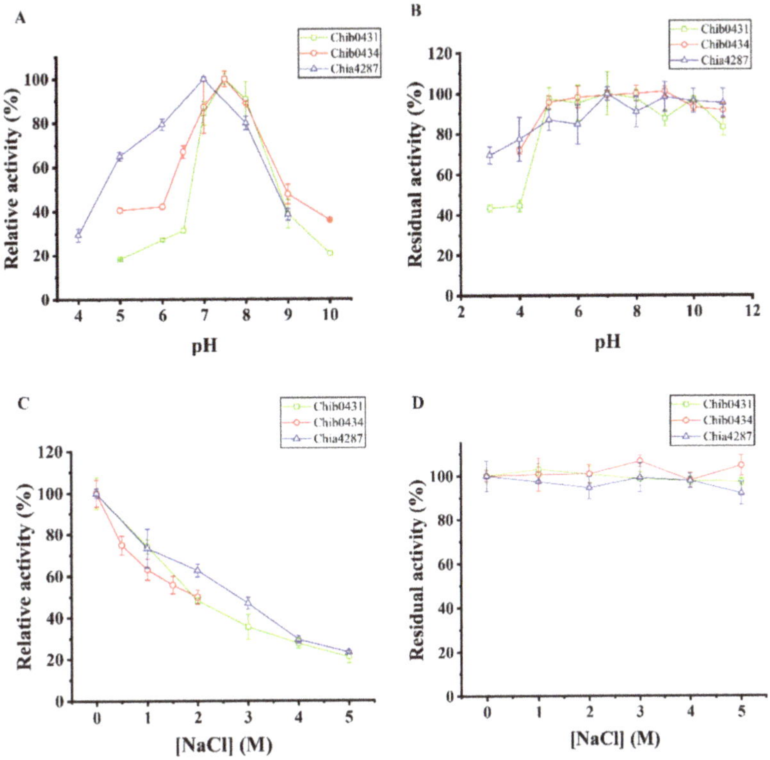

Figure 6. Effects of pH and NaCl on the activities and stabilities of chitinases Chib0431, Chib0434, and Chia4287. (**A**) Effect of pH on the activities of Chib0431, Chib0434, and Chia4287. The activities of each enzyme were measured at its optimal temperature with chitin powder as the substrate. The highest activity of each enzyme was defined as 100%. (**B**) Effect of pH on the stabilities of Chib0431, Chib0434, and Chia4287. The residual activities of each enzyme were measured at its optimal temperature and pH with chitin powder as the substrate. (**C**) Effect of NaCl concentration on the activities of Chib0431, Chib0434, and Chia4287. The activities of each enzyme were measured at its optimal temperature and pH with chitin powder as the substrate. The activity of each enzyme in 0 M NaCl was defined as 100%. (**D**) Effect of NaCl concentration on the stabilities of Chib0431, Chib0434, and Chia4287. The residual activities of each enzyme were measured at its optimal temperature and pH with chitin powder as the substrate. The highest activity of each enzyme was defined as 100%. The graphs show data from triplicate experiments (mean ± SD).

Many chitinases have been heterologously expressed and characterized with colloidal chitin or synthetic chitooligosaccharide analogs. As shown in Table 3, the temperature and pH optima of the reported chitinases and their thermostability are quite diverse. So far, several *Pseudoalteromonas* GH18 chitinases have been characterized (Table 3). The chitinase Chi23 from *P. aurantia* DSM6057 was reported to be thermostable but active toward crystalline chitin only in acidic conditions (pH of 3.0–6.0) [18]. Chitinases ChiA and ChiC from *Pseudoalteromonas* sp. DL-6 [27,37] and ChiB from *Pseudoalteromonas* sp. O-7 [38] are all cold-active enzymes with optimal activities at 20–30 °C and low thermostability. The 3 mesophilic chitinases, Chib0431, Chib0434, and Chia4287, characterized in this study are active toward crystalline chitin at neutral pH conditions (pH 7.0–7.5) and have good thermostability and pH- and salt-tolerance, which, therefore, may be good candidates for industrial application.

Table 3. Characteristics of bacterial chitinases.

Enzyme	Family	Molecular Weight (kDa)	pH Optimum	Temperature Optimum (°C)	NaCl Optimum (M)	Thermostability (Half-Life)	Substrate (Specific Activity)	Hydrolytic Products (Substrate)	References
Chib0431 from *Pseudoalteromonas flavipulchra* DSM 14401^T	GH18	87.51	7.5	50	0	>2 h at 50 °C	α-chitin (0.04 ± 0.002 U/mg)	GlcNAc and $(GlcNAc)_2$ (α-chitin)	This study
Chib0434 from *Pseudoalteromonas flavipulchra* DSM 14401^T	GH18	112.17	7.5	45	0	~80 min at 50 °C	α-chitin (0.01 ± 0.001 U/mg)	GlcNAc and $(GlcNAc)_2$ (α-chitin)	This study
Chia4287 from *Pseudoalteromonas flavipulchra* DSM 14401^T	GH18	50.86	7.0	50	0	<60 min at 50 °C	α-chitin (0.17 ± 0.005 U/mg)	GlcNAc and $(GlcNAc)_2$ (α-chitin)	This study
CHI II from *Glaciozyma antarctica* PI12	GH18	39 and 50	4.0	15	-	<30 min at 30 °C	Colloidal chitin (-)	-	[26]
MmChi60 from *Moritella marina*	GH18	60.8	5.0	28	-	~5 h at 50 °C	Colloidal chitin (0.016 U/mg)	-	[29]
ChiA from *Pseudoalteromonas* sp. DL-6	GH18	113.5	8.0	20	-	~1 h at 40 °C	α-chitin (0.128 ± 0.001 U/mL)	$(GlcNAc)_2$ (α-chitin)	[27]
ChiC from *Pseudoalteromonas* sp. DL-6	GH18	91	9.0	30	2	~1 h at 50 °C	α-chitin (4.8 ± 0.2 U/mg)	$(GlcNAc)_2$ (colloidal chitin)	[37]
Chi23 from *Pseudoalteromonas aurantia* DSM6057	GH18	30.4	5.0	60	3	~40 min at 70 °C	Crystalline Chitin (0.1 ± 0.01 U/mg)	$(GlcNAc)_2$ and $GlcNAc)_3$ (α-chitin)	[18]
ChiB from *Pseudoalteromonas* sp. O-7	GH18	90.2	6.0	30	-	-	pNP-$(GlcNAc)_2$ (30.8 U/mg)	-	[38]
ScChiC from *Streptomyces coelicolor* A3(2)	GH18	-	5	55	-	~1 h at 60 °C	$(GlcNAc)_6$ (4120 ± 80 U/mg)	$(GlcNAc)_2$ (crab shell chitin)	[19]
StmChiA from *Stenotrophomonas maltophilia*	GH18	70.5	5.0	40	-	>90% of initial activity at 30–50 °C (up to 1 h)	$(GlcNAc)_6$ (-)	GlcNAc and $(GlcNAc)_2$ (α-chitin)	[20]
StmChiB from *Stenotrophomonas maltophilia*	GH18	41.6	7.0	40	-	>90% of initial activity at 30–50 °C (up to 1 h)	$(GlcNAc)_6$ (-)	-	[20]

Table 3. *Cont.*

Enzyme	Family	Molecular Weight (kDa)	pH Optimum	Temperature Optimum (°C)	NaCl Optimum (M)	Thermostability (Half-Life)	Substrate (Specific Activity)	Hydrolytic Products (Substrate)	References
PbChi67 from *Paenicibacillus barengoltzii* CAU904	-	67.9	3.5	60	-	43 min at 65 °C	α-chitin (0.3 ± 0.04 U/mg)	$(GlcNAc)_2$, $(GlcNAc)_3$ and$(GlcNAc)_4$ (colloidal chitin)	[17]
A chitinase from *Bacillus* sp. R2	-	41.69	7.5	40	-	>30 min at 50 °C	Colloidal chitin (-)	-	[21]
A chitinase from *Citrobacter freundii* haritD11	-	64	8.0	35	-	~1 h at 60 °C	Colloidal chitin (140.55 U/mg)	-	[28]
A chitinase from *Micrococcus* sp. AG84	-	33	8.0	40	-	>1 h at 80 °C	Colloidal chitin (93.02 U/mg)	-	[22]
A chitinase from *Pseudoalteromonas* sp. DC14	-	65	9.0	40	10% (*w*/*v*)	>30 min at 60 °C	Colloidal chitin (5.6 U/mg)	-	[23]
A chitinase from *Streptomyces chilikensis* RC1830	-	10.5	7.0	60	-	-	Colloidal chitin (60.53 U/mg)	-	[24]
PtChi19 from *Pseudoalteromonas tunicata* CCUG 44952^T	GH19	53.5	7.5	45	2	>40 min at 50 °C	Crystalline Chitin (16.4 mU/ mg)	-	[25]

- Not available.

2.4. Analysis of the Products of the Chitinases on Crystalline Chitin

In order to investigate the application potential of the three chitinases in preparing COSs/GlcNAc from natural chitin, we analyzed the degradation products of Chia4287, Chib0431, and Chib0434 towards crystalline chitin. The reaction mixtures, containing chitin powder and chitinases, were incubated at their respective optimal temperatures for different time periods (15 min, 30 min, 1 h, and 3 h). The COSs/GlcNAc released from chitin in the supernatants of the mixtures were analyzed by gel filtration chromatography on a Superdex Peptide 10/300 GL column. For Chib0431 and Chib0434, during the 3 h degradation of crystalline chitin, $(GlcNAc)_2$ was always the predominant product, with only a slight amount of GlcNAc (Figure 7A,B). However, in the hydrolytic products of Chia4287 on crystalline chitin, although $(GlcNAc)_2$ was also the main product, the proportion of GlcNAc was much higher compared to that in the hydrolytic products of Chib0431 and Chib0434 (Figure 7C). Together, these results indicate that Chia4287, Chib0431, and Chib0434 can degrade crystalline chitin into $(GlcNAc)_2$ and GlcNAc, with $(GlcNAc)_2$ as the main product. These results imply that they may have potential in the preparation of $(GlcNAc)_2$ from natural crystalline chitin.

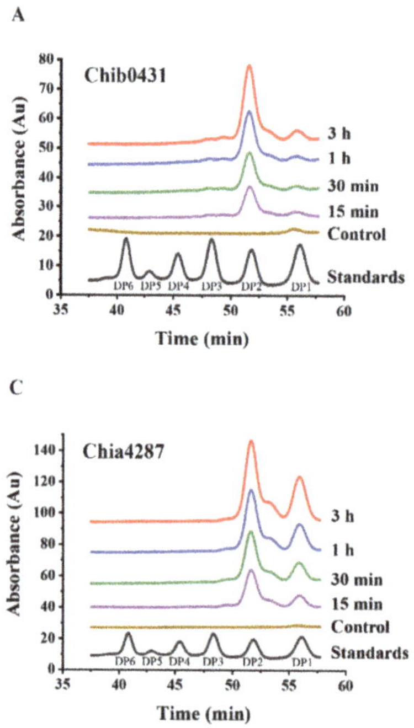

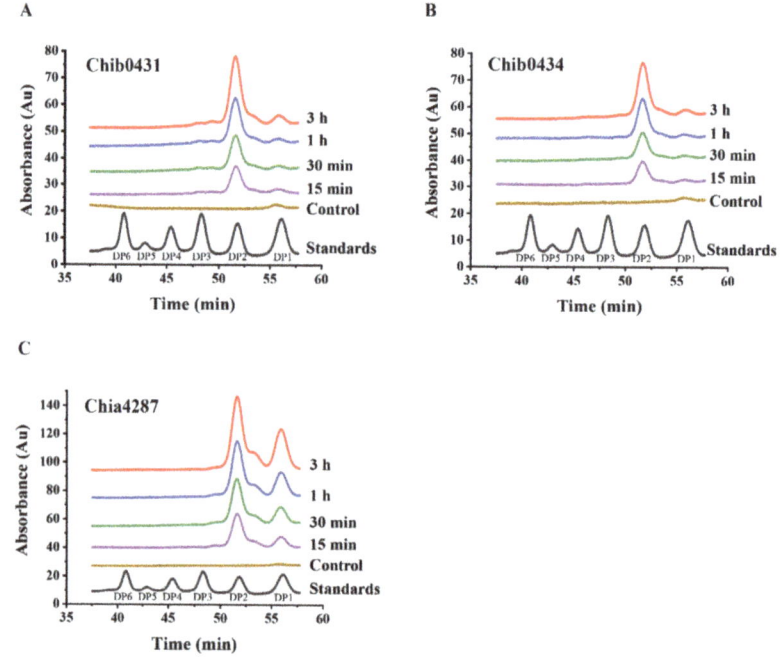

Figure 7. Analysis of the degradation products of the three chitinases on crystalline chitin. (**A**) The degradation product of Chib0431. (**B**) The degradation product of Chib0434. (**C**) The degradation product of Chia4287. Chitin powder was degraded by the chitinases at their respective optimal temperatures for different times (15 min, 30 min, 1 h, and 3 h). The reaction system with enzyme inactivated at 100 °C for 10 min was used as the control. The reaction was terminated by boiling at 100 °C for 10 min, and then the reaction mixtures were centrifuged at 17,949× *g* for 10 min. The products in the supernatants were analyzed by gel filtration chromatography on a Superdex Peptide10/300 GL column (GE Healthcare, Sweden), which were monitored at a wavelength of 210 nm. The injected volume was 10 µL. DP1-DP6 are chitooligosaccharide markers. DP1, GlcNAc; DP2, $(GlcNAc)_2$; DP3, $(GlcNAc)_3$; DP4, $(GlcNAc)_4$; DP5, $(GlcNAc)_5$; DP6, $(GlcNAc)_6$.

COSs/GlcNAc have been widely prepared with a variety of crude enzymes from wild strains and purified recombinant chitinases, most of which were prepared with colloidal chitin [17,58–61]. So far, however, there have been only a few chitinases used to prepare COSs/GlcNAc from natural crystalline chitin. The enzyme cocktail of strain *Paenibacillus* sp. LS1 can produce GlcNAc and $(GlcNAc)_2$ with minor $(GlcNAc)_3$ from crystalline α-chitin [30]. The crude enzyme of *Aeromonas hydrophila* H-2330 mainly produces GlcNAc from crystalline α-chitin [31]. The chitinase ChiA of strain *Pseudoalteromonas* sp. DL-6 is an endochitinase, and its products on crystalline α-chitin are a mixture of chitin COSs (DP 2–6), with $(GlcNAc)_2$ as the major product [27]. The mixture of purified chitinases SaChiB and SaHEX of strain *Streptomyces alfalfa* ACCC40021 can enhance the conversion of crystalline α-chitin to GlcNAc [62]. The chitinase of strain *Chitinibacter* sp. GC72 can degrade practical-grade chitin into GlcNAc [33]. The three chitinases characterized in this study can degrade crystalline α-chitin into $(GlcNAc)_2$, suggesting their potential in direct conversion of natural crystalline chitin into $(GlcNAc)_2$.

3. Materials and Methods

3.1. Bacterial Strains and Experimental Materials

The 26 type strains of genus *Pseudoalteromonas* were purchased from Deutsche Sammlung von Mikroorganismen and Zelkulturen (DSMZ) or Japan Collection of Microorganisms (JCM). Chitin powder (crystalline α-chitin), MUF-GlcNAc, MUF-$(GlcNAc)_2$, and MUF-$(GlcNAc)_3$ were purchased from Sigma-Aldrich (St. Louis, MO, USA). Chitin flakes, purchased from Yuan Cheng Group (Wuhan, China), are crystalline α-chitin. Colloidal chitin was prepared as previously described [18]. GlcNAc, $(GlcNAc)_2$, $(GlcNAc)_3$, $(GlcNAc)_4$, $(GlcNAc)_5$, and $(GlcNAc)_6$ were purchased from BZ Oligo Biotech Co., LTD (Qingdao, China). Chitosan was purchased from Sangon Biotech (Shanghai, China). BCA protein assay kit was purchased from Thermo Scientific (Boston, MA, USA). Other chemicals were of analytical grade and commercially available.

3.2. Screening of Strain DSM 14401

The 26 type strains of genus *Pseudoalteromonas* (Table S1) were cultivated at 25 °C and 180 rpm in the TYS medium composed of 0.5% (*w*/*v*) peptone, 0.1% (*w*/*v*) yeast powder, and artificial seawater (pH 7.8). When the OD_{600} of the culture was approximately 1.0, 2 mL cell suspension was collected and the cells were washed with the minimal medium (30 g/L NaCl, 0.5 g/L NH_4Cl, 3 g/L $MgCl_2{\cdot}6H_2O$, 2 g/L K_2SO_4, 0.2 g/L K_2HPO_4, 0.01 g/L $CaCl_2$, 0.006 g/L $FeCl_3{\cdot}6H_2O$, 0.005 g/L $Na_2MoO_4{\cdot}7H_2O$, 0.004 g/L $CuCl_2{\cdot}2H_2O$, 6 g/L Tris, pH 7.6) three times. Then, the washed cells were inoculated into the minimal medium supplemented with 0.05% (*w*/*v*) peptone, 0.01% (*w*/*v*) yeast powder, and 3% (*w*/*v*) chitin flakes and cultivated at 25 °C and 180 rpm for 5 days. Their growth and the degree of degradation of the chitin flakes were observed every day. Among them, strain DSM 14401 showed the highest degradation rate on crystalline α-chitin, which was then chosen for further study. The OD_{600} of the culture of this strain in the medium was measured at different time intervals, as indicated in Figure 1, to produce its growth curve. The washed cells were cultured in the same medium without chitin flakes and in the same conditions as the control.

3.3. Extracellular Chitinase Activity Assay of Strain DSM 14401

During the cultivation of strain DSM 14401 in the above liquid medium with or without chitin flakes, 1 mL of culture was taken out at different intervals, as indicated in Figure 1. The cultures were filtered with a 0.22 μm filter to remove the bacterial cells, and the filtrate was used for the extracellular chitinase activity assay. A 200 μL mixture consisting of 50 mM Tris-HCl (pH 7.0), 3% chitin powder, and 50 μL of filtrate was incubated at 50 °C for 2 h. The mixture was then centrifuged at 17,949× *g* for 2 min at 4 °C and the supernatant obtained was used for the reducing-sugar assay by the DNS method [63]. The control mixture contained a pre-boiled filtrate instead of the filtrate. Subsequently, the optical density at 550 nm was measured to quantify the released reducing sugar. The amount of reducing sugar generated was calculated using GlcNAc as a standard. One unit of enzyme activity was defined as the amount of enzyme that liberated 1 μmol of reducing sugar per minute.

3.4. Bioinformatics Analysis

The genome DNA of strain DSM 14401 was sequenced by our lab [64]. The putative chitinases of this strain were determined according to dbCAN [65] analyses. Signal peptides of the chitinases were predicted by SignalP 5.0 (http://www.cbs.dtu.dk/services/SignalP/ (accessed on 12 January 2022)) [66]. The domain architectures of the chitinases were predicted on the HMMER website (https://www.ebi.ac.uk/Tools/hmmer/search/hmmscan (accessed on 12 January 2022)) [67]. The phylogenetic tree was constructed based on the Neighbor-Joining method and using the Poisson model with MEGA X after multiple alignments of the sequences by MUCLE [68]. Sequences alignment results were visualized using the ESPript 3.0 server [69]. The molecular weights of the chitinases were predicted by the ExPASy Server (https://web.expasy.org/compute_pi/ (accessed on 12 January 2022)) [70].

3.5. Secretome Analysis

Strain DSM 14401 was cultured at 25 °C and 180 rpm in a medium containing the minimal medium and 3% chitin flakes. When approximately half of the chitin flakes were degraded, the culture was centrifuged at 8228× *g* at 4 °C for 6 min. The precipitates were resuspended using 20 mM Tris-HCl (pH 8.0) containing 1 M NaCl, and then centrifuged at 1157× *g* at 4 °C for 3 min. This step was repeated three times. The resultant precipitates were resuspended using 50 mM Tris-HCl (pH 8.0) containing 6 M Guanadine-HCl, and then centrifuged at 15,557× *g* at 4 °C for 10 min. The supernatant was moved into an ultrafiltration tube (15 mL, 3 kDa). The Guanadine-HCl in the supernatant was removed by adding 50 mM Tris-HCl to the ultrafiltration tube (molecular weight cut-off, 3 kDa) and centrifugation (4629× *g* for 10 min at 4 °C) for three times. Then, the proteins in the supernatant were precipitated by 50 mL acetone containing 10% trichloroacetic acid and 0.1% dithiothreitol overnight at −20 °C. The precipitates were harvested and washed by 80% acetone and 100% acetone successively, and then lyophilized. The lyophilized sample was successively denatured, reduced, and alkylated by denaturation buffer (0.5 M Tris-HCl, 2.75 mM EDTA, 6 M Guanadine-HCl), dithiothreitol (1 M), and iodoacetamide (1 M), respectively. The sample solution was further replaced with 25 mM NH_4HCO_3 solution by centrifugation ultrafiltration (15,294× *g* for 15 min at 4 °C) in an ultrafiltration tube (1 mL, 3 kDa). The sample was digested using trypsin at 37 °C for 12 h, and the resultant peptides were desalted on a C_{18} column (ZipTip C18, Millipore, Billerica, MA, USA). The desalted peptides were analyzed using the mass spectrometer Orbitrap Elite (Thermo Fisher Scientific, Bremen, Germany) coupled with Easy-nLC 1000 (Thermo Fisher Scientific, Bremen, Germany). Finally, the raw data was analyzed against the genome of strain DSM 14401 using Thermo Scientific Proteome Discoverer™ 1.4. The mass spectrometry proteomics data have been deposited to the ProteomeXchange [71] Consortium via the PRIDE [72] partner repository with the dataset identifier PXD030600. The reviewer account details: Username: reviewer_pxd030600@ebi.ac.uk; Password: 1QCP2jqI.

3.6. Expression and Purification of Chitinases Chib0431, Chib0434, Chia4287

The gene sequences of Chib0431, Chib0434, and Chia4287 without the signal peptide were cloned from the genomic DNA of strain DSM 14401 and inserted into the NdeI and XhoI sites of the expression vector pET-22b(+). The constructed recombinant plasmids were then transformed into *E. coli* BL21(DE3) for protein expression. The constructed recombinant *E. coli* BL21(DE3) strains were cultured at 37 °C in liquid LB medium containing 100 μg/mL ampicillin. When the OD_{600} of the cultures reached 0.6–1.0, 0.45 mM isopropyl thio-β-D-galactoside (IPTG), used as an inducer, was added into the cultures, and the cultures were incubated at 18 °C for 16 h. Then, the recombinant *E. coli* cells in the cultures were collected via centrifugation and crushed by sonication in the lysis buffer (100 mM NaCl, 5 mM imidazole, 50 mM Tris-HCl pH 8.0). The recombinant proteins of

Chib0431, Chib0434, and Chia4287 in the cell extracts were further purified by affinity chromatography with Ni-NTA agarose resins (Qiagen, Santa Clarita, CA, USA), followed by desalination on PD-10 Desalting Columns (GE Healthcare, Piscataway, NJ, USA), using 10 mM Tris-HCl containing 100 mM NaCl (pH 8.0) as the running buffer. The purified proteins were analyzed by sodium dodecyl sulfate polyacrylamide gel electrophoresis (SDS-PAGE) [73]. The protein concentrations were determined using a BCA protein assay kit with bovine serum albumin (BSA) as the standard.

3.7. Enzyme Assays

The activities of the three purified chitinases towards chitin powder, colloidal chitin, chitosan, microcrystalline cellulose, MUF-GlcNAc, MUF-$(GlcNAc)_2$ and MUF-$(GlcNAc)_3$ were assayed in 50 mM Tris-HCl at their respective optimal temperatures and pHs (50 °C and pH 7.0 for Chia4287, 50 °C and pH 7.5 for Chib0431, 45 °C and pH 7.5 for Chib0434). When the insoluble chitin powder, chitosan, or microcrystalline cellulose was used as the substrate, the reaction mixture contained 190 µL 50 mM Tris-HCl, 3% (*w*/*v*) substrate and 10 µL enzyme, which was incubated for 1 h for Chia4287 or 2 h for Chib0431 and Chib0434. When colloidal chitin was used as the substrate, the reaction mixture contained 190 µL 0.75% (*w*/*v*) colloidal chitin in 50 mM Tris-HCl and 10 µL enzyme, which was incubated for 40 min. After incubation, the activities of the chitinases towards these substrates were determined using the DNS method [63]. The enzyme activity (U) was defined as the amount of enzyme that required to release 1 µmol GlcNAc equivalent reducing sugar from the substrate per minute. When MUF- GlcNAc, MUF-$(GlcNAc)_2$, or MUF-$(GlcNAc)_3$ was used as the substrate, the enzyme activity was assayed for 15 min with the reaction mixture contained 790 µL 1 mM substrate in 50 mM Tris-HCl and 10 µL enzyme, which was incubated for 15 min and then terminated by an addition of 0.4 M $NaCO_3$. The enzyme activity (U) was defined as the amount of enzyme that required to release 1 µmol MUF from the substrate per minute.

3.8. Characterization of the Chitinases

The purified Chib0431, Chib0434, and Chia4287 were characterized with chitin powder as substrate. The effect of temperature on the enzyme activity was measured by assaying the enzyme activity at different temperatures (0–80 °C for Chia4287; 10–70 °C for Chib0431 and 20–60 °C for Chib0434) and their respective optimal pHs. The effect of pH on the enzyme activity was measured by assaying the enzyme activity in the Britton-Robinson buffer at different pHs (pH 4.0–9.0 for Chia4287; pH 5.0–10.0 for Chib0431 and Chib0434) and their respective optimal temperatures. Effect of salinity on the enzyme activity was assayed by assaying the enzyme activity in 50 mM Tris-HCl containing different concentrations of NaCl (0–5 M for Chib0431 and Chia4287; 0–2 M for Chib0434) at their respective optimal temperatures and pHs.

For the thermal stability assay, the purified chitinases were incubated at 40 °C, 50 °C, or 60 °C for 0–120 min, and the residual activities towards chitin powder were measured at an interval of 15 min under their respective optimal temperatures and pHs. For the pH stability assay, the purified chitinases were incubated in the Britton-Robinson buffers ranging from pH 3.0 to pH 11.0 at 4 °C for 10 h, and the residual activities towards chitin powder were measured at their respective optimal temperatures and pHs. For the halotolerance assay, the purified chitinases were incubated in 50 mM Tris-HCl containing different concentrations of NaCl (0–5 M) at 4 °C for 10 h, and the residual enzyme activities towards chitin powder were measured at their respective optimal temperatures and pHs.

3.9. Analysis of the Products Released from Crystalline Chitin by the Chitinases

The purified Chib0431, Chib0434, and Chia4287 (10 µL) were incubated with 3.0% chitin powder in 190 µL of 50 mM Tris-HCl (pH 7.0) for different times (15 min, 30 min, 1 h, and 3 h) at their respective optimal temperatures. The reaction was terminated by boiling at 100 °C for 10 min, and the reaction mixtures were centrifuged at 17,949× *g* for 10 min.

Then, the products in the supernatants were analyzed by gel filtration chromatography on a Superdex Peptide 10/300 GL column (GE Healthcare, Uppsala, Sweden), which were monitored at 210 nm using a UV detector. The injected volume was 10 μL. The products were eluted with 0.2 M ammonium hydrogen carbonate for 90 min with a flow rate of 0.3 mL/min. The reaction system containing 10 μL enzyme pre-heated at 100 °C for 10 min was used as the control. A mixture of GlcNAc, $(GlcNAc)_2$, $(GlcNAc)_3$, $(GlcNAc)_4$, $(GlcNAc)_5$, and $(GlcNAc)_6$ was used as the marker.

4. Conclusions

COSs have wide application in agriculture, medicine, cosmetics, and foods. While most COSs are now prepared with colloidal chitin, there are only a few reports of chitinases with potential in the preparation of COSs from natural crystalline chitin. In this study, three chitinases with activity on crystalline chitin were identified from a marine *Pseudoalteromonas* strain and characterized. These chitinases are all neutral mesophilic enzymes, which are most active at 45–50 °C and pH 7.0–7.5, and have high stability at 40 °C, pH 5.0–11.0, and in 5 M NaCl. The main products of the three chitinases on crystalline chitin are all $(GlcNAc)_2$, suggesting that these chitinases have potential in preparing $(GlcNAc)_2$ via direct degradation of natural crystalline chitin. Further studies such as improving the expression amount of these chitinases and their degradation efficiency on crystalline chitin are underway.

Supplementary Materials: The following supporting information can be downloaded at: https://www.mdpi.com/article/10.3390/md20030165/s1, Figure S1: Multiple sequence alignments of Chib0431, Chib0434, Chia4287, and Chia2822 with known GH18 chitinases.; Figure S2: Phylogenetic analysis of Chib0889 with other GH19 chitinases.; Table S1: General information of 26 type strains of Pseudoalteromonas.; Table S2: Purification of the recombinant enzymes Chib0431, Chib0434, and Chia4287. References [39,74–96] are cited in the supplementary materials.

Author Contributions: Conceptualization, X.-L.C. and Y.-Z.Z.; Investigation, Y.-J.W.; Methodology, X.-B.R., S.-S.L. and Y.-J.W.; Project administration, X.-L.C. and P.-Y.L.; Resources, X.-L.C. and Y.-Z.Z.; Software, Y.-R.D. and K.-X.H.; Supervision, Q.-L.Q., X.-L.C. and P.-Y.L.; Writing—original draft, X.-B.R.; Writing—review & editing, X.-L.C. and P.-Y.L. All authors have read and agreed to the published version of the manuscript.

Funding: This work was supported by the National Science Foundation of China (grants 42176229, 31870101, U2006205, 31870052 and awarded to P.-Y.L., Q.-L.Q., X.-L.C. and X.-L.C., respectively), the Major Scientific and Technological Innovation Project (MSTIP) of Shandong Province (2019JZZY010817 awarded to Y.-Z.Z.), Taishan Scholars Program of Shandong Province (tspd20181203 awarded to Y.-Z.Z.).

Institutional Review Board Statement: This article does not contain any studies involving human participants or animals performed by any of the authors.

Data Availability Statement: Proteomic data are available via ProteomeXchange with identifier PXD030600.

Acknowledgments: We would like to thank Andrew McMinn from the University of Tasmania, Australia, for editing this paper. We would like to thank Cai-Yun Sun and Rui Wang from State Key Laboratory of Microbial Technology of Shandong University for help and guidance in Bioscreen C Microbiology reader.

Conflicts of Interest: The authors declare no conflict of interest.

References

1. Rinaudo, M. Chitin and chitosan: Properties and applications. *Prog. Polym. Sci.* **2006**, *31*, 603–632. [CrossRef]
2. Jang, M.K.; Kong, B.G.; Jeong, Y.I.; Lee, C.H.; Nah, J.W. Physicochemical characterization of α-chitin, β-chitin, and γ-chitin separated from natural resources. *J. Polym. Sci. Part A Polym. Chem.* **2004**, *42*, 3423–3432. [CrossRef]
3. Johnstone, J. *Conditions of Life in the Sea*; Cambridge University Press: Cambridge, UK, 1908; p. 332.
4. Poulicek, M.; Jeauniaux, C. Chitin biomass in marine sediments. In *Chitin Chitosan*; Elsevier: London, UK, 1988; pp. 152–160.
5. Tokoro, A.; Kobayashi, M.; Tatewaki, N.; Suzuki, K.; Okawa, Y.; Mikami, T.; Suzuki, S.; Suzuki, M. Protective effect of *N*-acetyl chitohexaose on *Listeria monocytogenes* infection in mice. *Microbiol. Immunol.* **1989**, *33*, 357–367. [CrossRef]
6. Nishimura, K.; Nishimura, S.; Nishi, N.; Saiki, I.; Tokura, S.; Azuma, I. Immunological activity of chitin and its derivatives. *Vaccine* **1984**, *2*, 93–99. [CrossRef]
7. Kim, S.K.; Ravichandran, Y.D.; Khan, S.B.; Kim, Y.T. Prospective of the cosmeceuticals derived from marine organisms. *Biotechnol. Bioprocess Eng.* **2008**, *13*, 511–523. [CrossRef]
8. Bak, Y.K.; Lampe, J.W.; Sung, M.K. Effects of dietary supplementation of glucosamine sulfate on intestinal inflammation in a mouse model of experimental colitis. *J. Gastroenterol. Hepatol.* **2014**, *29*, 957–963. [CrossRef]
9. Tamai, Y.; Miyatake, K.; Okamoto, Y.; Takamori, Y.; Sakamoto, K.; Minami, S. Enhanced healing of cartilaginous injuries by *N*-acetyl-D-glucosamine and glucuronic acid. *Carbohydr. Polym.* **2003**, *54*, 251–262. [CrossRef]
10. Wang, Y.C.; Lien, T.S.; Chen, N.Y.; Hsu, T.H. Purification and characterization of β-*N*-acetylglucos-aminidase from Grifola frondosa. *BioResources* **2021**, *16*, 7234–7248. [CrossRef]
11. Jiang, S.; Jiang, H.; Zhou, Y.; Jiang, S.; Zhang, G. High-level expression of β-*N*-Acetylglucosaminidase BsNagZ in Pichia pastoris to obtain GlcNAc. *Bioprocess Biosyst. Eng.* **2019**, *42*, 611–619. [CrossRef]
12. Suginta, W.; Chuenark, D.; Mizuhara, M.; Fukamizo, T. Novel β-*N*-acetylglucosaminidases from Vibrio harveyi 650: Cloning, expression, enzymatic properties, and subsite identification. *BMC Biochem.* **2010**, *11*, 40. [CrossRef]
13. Kumar, M.; Brar, A.; Vivekanand, V.; Pareek, N. Bioconversion of Chitin to Bioactive Chitooligosaccharides: Amelioration and Coastal Pollution Reduction by Microbial Resources. *Mar. Biotechnol.* **2018**, *20*, 269–281. [CrossRef] [PubMed]
14. Liu, C.; Shen, N.; Wu, J.; Jiang, M.; Shi, S.; Wang, J.; Wei, Y.; Yang, L. Cloning, expression and characterization of a chitinase from *Paenibacillus chitinolyticus* strain UMBR 0002. *PeerJ* **2020**, *8*, e8964. [CrossRef] [PubMed]
15. Chung, D.; Baek, K.; Bae, S.S.; Jung, J. Identification and characterization of a marine-derived chitinolytic fungus, *Acremonium* sp. YS2-2. *J. Microbiol.* **2019**, *57*, 372–380. [CrossRef]
16. Song, Y.S.; Lee, S.H.; Cho, J.A.; Moon, C.; Seo, D.J.; Jung, W.J. Expression and degradation patterns of chitinase purified from Xuehuali (Pyrus bretschneiderilia) pollen. *Int. J. Biol. Macromol.* **2018**, *107*, 446–452. [CrossRef] [PubMed]
17. Fu, X.; Yan, Q.; Wang, J.; Yang, S.; Jiang, Z. Purification and biochemical characterization of novel acidic chitinase from *Paenicibacillus barengoltzii*. *Int. J. Biol. Macromol.* **2016**, *91*, 973–979. [CrossRef]
18. Wang, Y.J.; Jiang, W.X.; Zhang, Y.S.; Cao, H.Y.; Zhang, Y.; Chen, X.L.; Li, C.Y.; Wang, P.; Zhang, Y.Z.; Song, X.Y.; et al. Structural Insight into Chitin Degradation and Thermostability of a Novel Endochitinase from the Glycoside Hydrolase Family 18. *Front. Microbiol.* **2019**, *10*, 2457. [CrossRef] [PubMed]
19. Nguyen-Thi, N.; Doucet, N. Combining chitinase C and *N*-acetylhexosaminidase from *Streptomyces coelicolor* A3(2) provides an efficient way to synthesize *N*-acetylglucosamine from crystalline chitin. *J. Biotechnol.* **2016**, *220*, 25–32. [CrossRef] [PubMed]
20. Suma, K.; Podile, A.R. Chitinase A from *Stenotrophomonas maltophilia* shows transglycosylation and antifungal activities. *Bioresour. Technol.* **2013**, *133*, 213–220. [CrossRef]
21. Cheba, B.A.; Zaghloul, T.I.; EL-Mahdy, A.R.; EL-Massry, M.H. Effect of pH and Temperature on *Bacillus* sp. R2 Chitinase A activity and Stability. *Procedia Technol.* **2016**, *22*, 471–477. [CrossRef]
22. Neelamegam, A.; Sadhasivam, G.; Muthuvel, A.; Thangavel, B. Purification and characterization of chitinase from *micrococcus* sp.AG84 isolated from marine environment. *Afr. J. Microbiol. Res.* **2011**, *4*, 2822–2827.
23. Makhdoumi, A.; Dehghani-Joybari, Z.; Mashreghi, M.; Jamialahmadi, K.; Asoodeh, A. A novel halo-alkali-tolerant and thermo-tolerant chitinase from *Pseudoalteromonas* sp. DC14 isolated from the Caspian Sea. *Int. J. Environ. Sci. Technol.* **2015**, *12*, 3895–3904. [CrossRef]
24. Ray, L.; Panda, A.N.; Mishra, S.R.; Pattanaik, A.K.; Adhya, T.K.; Suar, M.; Raina, V. Purification and characterization of an extracellular thermo-alkali stable, metal tolerant chitinase from *Streptomyces chilikensis* RC1830 isolated from a brackish water lake sediment. *Biotechnol. Rep.* **2019**, *21*, e00311. [CrossRef] [PubMed]
25. Tsujibo, H.; Orikoshi, H.; Shiotani, K.; Hayashi, M.; Umeda, J.; Miyamoto, K.; Imada, C.; Okami, Y.; Inamori, Y. A novel family 19 chitinase from the marine-derived *Pseudoalteromonas tunicata* CCUG 44952^{T}: Heterologous expression, characterization and antifungal activity. *Biochem. Eng. J.* **2015**, *93*, 84–93.
26. Ramli, A.N.; Mahadi, N.M.; Rabu, A.; Murad, A.M.; Bakar, F.D.; Illias, R.M. Molecular cloning, expression and biochemical characterisation of a cold-adapted novel recombinant chitinase from *Glaciozyma antarctica* PI12. *Microb. Cell Fact.* **2011**, *10*, 94. [CrossRef]
27. Wang, X.H.; Zhao, Y.; Tan, H.D.; Chi, N.Y.; Zhang, Q.F.; Du, Y.G.; Yin, H. Characterisation of a chitinase from *Pseudoalteromonas* sp. DL-6, a marine psychrophilic bacterium. *Int. J. Biol. Macromol.* **2014**, *70*, 455–462. [CrossRef] [PubMed]
28. Meruvu, H.; Donthireddy, S.R. Purification and characterization of an antifungal chitinase from *Citrobacter freundii* str. nov. haritD11. *Appl. Biochem. Biotechnol.* **2014**, *172*, 196–205. [CrossRef]

29. Stefanidi, E.; Vorgias, C.E. Molecular analysis of the gene encoding a new chitinase from the marine psychrophilic bacterium *Moritella marina* and biochemical characterization of the recombinant enzyme. *Extremophiles* **2008**, *12*, 541–552. [CrossRef]
30. Mukherjee, S.; Behera, P.K.; Madhuprakash, J. Efficient conversion of crystalline chitin to *N*-acetylglucosamine and *N,N'*-diacetylchitobiose by the enzyme cocktail produced by *Paenibacillus* sp. LS1. *Carbohydr. Polym.* **2020**, *250*, 116889. [CrossRef]
31. Sashiwa, H.; Fujishima, S.; Yamano, N.; Kawasaki, N.; Nakayama, A.; Muraki, E.; Hiraga, K.; Oda, K.; Aiba, S. Production of *N*-acetyl-D-glucosamine from alpha-chitin by crude enzymes from *Aeromonas hydrophila* H-2330. *Carbohydr. Res.* **2002**, *337*, 761–763. [CrossRef]
32. Lv, C.Y.; Gu, T.Y.; Ma, R.; Yao, W.; Huang, Y.Y.; Gu, J.G.; Zhao, G.G. Biochemical characterization of a GH19 chitinase from *Streptomyces alfalfae* and its applications in crystalline chitin conversion and biocontrol. *Int. J. Biol. Macromol.* **2021**, *167*, 193–201. [CrossRef]
33. Gao, C.; Zhang, A.; Chen, K.; Hao, Z.; Tong, J.; Ouyang, P. Characterization of extracellular chitinase from *Chitinibacter* sp. GC72 and its application in GlcNAc production from crayfish shell enzymatic degradation. *Biochem. Eng. J.* **2015**, *97*, 59–64. [CrossRef]
34. Chen, X.L.; Wang, Y.; Wang, P.; Zhang, Y.Z. Proteases from the marine bacteria in the genus *Pseudoalteromonas*: Diversity, characteristics, ecological roles, and application potentials. *Mar. Life Sci. Technol.* **2020**, *2*, 309–323. [CrossRef]
35. Wietz, M.; Gram, L.; Jørgensen, B.; Schramm, A. Latitudinal Patterns in the Abundance of Major Marine Bacterioplankton Groups. *Aquat. Microb. Ecol.* **2010**, *61*, 179–189. [CrossRef]
36. Paulsen, S.S.; Strube, M.L.; Bech, P.K.; Gram, L.; Sonnenschein, E.C. Marine Chitinolytic *Pseudoalteromonas* Represents an Untapped Reservoir of Bioactive Potential. *mSystems* **2019**, *4*, e00060-19. [CrossRef]
37. Wang, X.; Chi, N.; Bai, F.; Du, Y.; Zhao, Y.; Yin, H. Characterization of a cold-adapted and salt-tolerant exo-chitinase (ChiC) from Pseudoalteromonas sp. DL-6. *Extremophiles* **2016**, *20*, 167–176. [CrossRef] [PubMed]
38. Orikoshi, H.; Baba, N.; Nakayama, S.; Kashu, H.; Miyamoto, K.; Yasuda, M.; Inamori, Y.; Tsujibo, H. Molecular analysis of the gene encoding a novel cold-adapted chitinase (ChiB) from a marine bacterium, Alteromonas sp. strain O-7. *J. Bacteriol.* **2003**, *185*, 1153–1160. [CrossRef]
39. Ivanova, E.P.; Shevchenko, L.S.; Sawabe, T.; Lysenko, A.M.; Svetashev, V.I.; Gorshkova, N.M.; Satomi, M.; Christen, R.; Mikhailov, V.V. *Pseudoalteromonas maricaloris* sp. nov., isolated from an Australian sponge, and reclassification of [*Pseudoalteromonas aurantia*] NCIMB 2033 as *Pseudoalteromonas flavipulchra* sp. nov. *Int. J. Syst. Evol. Microbiol.* **2002**, *52*, 263–271. [CrossRef] [PubMed]
40. Chen, W.; Qu, M.; Zhou, Y.; Yang, Q. Structural analysis of group II chitinase (ChtII) catalysis completes the puzzle of chitin hydrolysis in insects. *J. Biol. Chem.* **2018**, *29*, 2652–2660. [CrossRef]
41. Pantoom, S.; Vetter, I.R.; Prinz, H.; Suginta, W. Potent family-18 chitinase inhibitors: X-ray structures, affinities, and binding mechanisms. *J. Biol. Chem.* **2011**, *286*, 24312–24323. [CrossRef]
42. Houston, D.R.; Shiomi, K.; Arai, N.; Omura, S.; Peter, M.G.; Turberg, A.; Synstad, B.; Eijsink, V.G.; van Aalten, D.M. High-resolution structures of a chitinase complexed with natural product cyclopentapeptide inhibitors: Mimicry of carbohydrate substrate. *Proc. Natl. Acad. Sci. USA* **2002**, *99*, 9127–9132. [CrossRef]
43. Sun, X.; Li, Y.; Tian, Z.; Qian, Y.; Zhang, H.; Wang, L. A novel thermostable chitinolytic machinery of *Streptomyces* sp. F-3 consisting of chitinases with different action modes. *Biotechnol. Biofuels* **2019**, *12*, 136. [CrossRef] [PubMed]
44. Suzuki, K.; Taiyoji, M.; Sugawara, N.; Nikaidou, N.; Henrissat, B.; Watanabe, T. The third chitinase gene (chiC) of *Serratia marcescens* 2170 and the relationship of its product to other bacterial chitinases. *Biochem. J.* **1999**, *343*, 587–596. [CrossRef] [PubMed]
45. Liu, T.; Zhu, W.; Wang, J.; Zhou, Y.; Duan, Y.; Qu, M.; Yang, Q. The deduced role of a chitinase containing two nonsynergistic catalytic domains. *Acta Crystallogr. D Struct. Biol.* **2018**, *74*, 30–40. [CrossRef] [PubMed]
46. Bai, Y.; Eijsink, V.G.; Kielak, A.M.; van Veen, J.A.; de Boer, W. Genomic comparison of chitinolytic enzyme systems from terrestrial and aquatic bacteria. *Environ. Microbiol.* **2016**, *18*, 38–49. [CrossRef] [PubMed]
47. Orlando, M.; Pucciarelli, S.; Lotti, M. Endolysins from Antarctic Pseudomonas Display Lysozyme Activity at Low Temperature. *Mar. Drugs* **2020**, *18*, 579. [CrossRef] [PubMed]
48. Watanabe, T.; Ito, Y.; Yamada, T.; Hashimoto, M.; Sekine, S.; Tanaka, H. The roles of the C-terminal domain and type-Iii domains of chitinase A1 from *Bacillus Circulans* Wl-12 in chitin degradation. *J. Bacteriol.* **1994**, *176*, 4465–4472. [CrossRef]
49. Svitil, A.L.; Kirchman, D.L. A chitin-binding domain in a marine bacterial chitinase and other microbial chitinases: Implications for the ecology and evolution of 1,4-beta-glycanases. *Microbiology* **1998**, *144*, 1299–1308. [CrossRef]
50. Eijsink, V.G.H.; Vaaje-Kolstad, G.; Varum, K.M.; Horn, S.J. Towards new enzymes for biofuels: Lessons from chitinase research. *Trends. Biotechnol.* **2008**, *26*, 228–235. [CrossRef]
51. Nimlos, M.R.; Beckham, G.T.; Matthews, J.F.; Bu, L.T.; Himmel, M.E.; Crowley, M.F. Binding preferences, surface attachment, diffusivity, and orientation of a family 1 carbohydrate-binding module on cellulose. *J. Biol. Chem.* **2012**, *287*, 20603–20612. [CrossRef]
52. Wang, X.; Isbrandt, T.; Strube, M.L.; Paulsen, S.S.; Nielsen, M.W.; Buijs, Y.; Schoof, E.M.; Larsen, T.O.; Gram, L.; Zhang, S.D. Chitin Degradation Machinery and Secondary Metabolite Profiles in the Marine Bacterium *Pseudoalteromonas rubra* S4059. *Mar. Drugs* **2021**, *19*, 108. [CrossRef]

53. Monge, E.C.; Tuveng, T.R.; Vaaje-Kolstad, G.; Eijsink, V.G.H.; Gardner, J.G. Systems analysis of the glycoside hydrolase family 18 enzymes from *Cellvibrio japonicus* characterizes essential chitin degradation functions. *J. Biol. Chem.* **2018**, *293*, 3849–3859. [CrossRef] [PubMed]
54. Meibom, K.L.; Li, X.B.; Nielsen, A.T.; Wu, C.Y.; Roseman, S.; Schoolnik, G.K. The *Vibrio cholerae* chitin utilization program. *Proc. Natl. Acad. Sci. USA* **2004**, *101*, 2524–2529. [CrossRef]
55. O'Brien, M.; Colwell, R.R. A rapid test for chitinase activity that uses 4-methylumbelliferyl-N-acetyl-beta-D-glucosaminide. *Appl. Environ. Microbiol.* **1987**, *53*, 1718–1720. [CrossRef] [PubMed]
56. Howard, M.B.; Ekborg., N.A.; Taylor, L.E.; Weiner, R.M.; Hutcheson, S.W. Genomic analysis and initial characterization of the chitinolytic system of *Microbulbifer degradans* strain 2-40. *J. Bacteriol.* **2003**, *185*, 3352–3360. [CrossRef] [PubMed]
57. Reindl, M.; Stock, J.; Hussnaetter, K.P.; Genc, A.; Brachmann, A.; Schipper, K. A Novel Factor Essential for Unconventional Secretion of Chitinase Cts1. *Front. Microbiol.* **2020**, *11*, 1529. [CrossRef] [PubMed]
58. Lee, H.J.; Lee, Y.S.; Choi, Y.L. Cloning, purification, and characterization of an organic solvent-tolerant chitinase, MtCh509, from *Microbulbifer thermotolerans* DAU221. *Biotechnol. Biofuels* **2018**, *11*, 303. [CrossRef]
59. Pan, M.; Li, J.; Lv, X.; Du, G.; Liu, L. Molecular engineering of chitinase from *Bacillus* sp. DAU101 for enzymatic production of chitooligosaccharides. *Enzyme. Microb. Technol.* **2019**, *124*, 54–62. [CrossRef]
60. Le, B.; Yang, S.H. Characterization of a chitinase from *Salinivibrio* sp. BAO-1801 as an antifungal activity and a biocatalyst for producing chitobiose. *J. Basic Microbiol.* **2018**, *58*, 848–856. [CrossRef]
61. Hosny, A.; El-Shayeb, N.A.; Abood, A.; Abdel-Fattah, A.M. A Potent Chitinolytic Activity of Marine *Actinomycete* sp. and Enzymatic Production of Chitooligosaccharides. *Aust. J. Basic Appl. Sci.* **2010**, *4*, 615–623.
62. Lv, C.; Gu, T.; Xu, K.; Gu, J.; Li, L.; Liu, X.; Zhang, A.; Gao, S.; Li, W.; Zhao, G. Biochemical characterization of a β-*N*-acetylhexosaminidase from *Streptomyces alfalfae* and its application in the production of *N*-acetyl-D-glucosamine. *J. Biosci. Bioeng.* **2019**, *128*, 135–141. [CrossRef]
63. Miller, G.L. Use of dinitrosalicylic acid reagent for determination of reducing sugar. *Anal. Chem.* **1959**, *31*, 426–428. [CrossRef]
64. Xie, B.B.; Rong, J.C.; Tang, B.L.; Wang, S.; Liu, G.; Qin, Q.L.; Zhang, X.Y.; Zhang, W.; She, Q.; Chen, Y.; et al. Evolutionary Trajectory of the Replication Mode of Bacterial Replicons. *mBio* **2021**, *26*, e02745-20. [CrossRef] [PubMed]
65. Yin, Y.; Mao, X.; Yang, J.; Chen, X.; Mao, F.; Xu, Y. dbCAN: A web resource for automated carbohydrate-active enzyme annotation. *Nucleic Acids Res.* **2012**, *40*, W445–W451. [CrossRef] [PubMed]
66. Almagro Armenteros, J.J.; Tsirigos, K.D.; Sønderby, C.K.; Petersen, T.N.; Winther, O.; Brunak, S.; von Heijne, G.; Nielsen, H. SignalP 5.0 improves signal peptide predictions using deep neural networks. *Nat. Biotechnol.* **2019**, *37*, 420–423. [CrossRef] [PubMed]
67. Potter, S.C.; Luciani, A.; Eddy, S.R.; Park, Y.; Lopez, R.; Finn, R.D. HMMER web server: 2018 update. *Nucleic Acids Res.* **2018**, *46*, W200–W204. [CrossRef]
68. Kumar, S.; Stecher, G.; Li, M.; Knyaz, C.; Tamura, K. MEGA X: Molecular Evolutionary Genetics Analysis across Computing Platforms. *Mol. Biol. Evol.* **2018**, *35*, 1547–1549. [CrossRef] [PubMed]
69. Robert, X.; Gouet, P. Deciphering key features in protein structures with the new ENDscript server. *Nucleic Acids Res.* **2014**, *42*, W320–W324. [CrossRef] [PubMed]
70. Wilkins, M.R.; Gasteiger, E.; Bairoch, A.; Sanchez, J.C.; Williams, K.L.; Appel, R.D.; Hochstrasser, D.F. Protein identification and analysis tools in the ExPASy server. *Methods Mol. Biol.* **1999**, *112*, 531–552. [PubMed]
71. Deutsch, E.W.; Bandeira, N.; Sharma, V.; Perez-Riverol, Y.; Carver, J.J.; Kundu, D.J.; García-Seisdedos, D.; Jarnuczak, A.F.; Hewapathirana, S.; Pullman, B.S.; et al. The ProteomeXchange consortium in 2020: Enabling 'big data' approaches in proteomics. *Nucleic Acids Res.* **2020**, *48*, D1145–D1152. [CrossRef]
72. Perez-Riverol, Y.; Csordas, A.; Bai, J.; Bernal-Llinares, M.; Hewapathirana, S.; Kundu, D.J.; Inuganti, A.; Griss, J.; Mayer, G.; Eisenacher, M.; et al. The PRIDE database and related tools and resources in 2019: Improving support for quantification data. *Nucleic Acids Res.* **2019**, *47*, D442–D450. [CrossRef]
73. Laemmli, U.K. Cleavage of structural proteins during the assembly of the head of bacteriophage T4. *Nature* **1970**, *227*, 680–685. [CrossRef] [PubMed]
74. Romanenko, L.A.; Zhukova, N.V.; Rohde, M.; Lysenko, A.M.; Mikhailov, V.V.; Stackebrandt, E. *Pseudoalteromonas agarivorans* sp. nov., a novel marine agarolytic bacterium. Int. J. *Syst. Evol. Microbiol.* **2003**, *53*, 125–131. [CrossRef]
75. Ivanova, E.P.; Gorshkova, N.M.; Zhukova, N.V.; Lysenko, A.M.; Zelepuga, E.A.; Prokof'eva, N.G.; Mikhailov, V.V.; Nicolau, D.V.; Christen, R. Characterization of Pseudoalteromonas distincta-like sea-water isolates and description of *Pseudoalteromonas aliena* sp. nov. *Int. J. Syst. Evol. Microbiol.* **2004**, *54*, 1431–1437. [CrossRef]
76. Al Khudary, R.; Stosser, N.I.; Qoura, F.; Antranikian, G. *Pseudoalteromonas arctica* sp. nov., an aerobic, psychrotolerant,marine bacterium isolated from Spitzbergen. *Int. J. Syst. Evol. Microbiol.* **2008**, *58*, 2018–2024. [CrossRef]
77. Gauthier, M.; Breittmayer, V.A. A new antibiotic-producing bacterium from seawater: *Alteromonas aurantia* sp. nov. *Int. J. Syst. Evol. Microbiol.* **1979**, *29*, 366–372. [CrossRef]
78. Akagawa-Matsushita, M.; Matsuo, M.; Koga, Y.; Yamasato, K. *Alteromonas atlantica* sp. nov. and *Alteromonas carrageenovora* sp. nov., bacteria that decompose algal polysaccharides. *Int. J. Syst. Evol. Microbiol.* **1993**, *42*, 621–627. [CrossRef]
79. Gauthier, M. *Alteromonas citrea*, a new Gram-negative, yellow-pigmented species from seawater. *Int. J. Syst. Evol. Microbiol.* **1977**, *27*, 349–354. [CrossRef]

80. Chan, K.; Baumann, L.; Garza, M.; Baumann, P. Two new species of *Alteromonas*: *Alteromonas espejiana* and *Alteromonas undina*. *Int. J. Syst. Evol. Microbiol.* **1978**, *28*, 217–222. [CrossRef]
81. Ivanova, E.P.; Sawabe, T.; Alexeeva, Y.V.; Lysenko, A.M.; Gorshkova, N.M.; Hayashi, K.; Zukova, N.V.; Christen, R.; Mikhailov, V.V. *Pseudoalteromonas issachenkonii* sp. nov., a bacterium that degrades the thallus of the brown alga *Fucus evanescens*. *Int. J. Syst. Evol. Microbiol* **2002**, *52*, 229–234. [CrossRef]
82. Xu, X.W.; Wu, Y.H.; Wang, C.S.; Gao, X.H.; Wang, X.G.; Wu, M. *Pseudoalteromonas lipolytica* sp. nov., isolated from the Yangtze River estuary. *Int. J. Syst. Evol. Microbiol.* **2009**, *60*, 2176–2181. [CrossRef]
83. Gauthier, M. Validation of the name *Alteromonas luteoviolacea*. *Int. J. Syst. Evol. Microbiol.* **1982**, *32*, 82–86. [CrossRef]
84. Yoon, J.H.; Kim, I.G.; Kang, K.H.; Oh, T.K.; Park, Y.H. *Alteromonas marina* sp. nov., isolated from sea water of the East Sea in Korea. *Int. J. Syst. Evol. Microbiol.* **2003**, *53*, 1625–1630. [CrossRef] [PubMed]
85. Romanenko, L.A.; Zhukova, N.V.; Lysenko, A.M.; Mikhailov, V.V.; Stackebrandt, E. Assignment of '*Alteromonas marinoglutinosa*'NCIMB 1770 to *Pseudoalteromonas mariniglutinosa* sp. nov., nom. rev., comb. nov. *Int. J. Syst. Evol. Microbiol.* **2003**, *53*, 1105–1109. [CrossRef] [PubMed]
86. Ivanova, E.P.; Kiprianova, E.A.; Mikhailov, V.V.; Levanova, G.F.; Garagulya, A.D.; Gorshkova, N.M.; Yumoto, N. Characterization and identification of marine *Alteromonas nigrifaciens* strains and emendation of the description. *Int. J. Syst. Evol. Microbiol.* **1996**, *46*, 223–228. [CrossRef]
87. Ivanova, E.P.; Sawabe, T.; Lysenko, A.M.; Gorshkova, N.M.; Hayashi, K.; Zhukova, N.V.; Nicolau, D.V.; Christen, R.; Mikhailov, V.V. *Pseudoalteromonas translucida* sp. nov. and *Pseudoalteromonas paragorgicola* sp. nov., and emended description of the genus. *Int. J. Syst. Evol. Microbiol.* **2002**, *52*, 1759–1766.
88. Venkateswaran, K.; Dohmoto, N. *Pseudoalteromonas peptidolytica* sp. nov., a novel marine mussel-thread-degrading bacterium isolated from the Sea of Japan. *Int. J. Syst. Evol. Microbiol* **2000**, *50*, 565–574. [CrossRef] [PubMed]
89. Isnansetyo, A.; Kamei, Y. *Pseudoalteromonas phenolica* sp. nov., a novel marine bacterium that produces phenolic anti-methicillin-resistant *Staphylococcus aureus* substances. *Int. J. Syst. Evol. Microbiol.* **2003**, *53*, 583–588. [CrossRef]
90. Hansen, A.; Weeks, O.; Colwell, R. Taxonomy of *Pseudomonas piscicida* (Bein) Buck, Meyers, and Leifson. *J. Bacteriol.* **1965**, *89*, 752–761. [CrossRef]
91. Bowman, J.P. *Pseudoalteromonas prydzensis* sp. nov., a psychrotrophic, halotolerant bacterium from Antarctic sea ice. *Int. J. Syst. Evol. Microbiol.* **1998**, *48*, 1037–1041. [CrossRef]
92. Gauthier, M. *Alteromonas rubra* sp. nov., a new marine antibiotic-producing bacterium. *Int. J. Syst. Evol. Microbiol.* **1976**, *26*, 459–466. [CrossRef]
93. Lau, S.C.; Tsoi, M.M.; Li, X.; Dobretsov, S.; Plakhotnikova, Y.; Wong, P.-K.; Qian, P.Y. *Pseudoalteromonas spongiae* sp. nov., a novel member of the γ-Proteobacteria isolated from the sponge Mycale adhaerens in Hong Kong waters. *Int. J. Syst. Evol. Microbiol.* **2005**, *55*, 1593–1596. [CrossRef] [PubMed]
94. Ivanova, E.P.; Romanenko, L.A.; Matte, M.H.; Matte, G.R.; Lysenko, A.M.; Simidu, U.; Kita-Tsukamoto, K.; Sawabe, T.; Vysotskii, M.V.; Frolova, G.M.; et al. Retrieval of the species *Alteromonas tetraodonis* Simidu et al. 1990 as *Pseudoalteromonas tetraodonis* comb. nov. and emendation of description. *Int. J. Syst. Evol. Microbiol.* **2001**, *51*, 1071–1078. [CrossRef] [PubMed]
95. Holmström, C.; James, S.; Neilan, B.A.; White, D.C.; Kjelleberg, S. *Pseudoalteromonas tunicata* sp. nov., a bacterium that produces antifouling agents. *Int. J. Syst. Evol. Microbiol.* **1998**, *48*, 1205–1212. [CrossRef] [PubMed]
96. Egan, S.; Holmström, C.; Kjelleberg, S. *Pseudoalteromonas ulvae* sp. nov., a bacterium with antifouling activities isolated from the surface of a marine alga. *Int. J. Syst. Evol. Microbiol.* **2001**, *51*, 1499–1504. [CrossRef] [PubMed]

marine drugs

MDPI

Review

Ulva (*Enteromorpha*) Polysaccharides and Oligosaccharides: A Potential Functional Food Source from Green-Tide-Forming Macroalgae

Limin Ning [1,2], Zhong Yao [2] and Benwei Zhu [2,*]

[1] School of Medicine and Holistic Integrated Medicine, Nanjing University of Chinese Medicine, Nanjing 210023, China; ninglimin@njucm.edu.cn
[2] Laboratory of Marine Bioresource, College of Food Science and Light Industry, Nanjing Tech University, Nanjing 211816, China; yaozhong@njtech.edu.cn
* Correspondence: zhubenwei@njtech.edu.cn; Tel.: +86-25-58139419

Abstract: The high-valued utilization of *Ulva* (previously known as *Enteromorpha*) bioresources has drawn increasing attention due to the periodic blooms of world-wide green tide. The polysaccharide is the main functional component of *Ulva* and exhibits various physiological activities. The *Ulva* oligosaccharide as the degradation product of polysaccharide not only possesses some obvious activities, but also possesses excellent solubility and bioavailability. Both *Ulva* polysaccharides and oligosaccharides hold promising potential in the food industry as new functional foods or food additives. Studies on *Ulva* polysaccharides and oligosaccharides are increasing and have been the focus of the marine bioresources field. However, the comprehensive review of this topic is still rare and do not cover the recent advances of the structure, isolation, preparation, activity and applications of *Ulva* polysaccharides and oligosaccharides. This review systematically summarizes and discusses the recent advances of chemical composition, extraction, purification, structure, and activity of *Ulva* polysaccharides as well as oligosaccharides. In addition, the potential applications as new functional food and food additives have also been considered, and these will definitely expand the applications of *Ulva* oligosaccharides in the food and medical fields.

Keywords: *Ulva*; polysaccharide; oligosaccharide; structure; preparation; activity

Citation: Ning, L.; Yao, Z.; Zhu, B. *Ulva* (*Enteromorpha*) Polysaccharides and Oligosaccharides: A Potential Functional Food Source from Green-Tide-Forming Macroalgae. *Mar. Drugs* **2022**, *20*, 202. https://doi.org/10.3390/md20030202

Academic Editor: Hitoshi Sashiwa

Received: 17 February 2022
Accepted: 7 March 2022
Published: 10 March 2022

1. Introduction

The *Ulva* (previously known as *Enteromorpha Enteromorpha*), known as green-tide-forming macroalgae, has drawn increasing attention in both the marine environment protection and marine bioresources fields [1,2]. Recently, the green tide blooms more and more frequently due to the global seawater eutrophication and temperature rise [3–7]. The largest *Ulva*-forming green tide in history occurred in the Yellow Sea of China this year, and covered almost 1746 km^2, producing over 24 million tons of biomass [8]. The *Ulva* genus belongs to the Ulvaceae family and includes nearly 40 kinds of species such as *Ulva prolifera* (previously known as *Enteromorpha prolifera*), *Ulva linza* (previously known as *Enteromorpha linza*), and *Ulva intestinalis* (previously known as *Enteromorpha intestinalis*) (as shown in Figure 1) [9]. For a long time, the *Ulva* and *Enteromorpha* were considered as two different genera, but the molecular evidence indicated that *Ulva* and *Enteromorpha* are not distinct evolutionary entities and should not be recognized as separate genera [9]. Therefore, the taxonomic name "*Enteromorpha*" is currently regarded as a synonym for *Ulva*.

The *Ulva* polysaccharide constitutes the main component of the cell wall of *Ulva* species algae, and it accounts for nearly 18% of the dry weight. In addition, it possesses various physiological properties such as antioxidant, anticoagulant, antitumor, antiaging and immune regulatory activities [10–12]. Therefore, the *Ulva* polysaccharides could be widely used as medicine and chemical agents in the agricultural and medical fields [13,14].

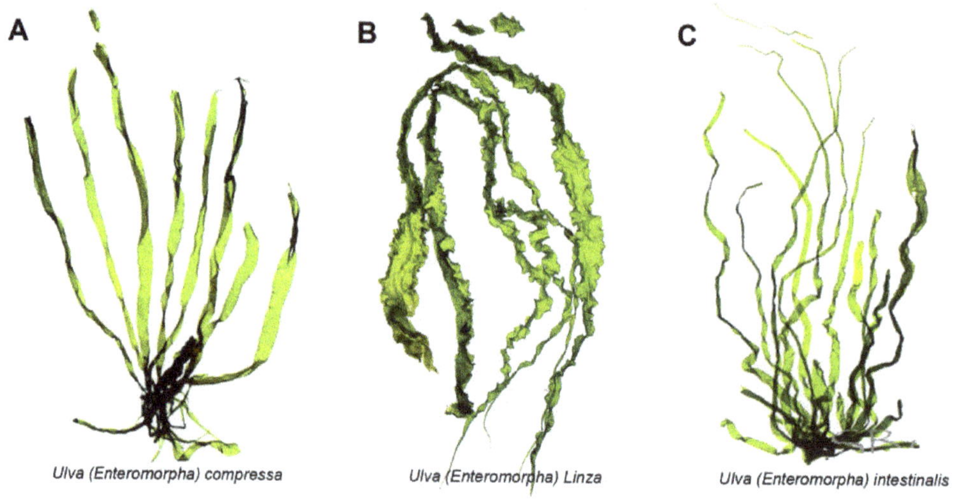

Figure 1. The morphology pictures of three kinds of *Ulva* species. (**A**). *Ulva compressa*; (**B**). *Ulva linza*; (**C**). *Ulva intestinalis*.

It is worth noting that another green algal polysaccharide, Ulvan, has also drawn increased attention, and its structure has been well characterized. The water-soluble sulfated polysaccharide is mainly extracted from *Ulva* sp. and consists of a linear backbone with L-rhamnose-3-sulfate (Rha3S), D-glucuronic acid (GlcUA), L-iduronic acid (IdoA) and D-xylose (Xyl), and the sulfate group is linked to the rhamnose. The two major repeating disaccharide units of ulvan are →4)-β-D-glucuronic acid (1→4)-α-L-rhamnose-3-sulfate (1→(A3S) and →4) α-L-iduronic acid (1→4)-α-L-rhamnose-3-sulfate (1→(B3S) [15]. However, the *Ulva* polysaccharide possesses a more complex chemical composition and fine structure. In addition, the *Ulva* polysaccharides exhibit great potential as functional foods and food additives due to their obvious metabolism-regulatory activity [16–18]. For instance, Guo et al. discovered that the polysaccharides extracted from *Ulva prolifera* could prevent high-fat diet-induced obesity in hamsters [19]. They also found that polysaccharides isolated from *Ulva prolifera* could protect against carbon tetrachloride-induced acute liver injury in mice via the activation of Nrf2/HO-1 signaling, and the suppression of oxidative stress, inflammation and apoptosis [20]. Li et al. found that the *Ulva* polysaccharides could improve blood glucose regulation, blood lipid metabolism and liver oxidative stress in T2DM cells [21]. However, the applications of the *Ulva* polysaccharide have been greatly limited by its poor solubility and low bioavailability [22]. In order to overcome this drawback, it is feasible to degrade the polysaccharide into oligosaccharide, which also possesses the biological activities but also has much better solubility and bioavailability [23]. The methods for polysaccharide degradation mainly include physicochemical or enzymatic methods [24–26]. In particular, the enzymatic method has drawn increasing attention due to its advantages, such as its mild reaction conditions and specific product distributions.

Studies of the *Ulva* polysaccharide and oligosaccharide have been increasing in the past two decades (Figure 2). Among these, most of them have focused on the structure and activity of the polysaccharides and oligosaccharides [14]. In addition, the preparation of oligosaccharides has drawn increasing attention [22]. However, there is not a comprehensive review which has summarized the recent advances in every aspect of the *Ulva* polysaccharide and oligosaccharide. In this review, we summarized and discussed the recent advances of chemical composition, extraction, purification, structure, activity and applications of *Ulva* polysaccharides as well as oligosaccharides. In addition, the potential applications as new functional foods and food additives have also been reviewed.

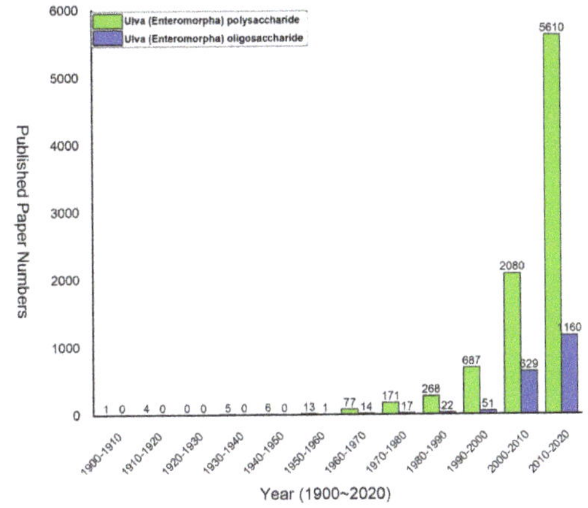

Figure 2. The numbers of published papers with keywords of *Ulva* polysaccharide and oligosaccharide between 1900 and 2020.

2. *Ulva* Polysaccharide

2.1. *Chemical Composition and Structure of* Ulva *Polysaccharide*

The chemical composition of the *Ulva* polysaccharide is more complex than other common algal polysaccharides such as alginate (Phaeophyceae), carrageenan and agar (Rhodophyta) (Figure 3) [22,27–29]. The monosaccharide composition of *Ulva* polysaccharide mainly includes glucose, rhamnose, arabinose, xylose, mannose, galactose, fucose, glucosamine and glucuronic acid [27,28], which is different from algal polysaccharides (such as agar, carrageenan, alginate and fucoidan) that originate from brown and red algae. In addition, the chemical composition of *Ulva* polysaccharide differs in growth condition, harvesting season and the types of original *Ulva* species [14,30]. Qi et al. characterized the chemical compositions of the polysaccharides isolated from *Ulva linza*, *Ulva prolifera* and *Ulva clathrata*, respectively [28,31,32]. The results suggested that the chemical compositions of the three kinds of polysaccharides differed from each other. For instance, the polysaccharide from *Ulva linza* was composed of much rhamnose and a small amount of galactose, xylose and glucuronic acid; while the polysaccharides from *Ulva clathrata* contained larger amounts of arabinose and galactose and a small amount of rhamnose, fucose and xylose.

In addition, the main component (rhamnose) of the polysaccharides from *Ulva prolifera* is similar to the polysaccharide from *Ulva linza*. However, it contains some mannose, glucuronic acid and glucosamine, which is very different from the monosaccharide composition of the polysaccharide from *Ulva linza*. Moreover, the harvest time of *Ulva* algae also could influence on the chemical composition of the polysaccharide [31]. Shi et al. investigated the monosaccharide composition of *Ulva* polysaccharides, which isolated from the *Ulva clathrata* with different harvesting times [33]. The results suggested that the kinds of monosaccharide for polysaccharides isolated from the *Ulva clathrata* with different harvesting times seemed to be same. However, the ratios of these monosaccharides were different from each other. For instance, the monosaccharide (mannose, rhamnose, glucose, galactose and xylose) ratios of polysaccharides isolated from *Ulva clathrata* harvested in January and June are 6.74:65.56:5.54:2.83:19.33 and 2.81:67.55:2.31:2.71:24.61, respectively. In addition, the growth conditions also could exert an influence on the chemical composition of *Ulva* polysaccharide. Ji et al. analyzed the composition of *Ulva clathrata* samples and found that the monosaccharide compositions of *Ulva clathrata* under normal and explosive states exhibited obviously different levels [34]. The polysaccharides isolated from the *Ulva clathrata* under an explosive state contained iduronic acid, which did not exist in the polysaccharides isolated from *Ulva clathrata* under normal conditions.

The structure of polysaccharides that originate from *Ulva clathrata* is much more complex than other algal polysaccharides such as alginate, agar and carrageenan due to its complexity of monosaccharide composition, glycosidic linkage and group modification [14]. In addition, many factors such as the growth condition, harvesting season, the types of original *Ulva* species, etc., could lead to diverse structures of polysaccharides. Therefore, it is difficult to elucidate the fine structure of *Ulva* polysaccharide. Qi et al. investigated the fine structures of polysaccharides isolated from different sources in detail [28,32] (Table 1). The results indicated the polysaccharide of *Ulva linza* consisted of five fractions, namely MCS, MHS, SCS, SH1S and SH2S. In addition, it also included some fragments such as [→4)-β-D-Xylp-(1→], [→2)-α-L-Rhap-(1→], [→3)-α-L-Rhap-(1→], [→3, 4)-α-L-Rhap-(1→], [→2, 3)-α-L-Rhap-(1→], and [→2, 4)-α-L-Rhap-(1→]. The MCS and MHS fractions mainly contained [→4)-α-L-Rhap-(1→], [→2,4)-α-L-Rhap-(1→], [→4)-β-D-Xylp-(1→], [→4)-β-D-GlcAp-(1→], [→3)-α-L-Rhap-(1→] and [→2)-α-L-Rhap-(1→]. The SCS was consisted of [→3)-α-L-Rhap-(1→], [→2)-α-L-Rhap-(1→], [→4)-β-D-Xylp-(1→], [→4)-α-L-Rhap-(1→] and [→2,4)-α-L-Rhap-(1→], while the SH1S fraction composed of [→4)-α-L-Rhap-(1→], [→3)-α-L-Rhap-(1→], [→2,4)-α-L-Rhap-(1→], [→4)-β-D-Xylp-(1→] and [→4)-β-D-GlcAp-(1→]. The last fraction SH2S included [→4)-α-L-Rhap-(1→], [→4)-β-D-Xylp-(1→], [→2)-α-L-Rhap-(1→], [→3)-α-L-Rhap-(1→], [→3,4)-α-L-Rhap-(1→], [→2,3)-α-L-Rhap-(1→] and [→2,4)-α-L-Rhap-(1→]. They obtained four polysaccharide fractions (QC1S, QCQ2, QCQ3, and QHS) from *Ulva prolifera* and found that it mainly consisted of two disaccharide units, namely [→4)-β-D-GlcAp-(1→4)-α-L-Rhap3S-(1→] and [→4)-β-D-Xylp-(1→4)-α-L-Rhap3S-(1→]. The QC1S fraction contained [→4)-α-L-Rhap-(1→], [→4)-β-D-Xylp-(1→], [→2)-α-L-Rhap4S-(1→], [→3)-α-L-Rha4S-(1→], [→4)-α-L-Rhap2S-(1→] and [→3,4)-α-L-Rhap-(1→]. The QHS fraction mainly consisted of [→4)-α-L-Rhap-(1→], [→4)-β-D-Xylp-(1→], [→4)-β-D-GlcAp-(1→], [→3)-α-L-Rhap-(1→] and [→2,4)-α-L-Rhap-(1→]. In addition, three fractions (XCS, XH1S, XH2S) were isolated and characterized, the XCS fraction has been identified to have [→2)-β-D-Galp-(1→], [→3)-β-D-Galp-(1→], [→4)-β-D-Galp-(1→], [→6)-β-D-Galp-(1→], [→4)-β-L-Arap-(1→], [→2)-α-L-Rhap-(1→], [→3)-α-L-Rhap-(1→] and [→2)-α-L-Rhap-(1→]. Moreover, the XH1S fraction consisted of [→4)-β-L-Arap-(1→], [→3)-β-D-Galp-(1→], [→4)-β-D-Galp-(1→] and [→6)-β-D-Galp-(1→]. However, the XH2S fraction possessed new structures of [→4)-β-L-Arap3S-(1→], [→4)-β-L-Arap-(1→], [→3)-α-L-Rhap4S-(1→]. Jiao et al. characterized the fine structure of *Ulva intestinalis* polysaccharide and found that it mainly included the (1→)-Rha, (1→4)-Rha, (1→2, 4)-Rha, (1→) –Xyl, (1→2,3)-Xyl, (1→3)-Xyl, (1→4)-Glc and (1→3)-Gal structural units (Jiao et al., 2010; Jiao et al., 2009). They also determined the position of sulfate groups for different polysaccharide fractions and found that the position information is also very complicated and that there is not a uniform formula to describe the structures of *Ulva* polysaccharides [10,32,35].

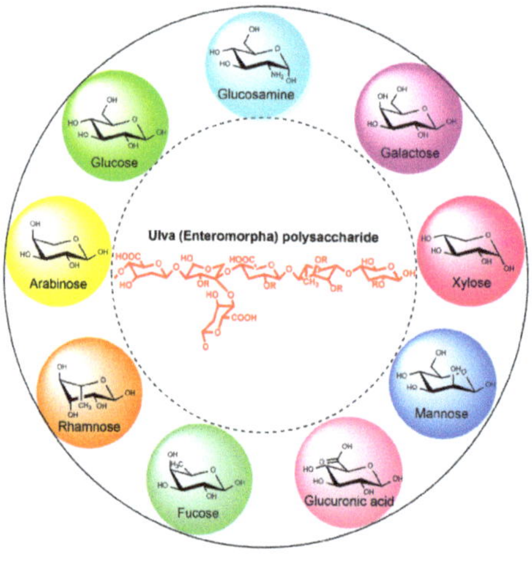

Figure 3. The main monosaccharide composition of *Ulva* polysaccharides.

Table 1. The summary of structures of polysaccharides originated from different species.

Ulva linza

Fraction			
MCS	Main components	[→4)-α-L-Rhap-(1→] [→2,4)-α-L-Rhap-(1→] [→4)-β-D-Xylp-(1→] [→4)-β-D-GlcUAp-(1→]
	Other components	[→3)-α-L-Rhap-(1→] [→2)-α-L-Rhap-(1→]
	Sulfated position	The C_3 of [→4)-α-L-Rhap-(1→]
MHS	Main components	[→4)-α-L-Rhap-(1→] [→2,4)-α-L-Rhap-(1→] [→4)-β-D-Xylp-(1→] [→4)-β-D-GlcUAp-(1→]
	Other components	[→3)-α-L-Rhap-(1→] [→2)-α-L-Rhap-(1→]
	Sulfated position	The C_3 of [→4)-α-L-Rhap-(1→]
SCS	Main components	[→3)-α-L-Rhap-(1→] [→2)-α-L-Rhap-(1→] [→4)-β-D-Xylp-(1→] [→4)-α-L-Rhap-(1→] [→2,4)-α-L-Rhap-(1→]
	Sulfated position	The C_2 or C_4 of [→3)-α-L-Rhap-(1→], the C_3 or C_4 [→2)-α-L-Rhap-(1→], the C_2 of [→4)-α-L-Rhap-(1→]

Ulva prolifera

Fraction		
QC1S	Main components	[→4)-α-L-Rhap-(1→] [→4)-β-D-Xylp-(1→]
	Other components	[→2)-α-L-Rhap4S-(1→] [→3)-α-L-Rha4S-(1→] [→4)-α-L-Rhap2S-(1→] [→3,4)-α-L-Rhap-(1→]
QHS	Main components	[→4)-α-L-Rhap-(1→] [→4)-β-D-Xylp-(1→] [→4)-β-D-GlcUAp-(1→]
	Other components	[→3)-α-L-Rhap-(1→] [→2,4)-α-L-Rhap-(1→]
	Sulfated position	The C_3 of [→4)-α-L-Rhap-(1→]
QCQ2		-

Ulva clathrata

Fraction		
XCS	Main components	[→2)-β-D-Galp-(1→] [→3)-β-D-Galp-(11→] [→4)-β-D-Galp-(1→] [→6)-β-D-Galp-(1→]
	Other components	[→4)-β-L-Arap-(1→] [→2)-α-L-Rhap-(1→] [→3)-α-L-Rhap-(1→] [→2)-α-L-Rhap-(1→]
	Sulfated position	The C_6 or C_2 [→4)-β-D-Galp-(1→], the C_4 or C_2 of [→6)-β-D-Galp-(1→]
XH1S	Main components	[→4)-β-L-Arap-(1→]
	Other components	[→3)-β-D-Galp-(1→] [→4)-β-D-Galp-(1→] [→6)-β-D-Galp-(1→]
	Sulfated position	The C_3 of [→4)-β-L-Arap-(1→]
XH2S	Main components	[→4)-β-L-Arap3S-(1→]
	Other components	[→4)-β-L-Arap-(1→] [→3)-α-L-Rhap4S-(1→]

Table 1. *Cont.*

Ulva linza				***Ulva prolifera***		***Ulva clathrata***
	SH1S	Main components	[→4)-α-L-Rhap-(1→] [→3)-α-L-Rhap-(1→] [→2,4)-α-L-Rhap-(1→] [→4)-β-D-Xylp-(1→] [→4)-β-D-Glc UAp-(1→]	QCQ3	-	
		Sulfated position	The C_3 of [→4)-α-L-Rhap-(1→]			
	SH2S	Main components	[→4)-α-L-Rhap-(1→] [→4)-β-D-Xylp-(1→]			
		Other components	[→2)-α-L-Rhap-(1→] [→3)-α-L-Rhap-(1→] [→3,4)-α-L-Rhap-(1→] [→2,3)-α-L-Rhap-(1→] [→2,4)-α-L-Rhap-(1→]			
		Sulfated position	The C_3 of [→4)-α-L-Rhap-(1→]			
	[→4)-β-D-Xylp-(1→]					
Other components	[→2)-α-L-Rhap-(1→] [→3)-α-L-Rhap-(1→] [→3,4)-α-L-Rhap-(1→] [→2,3)-α-L-Rhap-(1→] [→2,4)-α-L-Rhap-(1→]					

2.2. Extraction and Purification of *Ulva* Polysaccharide

The extraction of the *Ulva* polysaccharide mainly used the common methods which were usually employed in the extraction of plant polysaccharides, especially the hot water extraction method [12,36]. The methods for extraction of *Ulva* polysaccharide have been summarized in Table 2. Xu et al. extracted the polysaccharide by incubation in hot water (90 °C) for 4 h and obtained 21.96% of polysaccharide [25]. Chattopadhyay et al. incubated the algal powder-water mixture at 80 °C for 1.5 h and extracted 18% of the crude polysaccharide [12]. The hot water extraction is the most commonly used method for preparation of plant polysaccharides. It could be operated easily and suitably for industrial scale application. However, the hot water extraction is time-consuming, and the extracted polysaccharides contained some soluble impurities. In order to improve the polysaccharide's purity, alcohol was usually added remove the impurity before the hot water extraction. Wu et al. incubated the algal powder with 95% of alcohol at 80 °C for 2 h to remove the substance with low molecular weight and the purity reached 70% [37]. In addition, pH change also could remove the small molecules and further improve the polysaccharide's purity. For instance, Sun et al. extracted the algal powder in 0.5 M of NaOH solution and incubated the mixture at 90 °C for 2 h. Finally, 33.3% of polysaccharide was obtained [38]. Song et al. incubated the sample in 0.05 M of HCl for 2 h and obtained 86.1% of soluble polysaccharide [39]. The addition of alcohol, acid or alkali could improve the purity of polysaccharide. Therefore, a combination of these agents could be tried in order to enhance the purity and improve the extraction efficiency. The ultrasonication could promote the dissolution of polysaccharide and has been widely used for extraction of *Ulva* polysaccharide [40]. Guo et al. extracted the polysaccharide under ultrasonication-treatment for 28 min and obtained 25.84 mg/g of crude polysaccharide [41]. Tang et al. obtained 17.42% of polysaccharide by incubation with ultrasonication of 531.17 W for 4.8 min [15]. However, the extraction efficiency of the ultrasonication method was not stable due to its short extraction time [42]. Furthermore, the microwave also has been used for extraction of *Ulva* polysaccharide due to its promotion of molecular motion [43]. Wang et al. used 610 W of microwave to assist the polysaccharide extraction and obtained 7.58% of crude polysaccharide [44]. Yuan et al. isolated the *Ulva* polysaccharide under 800 W of microwave and 95 °C, but only 4.04% of polysaccharide was obtained [45]. Therefore, microwave assistance could greatly reduce the extraction time, but could not promote the extraction yield and the purity of the polysaccharide [46,47]. The enzyme-assisted extraction method has drawn increasing attention due to its mild reaction condition and excellent extraction efficiency [48–50]. The protease and polysaccharide-degrading enzymes such as cellulase and pectin lyase could destroy the cell wall structure and promote the dissolution of polysaccharide [51]. Lü et al. added the protease into the extraction solution and obtained 27.75% of the polysaccharide [52]. Xu et al. used the cellulase to assist the extraction and the extraction ratio reached 20.22% [25]. However, a combination of different enzymes is needed to promote the extraction efficiency, and it also could increase the complexity of the reaction system. In conclusion, there are various methods for *Ulva* polysaccharide extraction and they all possess advantages and drawbacks. Therefore, it is reliable to combine these methods together to obtain the *Ulva* polysaccharide for further research. Because of the addition of enzymes, acid or alkali solution, the polysaccharide obtained by extraction needed to be purified for further structural characterization and activity investigation. At first, the protein could be removed by protease hydrolysis and Savage methods [40]. Then, the small substances produced by protein hydrolysis could be removed by dialysis. In order to obtain the purified polysaccharides, the ion exchange chromatography (IEC) and gel permeation chromatography (GPC) have usually been employed (Table 3) [53]. Qi et al. purified the *Ulva* polysaccharide from *Ulva linza* by Q Sepharose Fast Flow with NaCl as mobile phase and obtained five fractions [28,32]. Pan et al. purified four polysaccharide fractions from *Ulva intestinalis* by DEAE Sepharose Fast Flow with 0.5~1 M NaCl [54]. Jiao et al. used DEAE Sepharose CL-6B to purify the polysaccharide from *Ulva intestinalis*. In addition, the GPC has also been used for purification of *Ulva* polysaccharide [10]. Lü et al. purified two fractions by Sephadex G-100 with water as eluent [52] and Xu et al. used Sephadex G-75 to isolate the polysaccharide fractions by 1.0 mL·min^{-1} of H_2O [25]. In practice, the ICE and GPC have usually been used together to purify the polysaccharide with higher purity. Lin et al. first separated the polysaccharide by DEAE-Cellulose 52 with 0.7 M NaCl and then the eluate was further purified by Bio-Gel P-2 with 0.85 mL·min^{-1} of H_2O [55]. Tang et al. isolated the polysaccharide by DEAE-Sepharose CL-6B with 0.2~1.5 M NaCl and Sephadex G-200 with 0.85 mL·min^{-1} of H_2O, respectively [11]. In addition, with the development of chemical engineering, more new technologies have been employed to purify the *Ulva* polysaccharide [56,57]. For instance, an integrated membrane separation process combining the tubular ceramic microfiltration (MF) membrane and the flat-sheet ultrafiltration (UF) membrane was developed to purify polysaccharides from *Ulva prolifera,* and the results suggested that the content of oligosaccharides reached 96.3% after purification by this integrated membrane separation process [56]. However, there is no report of polysaccharide purification on a large scale, and commercial polysaccharide is very expensive. It is essential to develop appropriate methods for adequate separation and purification of *Ulva* polysaccharide for commercial and industrial applications.

Table 2. The summary of extraction of *Ulva* polysaccharide.

Extraction Method	Procedure Time	Yield	Recovery	Reference
Hot water extraction with Hot water (90 °C)	4 h	21.96%	-	[25]
Hot water extraction with Hot water (80 °C)	1.5 h	18%	-	[12]
Hot solution extraction with 95% of alcohol (80 °C)	2 h	-	70%	[37]
Hot alkaline solution extraction with 0.5 M NaOH (90 °C)	2 h	33.3%	-	[38]
Acidic solution extraction with 0.05 M HCl	2 h	86.1%		[39]
Ultrasonication treatment Ultrasonication treatment	28 min	25.84%	-	[41]
Ultrasonication treatment Ultrasonication (531.17 W)	4.8 min	17.42%	-	[15]
Ultrasonication treatment Ultrasonication (610 W)	-	-	7.58%	[44]
Ultrasonication treatment Ultrasonication (610 W)	-	-	4.04%	[45]
Enzymatic extraction with Protease	-	27.75%	-	[52]
Enzymatic extraction with Cellulase	-	20.22%	-	[25]

Table 3. The summary of purification of *Ulva* polysaccharide.

Purification Method	Column	Mobile Phase	Speed	Reference
IEC	Q Sepharose Fast Flow	0~2 M NaCl	0.5~2 mL/min	[31]
IEC	DEAE Sepharose Fast Flow	0~2 M NaCl	0.92 mL/min	[33]
IEC	DEAE Sepharose CL-6B	0.9%NaCl	0.18 mL/min	[35]
IEC	DEAE Cellulose 52	0.2~0.8 M NaCl	0.5 mL/min	[25]
IEC	DEAE Sephadex A-25	0~4 M NaCl	0.5 mL/min	[58]
GPC	Sephadex G-75	H_2O	1.0 mL/min	[25]
GPC	Sephadex G-100	H_2O	0.4 mL/min	[52]
GPC	SephacryTm S-300 HR	0.9% NaCl	0.5 mL/min	[58]
GPC	Sephacryl S-300 HR	0.2 M NH_4HCO_3	0.5 mL/min	[30]
GPC	Sephacryl S-400/HR	0.2 M NH_4HCO_3	0.3 mL/min	[28]
IEC+GPC	DEAE Cellulose 52, Bio-Gel P-2	0.7 M NaCl	0.85 mL/min	[40]
IEC+GPC	DEAE-Sepharose CL-6B, Sephadex G-200	0.2~1.5 M NaCl	0.8 mL/min	[11]

2.3. *Activity of Ulva Polysaccharide*

The activity of *Ulva* polysaccharide has been symmetrically investigated and characterized, and this green algal polysaccharide exhibited diverse biological activities such as antioxidant, antitumor, immunomodulatory, anticoagulant and hypolipidemic activities [11].

2.3.1. Antioxidant Activity

Many algal polysaccharides such as alginate, carrageenan and agar possessed obvious antioxidant activity by cleaning the oxidant radicals and improving antioxidant enzymes' activity [22]. Xu et al. evaluated the antioxidant activities of *Ulva* polysaccharide by determining their ability to scavenge 1, 1-diphenyl-2-picrylhydrazyl (DPPH), hydroxyl ($OH^{\bullet}$), and superoxide anion ($O_2^{\bullet-}$) radicals [25]. The results suggested that the *Ulva* polysaccharide could clean up DPPH, $OH^{\bullet}$, and $O_2^{\bullet-}$ [25]. It could also improve the activities of endogenous antioxidant enzymes such as catalase, glutathione peroxidase, and superoxide dismutase, which have been viewed as the major defense system against ROS during oxidative stress [40]. Moreover, Tang et al. found that the polysaccharides could reduce the content of maleic dialdehyde (MDA) in serum. The low MDA levels resulted in lower oxidant stress and lipid peroxidation [11].

2.3.2. Antitumor Activity

The antitumor activity of *Ulva* polysaccharide has aroused increasing interest due to the tumor's multiplicity worldwide [59,60]. Jiao et al. found that polysaccharides could inhibit tumor growth in S180 tumor-bearing mice, and could increase the relative spleen and thymus weight [10]. They also promoted the expression of tumor necrosis factor-alpha (TNF-α) in serum and induced lymphocyte proliferation, induced the production of TNF-α in macrophages, and stimulated macrophages to produce nitric oxide dose-dependently through the up-regulation of inducible NO synthase activity [35]. The *Ulva* polysaccharide could motivate modulation of the immune system to indirectly inhibit tumor cells without direct cytotoxicity [61].

2.3.3. Immune Regulatory Activity

The immune system includes nonspecific and specific immunity [62]. Nonspecific immunity can immediately respond to invaders without encountering previous pathogens, and gives signals to subsequently activate adaptive specific immunity [63]. Specific immunity involves B- and T-lymphocytes, and its function is activated immediately after the initial antigenic stimulus [64]. The *Ulva* polysaccharide can significantly increase the relative spleen and thymus weight of tumor-bearing animals, promote the secretion of tumor necrosis factor alpha (TNF-α), stimulate lymphocyte proliferation, and augment phagocytosis and secretion of NO and TNF-α in peritoneal macrophages [65]. In addition, the *Ulva* polysaccharide could promote the proliferation of B lymphocytes and T lymphocytes, activate the NK cell and induce the delayed apoptosis of neutrophils, as shown in Figure 4. More specifically, the polysaccharides could increase the production of reactive oxygen species (ROS), IL-6, and TNF-α through regulating the expressions of iNOS, IL-6, and TNF-α. In addition, the polysaccharides can strengthen the macrophage phagocytic activity, activate NK cells, increase thymus and spleen indices, and delay neutrophil apoptosis [7,66] (Figure 4).

2.3.4. Anticoagulant Activity

It has been reported that polysaccharides from green alga have been investigated, showing stronger anticoagulant activities than those from brown and red alga [28,67,68]. Wang et al. investigated and elucidated the anticoagulant activity of polysaccharide from green algae *Ulva linza* in the coagulation assays, and activated partial thromboplastin time (APTT), thrombin time (TT) and prothrombin time (PT) [69]. The results suggested that the sulfated polysaccharides could prolong APTT and TT, but not TP. These activities strongly depended on the degree of sulfation (DS), the molecular weights (MW) and the branching structure of polysaccharides [69]. Qi et al. evaluated the anticoagulant activity of polysaccharides from *Ulva clathrata* and an in vitro anticoagulant assay indicated that FEP effectively prolonged the activated partial thromboplastin time and thrombin time [28,32].

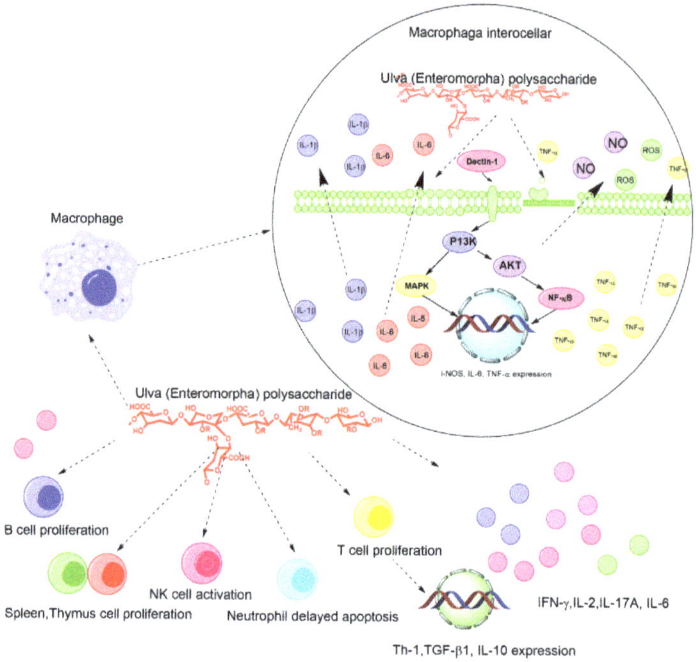

Figure 4. The schematic diagram of the immune regulatory and antitumor mechanism of *Ulva* polysaccharides on the molecular and cellular level.

2.3.5. Hypolipidemic Activity

Hyperlipidemia, as a common endocrine disease, induces cerebrovascular and cardiovascular activity and atherosclerosis [70,71]. While hypolipidemic drugs such as statins prevent and cure hyperlipidemia, their side effects cannot be ignored [70]. Teng et al. reported that *Ulva prolifera* polysaccharides presented high anti-hyperlipidemic activities which inhibited the body weight gain and also decreased triacylglycerol (TG), the total cholesterol (TC), and low-density lipoprotein cholesterol (LDL-C) levels of plasma and liver [72]. They also inhibited the expressions of sterol regulatory element-binding protein-1c (SREBP-1c) and hepatic acetyl-CoA carboxylase (ACC) in high-fat diet rats. SREBP-1c enhances the transcription of the required genes for fatty acid synthesis [72]. ACC, as the rate-limiting enzyme in de-novo lipogenesis, controls the β-oxidation of fatty acids in the mitochondria. Moreover, *Ulva prolifera* polysaccharides showed pancreatic lipase inhibition activity [45]. The polysaccharide from *Ulva prolifera* exhibited a stronger hypolipidemic effect than simvastatin and enhanced endogenous antioxidant enzymes and decreased MDA content and lipid peroxidation in serum [72,73].

3. Ulva Oligosaccharides

The *Ulva* polysaccharide which acted as the main component of *Ulva* sp. has attracted increasing attention in the algal bioresources field. As discussed above, the reports of extraction, isolation, purification, structural characterization and physiological activity of this polysaccharide have increased year after year. In addition, the techniques for extracting the polysaccharide have developed rapidly on an industrial scale, and this advance established a solid foundation for the wide application of *Ulva* polysaccharides. However, the applications of polysaccharide for the food and medical industries have been greatly restricted by its high molecular weight and low solubility, so the degradation of polysaccharide into oligosaccharides has been the area of emerging focus in utilization of *Ulva* polysaccharide bioresources.

3.1. Preparation of *Ulva* Oligosaccharides

The *Ulva* oligosaccharides retained the versatile activities of polysaccharide and were found to possess excellent solubility and bioavailability, and they have drawn increasing attention from scientists from the food and medical fields [23]. The preparation of *Ulva* oligosaccharides mainly depended on physical degradation, chemical hydrolysis and enzymatic preparation, as shown in Table 4 [22]. Similar to the preparation of other algal oligosaccharides such as alginate oligosaccharides and carrageenan oligosaccharides, the microwave-assisted method has been widely used. Li et al. prepared *Ulva* oligosaccharides by a microwave-assisted acid hydrolysis method and the results showed that only glycosidic linkages were left without breaking significant structural units [74]. Duan et al. degraded *Ulva* polysaccharide with HCl and assisted by microwave. The optimal degradation conditions were 900 W at 50 °C for 10 min with 5% H_2O_2 in 1 mol/L hydrochloric acid solution by single factor and orthogonal experiments [75]. Zhang et al. used the ascorbic acid and H_2O_2 as degradation reagents to degrade the polysaccharides in order to obtain the lower molecular weight products. The enzymatic preparation of *Ulva* oligosaccharides has been the research focus due to its advantages such as mild reaction conditions, specific products' distribution, etc [26].

Table 4. The summary of methods for preparation of *Ulva* oligosaccharides.

Preparation Method	Structure	Molecular Weight	Bioactivities	Reference
Microwave-assisted acid hydrolysis	-	3.1 kDa	Antioxidant activity	[76]
Microwave-assisted acid hydrolysis	-	53.59 kDa	Antioxidant activity	[75]
H_2O_2 degradation	-	-	Antioxidant activity	[26]
Enzymatic degradation	-	243, 341, 401, 503, 665 Da	-	[77]
Enzymatic degradation	-	103, 45.4, 9.8 kDa	Antioxidant activity	[25]
Enzymatic degradation	$Rha_1(SO_3H)_1$, $Rha_1(SO_3H)_1Glc_1$, $Rha_2(SO_3H)_2Glc_1$, $Rha_3(SO_3H)_3Glc_1Xyl_1$	244, 402, 628, 760 Da	-	[78]

Zhang et al. degraded the *Ulva* polysaccharide by degrading enzymes produced by *Alteromonas* sp. A321 and the oligosaccharides yield reached 61.21% [77]. Xu et al. degraded *Ulva* polysaccharide by the addition of pectin lyase (9.6 U/mL) and obtained oligosaccharides with different molecular weights [25]. Surprisingly, there are no reports of the gene information for specific enzymes which could degrade the *Ulva* polysaccharide. As we know, other algal polysaccharides such as alginate, agar, and carrageenan could be specifically degraded by the respective enzymes, namely alginate lyases, agarases and carrageenases. Li et al. screened and identified a new *Ulva* polysaccharide-degrading strain *Alteromonas* sp. A321 from the rotten green algae [76,78]. They characterized the enzymes produced by *Alteromonas* sp. A321 and sequenced the N-terminal of them [76,78]. However, it was unable to be determined whether the two enzymes belonged to polysaccharide lyase or glycosidic hydrolase. Therefore, further and systematic research is required to investigate and elucidate this question.

3.2. Separation and Purification of *Ulva* Oligosaccharides

The methods used for separation and purification of *Ulva* oligosaccharides are similar with the methods for purification of *Ulva* polysaccharides. Xu et al. sequentially purified the *Ulva* oligosaccharides by DEAE Cellulose-52 chromatography and Sephadex G-100 chromatography. In addition, the molecular weights of these three fractions were measured to be 103, 45.4, and 9.8 kDa, respectively, using high performance gel permeation chromatography (HPGPC) [25]. Lü et al. purified the degraded polysaccharide by Sephadex G-100 with water as eluent, and obtained a yield of 40.00% [52]. Li et al. employed a TSK G4000-PWxl column, using 0.05 M $NaNO_3$ aqueous solution as the mobile phase at a flow rate of 0.5 mL/min with a column temperature of 30 °C to purify the degraded *Ulva* [76].

According to the examples discussed above, the purification methods of *Ulva* oligosaccharides seemed similar to the polysaccharides purification procedure, but the purpose of polysaccharide purification is to remove the impurities from the polysaccharide system, while the target of oligosaccharide purification is to separate the oligosaccharide fraction from the mixture. Therefore, it is more difficult to obtain the oligosaccharide monomer since the methods for polysaccharides' purification have developed, and it is promising for researchers to find more suitable methods for purification of *Ulva* oligosaccharides.

3.3. Activity of Ulva Oligosaccharides

So far, more and more studies are focusing on the activity of *Ulva* oligosaccharides [22,23]. However, the current reports are still very scattered with the mechanism of related activity and the structural-activity relationship of oligosaccharides was still undefined due to the complexity of the *Ulva* oligosaccharides' structure. Lü et al. evaluated the antibacterial activity of *Ulva* oligosaccharides and their selenized derivatives prepared by acid method [52]. They found that the selenized *Ulva* oligosaccharides showed stronger inhibitory activity towards *Eschetichia coli* and plant pathogenic fungi than that to *Staphylococcus aureus* [52,79]. Liu et al. studied the anti-aging and anti-oxidation effects of *Ulva* oligosaccharides in SAMP8 mice [23]. They found that *Ulva* oligosaccharides can protect neurons in the hippocampus by significantly reducing the secretion of inflammatory factors such as IFN-γ, TNF-α and IL-6, and improving the brain-derived neurotrophic factor (BDNF) [23]. Liu et al. evaluated the immunoregulatory effect of *Ulva* oligosaccharides in a cyclophosphamide-induced immunosuppression mouse model [80]. It can be found that *Ulva* oligosaccharides can activate the immune system by promoting the secretion of NO, up-regulating the expression of cytokines such as IL-1β, IL-6 and TNF-α, and activating inflammatory bodies such as iNOS, COX2 and NLRP3 [80]. Xu et al. studied the antioxidant activities of three *Ulva* oligosaccharides, and found that *Ulva* oligosaccharides can effectively eliminate the DPPH, $OH^{\bullet}$, and $O_2{}^{\bullet-}$ [25]. Li et al. investigated the antioxidant capacity of *Ulva* oligosaccharides and found that the activity was closely related to molecular weight [74]. Specifically, *Ulva* oligosaccharides with low molecular weight can scavenge superoxide anion and hydroxyl radicals with an IC50 of 0.39 mg/mL [74]. Zhang et al. found that 2.28 mg/mL of *Ulva* oligosaccharides prepared by an H_2O_2 oxidation method can scavenge 92.2% of the hydroxyl radical, which is higher than *Ulva* polysaccharides with the same concentration [26]. That is probably because there were more hydroxyl groups in the oligosaccharides' structure [26]. Cui et al. prepared complexes of Fe^{2+} ions and *Ulva* oligosaccharides, which can be used to treat iron deficiency anemia as a nutritional supplement for iron [81]. Wang et al. discovered that *Ulva* oligosaccharides possessed an anticoagulant activity which was closely related to the number and distribution of sulfuric acid groups in oligosaccharides [69]. Jin et al. prepared ep-3-H, a glucuronic-xylo-rhamnose-component, from *Ulva* prolifera, and found that EP-3-H could inhibit cell proliferation of human lung cancer cells by interacting with the fibroblast growth factors FGF1 and FGF2 [82]. In addition, the physiological activities may differ in *Ulva* oligosaccharides and polysaccharides, but the specific mechanism still remains unclear. However, we could propose the possible reasons based on some experience. The active groups appeared after the linkage of the polysaccharide was broken down by physical, chemical or enzymatic hydrolysis, and therefore the activities of *Ulva* oligosaccharide became more obvious than the polysaccharide. To sum up, the current studies on the activity of *Ulva* oligosaccharides are relatively superficial since there is still no appropriate method to obtain oligosaccharides with a fine structure for studying the structure-activity relationship of oligosaccharides due to their quite complex structure.

4. Conclusions and Future Perspective

In recent years, the biomass of *Ulva* has increased rapidly worldwide, resulting in a large number of green tides [4,80,83]. Actually, *Ulva prolifera* has invaded the Yellow Sea for 15 consecutively years, which has damaged the marine ecological environment in

Qingdao and the coastal cities of Shandong Province. It is therefore urgent to effectively curb the growth of *Ulva prolifera* and achieve the harmless and high-value utilization of *Enteromorpha prolifera* [84–86] (as shown in Figure 5). For instance, the *Ulva* polysaccharide and oligosaccharide could eliminate the oxidative radicals such as DPPH, $OH^{\bullet}$, and $O_2^{\bullet-}$, and they could also promote the proliferation of probiotics of intestinal microbiome composition. In addition, the *Ulva* polysaccharide exhibited obvious hypolipidemic activity; therefore, the *Ulva* polysaccharide and oligosaccharide can be used as a functional food, a food additive, an antioxidant agent, and animal feed. Due to its excellent rheological properties, gelling behavior, texture characteristics and antibacterial activity, the *Ulva* polysaccharide could be developed as a novel medical dressing to prevent bacterial infection. More importantly, the *Ulva* polysaccharide and oligosaccharide both possess obvious physiological activities such as immune regulatory, antitumor, anticoagulant and hypolipidemic activities, they are important resources for developing novel marine drugs for curing various malignant tumors, and they are used in the treatment of hyperlipidemia, hypertension and other metabolic diseases. This kind of carbohydrate that originated from green algae has drawn increasing attentions and became a topic of much discussion in the marine bioresources and functional foods fields.

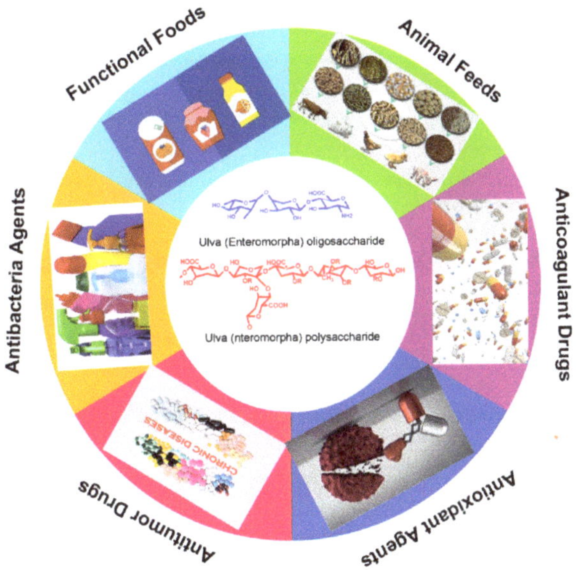

Figure 5. The potential and promising applications of *Ulva* polysaccharide and oligosaccharides.

Ulva polysaccharide, as the main active ingredient of the *Ulva* species, can be used to develop new foods, medicine and health care products. At present, it is easy to extract *Ulva* polysaccharides at a large-scale level. Nevertheless, it still cannot meet the requirements of high-value utilization due to its low purity. So it is now one of the areas of intensive research to find out how to prepare *Ulva* polysaccharides with high purity. On the other hand, the solubility and bioavailability of *Ulva* polysaccharides is restrained by their high molecular weight (>400 kDa), which has further limited the biological activity and application of *Ulva* polysaccharides. It is therefore another area of focus to prepare *Ulva* oligosaccharides with *Ulva* polysaccharides degrading enzymes. In addition, it is still a great challenge to analyze the structure of *Ulva* polysaccharides and *Ulva* oligosaccharides due to the complex and diverse monosaccharide composition and glycosidic bond connection modes in *Ulva* polysaccharides. Therefore, it is of great significance to accurately analyze the fine structure of *Ulva* polysaccharides and oligosaccharides, which will promote the study of the structure-activity relationship and the high value utilization of *Ulva* polysaccharides and oligosaccharides. In addition there is a long history of humans utilizing the *Ulva* bioresources for food, and some beneficial foods such as biscuits, noodles and vegetarian meatballs have been developed. However, the applications of *Ulva* polysaccharide and oligosaccharide as functional foods have not been realized until now because the studies of the activity and function of the *Ulva* polysaccharide and oligosaccharide are ongoing. We believe that the *Ulva* polysaccharide and oligosaccharide could be used as a functional food such as the alginate oligosaccharides in the near future when we have obtained an adequate understanding of them.

Author Contributions: L.N. and B.Z.: Conceptualization, Writing-original draft. B.Z.: Funding acquisition. B.Z. and Z.Y.: Writing-review & editing. Z.Y.: Supervision. All authors have read and agreed to the published version of the manuscript.

Funding: The work was supported by the Jiangsu Government Scholarship for Overseas Studies, the Postdoctoral Research Foundation of Jiangsu Province (2021K374C), National Natural Science Foundation of China (31601410), The Suqian City Science and Technology Project (L201906).

Institutional Review Board Statement: This article does not contain any studies involving human participants or animals performed by any of the authors.

Data Availability Statement: Not applicable.

Acknowledgments: Ning Limin gratefully acknowledges the support of Jiangsu Government Scholarship for Overseas Studies, and Zhu Benwei gratefully acknowledges the support of Jiangsu Overseas Visiting Scholar Program for University Prominent Young and Mid-aged Teachers and Presidents.

Conflicts of Interest: The authors declare that they have no known competing financial interests or personal relationships that could have appeared to influence the work reported in this paper.

References

1. Blomster, J.; Bäck, S.; Fewer, D.P.; Kiirikki, M.; Lehvo, A.; Maggs, C.A.; Stanhope, M.J. Novel morphology in *Enteromorpha* (Ulvophyceae) forming green tides. *Am. J. Bot.* **2002**, *89*, 1756–1763. [CrossRef]
2. Zhong, L.; Zhang, J.; Ding, Y. Energy Utilization of Algae Biomass Waste Enteromorpha Resulting in Green Tide in China: Pyrolysis Kinetic Parameters Estimation Based on Shuffled Complex Evolution. *Sustainability* **2020**, *12*, 2086. [CrossRef]
3. Silveira Coelho, M.; da Silva Menezes, B.; Rivero Meza, S.L.; Lainetti Gianasi, B.; de las Mercedes Salas-Mellado, M.; Copertino, M.; da Rosa Andrade Zimmermann de Souza, M. Potential Utilization of Green Tide-Forming Macroalgae from Patos Lagoon, Rio Grande-RS, Brazil. *J. Aquat. Food Prod. Technol.* **2016**, *25*, 1096–1106. [CrossRef]
4. Van Alstyne, K.L.; Nelson, T.A.; Ridgway, R.L. Environmental Chemistry and Chemical Ecology of "Green Tide" Seaweed Blooms. *Integr. Comp. Biol.* **2015**, *55*, 518–532. [CrossRef]
5. Wang, Z.; Xiao, J.; Fan, S.; Li, Y.; Liu, X.; Liu, D. Who made the world's largest green tide in China?—An integrated study on the initiation and early development of the green tide in Yellow Sea. *Limnol. Oceanogr.* **2015**, *60*, 1105–1117. [CrossRef]
6. Yabe, T.; Ishii, Y.; Amano, Y.; Koga, T.; Hayashi, S.; Nohara, S.; Tatsumoto, H. Green tide formed by free-floating Ulva spp. at Yatsu tidal flat, Japan. *Limnology* **2009**, *10*, 239–245. [CrossRef]
7. Zhang, W.; Oda, T.; Yu, Q.; Jin, J.-O. Fucoidan from Macrocystis pyrifera Has Powerful Immune-Modulatory Effects Compared to Three Other Fucoidans. *Mar. Drugs* **2015**, *13*, 1084–1104. [CrossRef]
8. Xiao, J.; Wang, Z.; Liu, D.; Fu, M.; Yuan, C.; Yan, T. Harmful macroalgal blooms (HMBs) in China's coastal water: Green and golden tides. *Harmful Algae* **2021**, *107*, 102061. [CrossRef]
9. Hayden, H.S.; Blomster, J.; Maggs, C.A.; Silva, P.C.; Stanhope, M.J.; Waaland, J.R. Linnaeus was right all along: Ulva and Enteromorpha are not distinct genera. *Eur. J. Phycol.* **2003**, *38*, 277–294. [CrossRef]
10. Jiao, L.; Jiang, P.; Zhang, L.; Wu, M. Antitumor and immunomodulating activity of polysaccharides from Enteromorpha intestinalis. *Biotechnol. Bioprocess Eng.* **2010**, *15*, 421–428. [CrossRef]
11. Tang, Z.; Gao, H.; Wang, S.; Wen, S.; Qin, S. Hypolipidemic and antioxidant properties of a polysaccharide fraction from Enteromorpha prolifera. *Int. J. Biol. Macromol.* **2013**, *58*, 186–189. [CrossRef]
12. Chattopadhyay, K.; Mandal, P.; Lerouge, P.; Driouich, A.; Ghosal, P.; Ray, B. Sulphated polysaccharides from Indian samples of *Enteromorpha compressa* (Ulvales, Chlorophyta): Isolation and structural features. *Food Chem.* **2007**, *104*, 928–935. [CrossRef]
13. Jiang, F.; Chi, Z.; Ding, Y.; Quan, M.; Tian, Y.; Shi, J.; Liu, C. Wound Dressing Hydrogel of Enteromorpha prolifera Polysaccharide–Polyacrylamide Composite: A Facile Transformation of Marine Blooming into Biomedical Material. *ACS Appl. Mater. Interfaces* **2021**, *13*, 14530–14542. [CrossRef]
14. Zhong, R.; Wan, X.; Wang, D.; Zhao, C.; Liu, D.; Gao, L.; Cao, H. Polysaccharides from Marine Enteromorpha: Structure and function. *Trends Food Sci. Technol.* **2020**, *99*, 11–20. [CrossRef]

15. Tang, Z.; Yu, Z.; Zhao, W.; Guo, J.; Gao, L.; Qin, S. Ultrasonic extraction of polysaccharides from Enteromorpha. *Mod. Food Sci. Technol.* **2011**, *27*, 56–59.
16. Liu, W.; Zhou, S.; Balasubramanian, B.; Zeng, F.; Sun, C.; Pang, H. Dietary seaweed (Enteromorpha) polysaccharides improves growth performance involved in regulation of immune responses, intestinal morphology and microbial community in banana shrimp Fenneropenaeus merguiensis. *Fish Shellfish. Immunol.* **2020**, *104*, 202–212. [CrossRef]
17. Shang, Q.; Wang, Y.; Pan, L.; Niu, Q.; Li, C.; Jiang, H.; Cai CHao, J.; Li, G.; Yu, G. Dietary Polysaccharide from Enteromorpha Clathrata Modulates Gut Microbiota and Promotes the Growth of Akkermansia muciniphila, Bifidobacterium spp. and Lactobacillus spp. *Mar. Drugs* **2018**, *16*, 167. [CrossRef]
18. Xie, C.; Zhang, Y.; Niu, K.; Liang, X.; Wang, H.; Shan, J.; Wu, X. Enteromorpha polysaccharide-zinc replacing prophylactic antibiotics contributes to improving gut health of weaned piglets. *Anim. Nutr.* **2021**, *7*, 641–649. [CrossRef]
19. Guo, F.; Han, M.; Lin, S.; Ye, H.; Chen, J.; Zhu, H.; Lin, W. Enteromorpha prolifera polysaccharide prevents high-fat diet-induced obesity in hamsters: A NMR-based metabolomic evaluation. *J. Food Sci.* **2021**, *86*, 3672–3685. [CrossRef]
20. Guo, F.; Zhuang, X.; Han, M.; Lin, W. Polysaccharides from Enteromorpha prolifera protect against carbon tetrachloride-induced acute liver injury in mice via activation of Nrf2/HO-1 signaling, and suppression of oxidative stress, inflammation and apoptosis. *Food Funct.* **2020**, *11*, 4485–4498. [CrossRef]
21. Li, X.; Guozhu, Z.; Zhifei, L.; Yang, S.; Peijun, L.; Jing, L. Hypoglycemic activity of Enteromorpha intestinalis polysaccharide. *Sci. Technol. Food Ind.* **2021**, *42*, 321–326. [CrossRef]
22. Zhu, B.; Ni, F.; Xiong, Q.; Yao, Z. Marine oligosaccharides originated from seaweeds: Source, preparation, structure, physiological activity and applications. *Crit. Rev. Food Sci. Nutr.* **2021**, *61*, 60–74. [CrossRef]
23. Liu, X.; Liu, D.; Lin, G.; Wu, Y.; Gao, L.; Ai, C.; Zhao, C. Anti-ageing and antioxidant effects of sulfate oligosaccharides from green algae Ulva lactuca and Enteromorpha prolifera in SAMP8 mice. *Int. J. Biol. Macromol.* **2019**, *139*, 342–351. [CrossRef]
24. Shao, L.; Xu, J.; Shi, M.; Wang, X.; Li, Y.; Kong, L.; Hider, R.; Zhou, T. Preparation, antioxidant and antimicrobial evaluation of hydroxamated degraded polysaccharides from Enteromorpha prolifera. *Food Chem.* **2017**, *237*, 481–487. [CrossRef]
25. Xu, J.; Xu, L.; Zhou, Q.; Hao, S.; Zhou, T.; Xie, H. Isolation, purification, and antioxidant activities of degraded polysaccharides from Enteromorpha prolifera. *Int. J. Biol. Macromol.* **2015**, *81*, 1026–1030. [CrossRef]
26. Zhang, Z.; Wang, X.; Mo, X.; Qi, H. Degradation and the antioxidant activity of polysaccharide from *Enteromorpha linza*. *Carbohydr. Polym.* **2013**, *92*, 2084–2087. [CrossRef]
27. Cho, M.; Yang, C.; Kim, S.M.; You, S. Molecular characterization and biological activities of watersoluble sulfated polysaccharides from *Enteromorpha prolifera*. *Food Sci. Biotechnol.* **2010**, *19*, 525–533. [CrossRef]
28. Qi, X.; Mao, W.; Gao, Y.; Chen, Y.; Chen, Y.; Zhao, C.; Shan, J. Chemical characteristic of an anticoagulant-active sulfated polysaccharide from *Enteromorpha clathrata*. *Carbohydr. Polym.* **2012**, *90*, 1804–1810. [CrossRef]
29. Ray, B. Polysaccharides from *Enteromorpha compressa*: Isolation, purification and structural features. *Carbohydr. Polym.* **2006**, *66*, 408–416. [CrossRef]
30. Yu, Y.; Li, Y.; Du, C.; Mou, H.; Wang, P. Compositional and structural characteristics of sulfated polysaccharide from *Enteromorpha prolifera*. *Carbohydr. Polym.* **2017**, *165*, 221–228. [CrossRef]
31. Qi, X.; Li, H.; Guo, S.; Chen, Y.; Chen, Y.; Xu, J.; Mao, W. Isolation and composition analysis of the polysaccharides from the green algae *Enteromorpha prolifera* collected in different seasons and sea areas. *Period. Ocean. Univ. China* **2010**, *40*, 7–12.
32. Qi, X.; Mao, W.; Chen, Y.; Chen, Y.; Zhao, C.; Li, N.; Wang, C. Chemical characteristics and anticoagulant activities of two sulfated polysaccharides from *Enteromorpha linza* (Chlorophyta). *J. Ocean. Univ. China* **2013**, *12*, 175–182. [CrossRef]
33. Shi, X. *Investigation of Chemical Composition and Biological Activities of Polysaccharides from Enteromorpha*; Institute of Oceanology, Chinese Academy of Sciences: Qingdao, China, 2009.
34. Ji, G.; Yu, G.; Wu, J.; Zhao, X.; Yang, B.; Wang, L.; Mei, X. Extraction, isolation and physiochemical character studies of polysaccharides from *Enteromorpha clathrata* in outbreak period. *Chin. J. Mar. Drugs* **2009**, *28*, 7–12.
35. Jiao, L.; Li, X.; Li, T.; Jiang, P.; Zhang, L.; Wu, M.; Zhang, L. Characterization and anti-tumor activity of alkali-extracted polysaccharide from *Enteromorpha intestinalis*. *Int. Immunopharmacol.* **2009**, *9*, 324–329. [CrossRef] [PubMed]
36. Li, X.; Xiong, F.; Liu, Y.; Liu, F.; Hao, Z.; Chen, H. Total fractionation and characterization of the water-soluble polysaccharides isolated from *Enteromorpha intestinalis*. *Int. J. Biol. Macromol.* **2018**, *111*, 319–325. [CrossRef]
37. Wu, M.; Jiao, L.; Sun, Y.; Li, T.; Zhang, L. Isolation purification and analysis on the EPIII of polysaccharide of *Enteromorpha*. *J. Northeast Nor. Univ.* **2007**, *39*, 97–100.
38. Sun, S. Study on lowering blood lipid of Polysaccharide from *Enteromorpha prolifera* by alkali extraction. *Chin. J. Mod. Drug Appl.* **2010**, *4*, 118–119.
39. Song, X.; Guo, X.; Zhou, W.; Wen, Y.; Zhu, C.; Yang, H. Composition and biological activity of water-soluble polysaccharide from *Enteromorpha prolifera*. *Lishizhen Med. Mater. Med. Res.* **2010**, *21*, 2448–2450.
40. Lin, G.; Wu, D.; Xiao, X.; Huang, Q.; Chen, H.; Liu, D.; Zhao, C. Structural characterization and antioxidant effect of green alga Enteromorpha prolifera polysaccharide in *Caenorhabditis elegans* via modulation of microRNAs. *Int. J. Biol. Macromol.* **2020**, *150*, 1084–1092. [CrossRef]
41. Guo, L.; Chen, Y. Optimization of ultrasonic-assisted extraction of polysaccharides from *Enteromorpha prolifera* by response surface methodology. *Food Sci.* **2010**, *31*, 117–121.

42. Yang, B.; Zhao, M.; Jiang, Y. Anti-glycated activity of polysaccharides of longan (*Dimocarpus longan Lour.*) fruit pericarp treated by ultrasonication. *Food Chem.* **2009**, *114*, 629–633. [CrossRef]
43. Zhou, C.; Ma, H. Ultrasonic Degradation of Polysaccharide from a Red Algae (*Porphyra yezoensis*). *J. Agric. Food Chem.* **2006**, *54*, 2223–2228. [CrossRef] [PubMed]
44. Wang, B.; Tong, G.Z.; Qu, Y.L.; Li, L. Microwave-Assisted Extraction and In Vitro Antioxidant Evaluation of Polysaccharides from *Enteromorpha prolifera*. *Appl. Mech. Mater.* **2011**, *79*, 204–209. [CrossRef]
45. Yuan, Y.; Xu, X.; Jing, C.; Zou, P.; Zhang, C.; Li, Y. Microwave assisted hydrothermal extraction of polysaccharides from *Ulva prolifera*: Functional properties and bioactivities. *Carbohydr. Polym.* **2018**, *181*, 902–910. [CrossRef] [PubMed]
46. Abdullah Al-Dhabi, N.; Ponmurugan, K. Microwave assisted extraction and characterization of polysaccharide from waste jamun fruit seeds. *Int. J. Biol. Macromol.* **2020**, *152*, 1157–1163. [CrossRef]
47. Rostami, H.; Gharibzahedi, S.M.T. Microwave-assisted extraction of jujube polysaccharide: Optimization, purification and functional characterization. *Carbohydr. Polym.* **2016**, *143*, 100–107. [CrossRef]
48. Guo, Y.; Shang, H.; Zhao, J.; Zhang, H.; Chen, S. Enzyme-assisted extraction of a cup plant (*Silphium perfoliatum* L.) Polysaccharide and its antioxidant and hypoglycemic activities. *Process Biochem.* **2020**, *92*, 17–28. [CrossRef]
49. Nadar, S.S.; Rao, P.; Rathod, V.K. Enzyme assisted extraction of biomolecules as an approach to novel extraction technology: A review. *Food Res. Int.* **2018**, *108*, 309–330. [CrossRef]
50. Song, X.; Xu, Q.; Zhou, Y.; Lin, C.; Yang, H. Growth, feed utilization and energy budgets of the sea cucumber Apostichopus japonicus with different diets containing the green tide macroalgae *Chaetomorpha linum* and the seagrass *Zostera marina*. *Aquaculture* **2017**, *470*, 157–163. [CrossRef]
51. Xiong, Q.; Song, Z.; Hu, W.; Liang, J.; Jing, Y.; He, L.; Li, S. Methods of extraction, separation, purification, structural characterization for polysaccharides from aquatic animals and their major pharmacological activities. *Crit. Rev. Food Sci. Nutr.* **2020**, *60*, 48–63. [CrossRef]
52. Lü, H.; Gao, Y.; Shan, H.; Lin, Y. Preparation and antibacterial activity studies of degraded polysaccharide selenide from *Enteromorpha prolifera*. *Carbohydr. Polym.* **2014**, *107*, 98–102. [CrossRef] [PubMed]
53. Ren, R.; Yang, Z.; Zhao, A.; Huang, Y.; Lin, S.; Gong, J.; Lin, W. Sulfated polysaccharide from *Enteromorpha prolifera* increases hydrogen sulfide production and attenuates non-alcoholic fatty liver disease in high-fat diet rats. *Food Funct.* **2018**, *9*, 4376–4383. [CrossRef] [PubMed]
54. Pan, X.; Wu, H.; Pan, M.; Zhang, Y.; Wei, X.; Cheng, J. Separation, purification and component analysis of *Enteromorpha polysaccharides* from Jiangsu. *Chin. J. New Drugs* **2019**, *28*, 2274–2278.
55. Lin, W.; Wang, W.; Liao, D.; Chen, D.; Zhu, P.; Cai, G.; Kiyoshi, A. Polysaccharides from *Enteromorpha prolifera* improve glucose metabolism in diabetic rats. *J. Diabetes Res.* **2015**, *2015*, 675201. [CrossRef] [PubMed]
56. Shao, W.; Zhang, H.; Duan, R.; Xie, Q.; Hong, Z.; Xiao, Z. A rapid and scalable integrated membrane separation process for purification of polysaccharides from *Enteromorpha prolifera*. *Nat. Prod. Res.* **2019**, *33*, 3109–3119. [CrossRef] [PubMed]
57. Zhao, S.; Gao, B.; Yue, Q.; Song, W.; Jia, R.; Liu, P. RETRACTED: Evaluation of floc properties and membrane fouling in coagulation–ultrafiltration system: The role of *Enteromorpha* polysaccharides. *Desalination* **2015**, *367*, 126–133. [CrossRef]
58. Xu, J.; Xu, L.-L.; Zhou, Q.-W.; Hao, S.-X.; Zhou, T.; Xie, H.-J. Enhanced in Vitro Antioxidant Activity of Polysaccharides From Enteromorpha Prolifera by Enzymatic Degradation. *J. Food Biochem.* **2016**, *40*, 275–283. [CrossRef]
59. Minton, N.P. Clostridia in cancer therapy. *Nat. Rev. Microbiol.* **2003**, *1*, 237–242. [CrossRef]
60. Sawyers, C. Targeted cancer therapy. *Nature* **2004**, *432*, 294–297. [CrossRef]
61. Kim, J.-K.; Cho, M.L.; Karnjanapratum, S.; Shin, I.-S.; You, S.G. In vitro and in vivo immunomodulatory activity of sulfated polysaccharides from *Enteromorpha prolifera*. *Int. J. Biol. Macromol.* **2011**, *49*, 1051–1058. [CrossRef]
62. Delves, P.J.; Roitt, I.M. The Immune System. *N. Engl. J. Med.* **2000**, *343*, 37–49. [CrossRef] [PubMed]
63. Parkin, J.; Cohen, B. An overview of the immune system. *Lancet* **2001**, *357*, 1777–1789. [CrossRef]
64. Levy, M.; Kolodziejczyk, A.A.; Thaiss, C.A.; Elinav, E. Dysbiosis and the immune system. *Nat. Rev. Immunol.* **2017**, *17*, 219–232. [CrossRef] [PubMed]
65. Ren, X.; Liu, L.; Gamallat, Y.; Zhang, B.; Xin, Y. Enteromorpha and polysaccharides from *Enteromorpha* ameliorate loperamide-induced constipation in mice. *Biomed. Pharmacother.* **2017**, *96*, 1075–1081. [CrossRef] [PubMed]
66. Zou, M.; Chen, Y.; Sun-Waterhouse, D.; Zhang, Y.; Li, F. Immunomodulatory acidic polysaccharides from *Zizyphus jujuba* cv. *Huizao*: Insights into their chemical characteristics and modes of action. *Food Chem.* **2018**, *258*, 35–42. [CrossRef]
67. Mao, W.; Zang, X.; Li, Y.; Zhang, H. Sulfated polysaccharides from marine green algae *Ulva conglobata* and their anticoagulant activity. *J. Appl. Phycol.* **2006**, *18*, 9–14. [CrossRef]
68. Yasantha, A.; KiWan, L.; SeKwon, K.; YouJin, J. Anticoagulant activity of marine green and brown algae collected from Jeju Island in Korea. *Bioresour. Technol.* **2007**, *98*, 1711–1716. [CrossRef]
69. Wang, X.; Zhang, Z.; Yao, Z.; Zhao, M.; Qi, H. Sulfation, anticoagulant and antioxidant activities of polysaccharide from green algae *Enteromorpha linza*. *Int. J. Biol. Macromol.* **2013**, *58*, 225–230. [CrossRef]
70. Jain, K.S.; Kathiravan, M.K.; Somani, R.S.; Shishoo, C.J. The biology and chemistry of hyperlipidemia. *Bioorganic Med. Chem.* **2007**, *15*, 4674–4699. [CrossRef]
71. Ross, R.; Harker, L. Hyperlipidemia and Atherosclerosis: Chronic hyperlipidemia initiates and maintains lesions by endothelial cell desquamation and lipid accumulation. *Science* **1976**, *193*, 1094–1100. [CrossRef]

72. Teng, Z.; Qian, L.; Zhou, Y. Hypolipidemic activity of the polysaccharides from *Enteromorpha prolifera*. *Int. J. Biol. Macromol.* **2013**, *62*, 254–256. [CrossRef] [PubMed]
73. Jiang, C.; Xiong, Q.; Gan, D.; Jiao, Y.; Liu, J.; Ma, L.; Zeng, X. Antioxidant activity and potential hepatoprotective effect of polysaccharides from *Cyclina sinensis*. *Carbohydr. Polym.* **2013**, *91*, 262–268. [CrossRef] [PubMed]
74. Li, B.; Liu, S.; Xing, R.; Li, K.; Li, R.; Qin, Y.; Li, P. Degradation of sulfated polysaccharides from *Enteromorpha prolifera* and their antioxidant activities. *Carbohydr. Polym.* **2013**, *92*, 1991–1996. [CrossRef] [PubMed]
75. Duan, K.; Shan, H.; Lin, Y.; Lv, H. Degradation of polysaccharide from *Enteromorpha prolifera* with hydrochloric acid and hydrogen peroxide assisted by microwave and its antioxidant activity. *Food Sci. Technol.* **2015**, *40*, 141–147.
76. Li, Y.; Wang, J.; Yu, Y.; Li, X.; Jiang, X.; Hwang, H.; Wang, P. Production of enzymes by Alteromonas sp. A321 to degrade polysaccharides from *Enteromorpha prolifera*. *Carbohydr. Polym.* **2013**, *98*, 988–994. [CrossRef]
77. Zhang, Z.; Han, X.; Xu, Y.; Li, J.; Li, Y.; Hu, Z. Biodegradation of *Enteromorpha* polysaccharides by intestinal micro-community from *Siganus oramin*. *J. Ocean Univ. China* **2016**, *15*, 1034–1038. [CrossRef]
78. Li, Y.; Li, W.; Zhang, G.; Lü, X.; Hwang, H.; Aker, W.G.; Wang, P. Purification and characterization of polysaccharides degradases produced by *Alteromonas* sp. A321. *Int. J. Biol. Macromol.* **2016**, *86*, 96–104. [CrossRef]
79. Patra, J.K.; Baek, K.-H. Antibacterial Activity and Action Mechanism of the Essential Oil from *Enteromorpha linza* L. against Foodborne Pathogenic Bacteria. *Molecules* **2016**, *21*, 388. [CrossRef]
80. Liu, D.; Keesing, J.K.; Dong, Z.; Zhen, Y.; Di, B.; Shi, Y.; Shi, P. Recurrence of the world's largest green-tide in 2009 in Yellow Sea, China: Porphyra yezoensis aquaculture rafts confirmed as nursery for macroalgal blooms. *Mar. Pollut. Bull.* **2010**, *60*, 1423–1432. [CrossRef]
81. Cui, J.; Li, Y.; Wang, S.; Chi, Y.; Hwang, H.; Wang, P. Directional preparation of anticoagulant-active sulfated polysaccharides from *Enteromorpha prolifera* using artificial neural networks. *Sci. Rep.* **2018**, *8*, 3062. [CrossRef]
82. Jin, W.; He, X.; Long, L.; Fang, Q.; Wei, B.; Sun, J.; Linhardt, R.J. Structural characterization and anti-lung cancer activity of a sulfated glucurono-xylo-rhamnan from *Enteromorpha prolifera*. *Carbohydr. Polym.* **2020**, *237*, 116143. [CrossRef] [PubMed]
83. Zhang, Y.; He, P.; Li, H.; Li, G.; Liu, J.; Jiao, F.; Jiao, N. Ulva prolifera green-tide outbreaks and their environmental impact in the Yellow Sea, China. *Natl. Sci. Rev.* **2019**, *6*, 825–838. [CrossRef] [PubMed]
84. De Paula Silva, P.H.; McBride, S.; de Nys, R.; Paul, N.A. Integrating filamentous 'green tide' algae into tropical pond-based aquaculture. *Aquaculture* **2008**, *284*, 74–80. [CrossRef]
85. Song, Y.; Han, A.; Park, S.; Cho, C.; Rhee, Y.; Hong, H. Effect of enzyme-assisted extraction on the physicochemical properties and bioactive potential of lotus leaf polysaccharides. *Int. J. Biol. Macromol.* **2020**, *153*, 169–179. [CrossRef] [PubMed]
86. Liu, Y.; Wu, X.; Jin, W.; Guo, Y. Immunomodulatory Effects of a Low-Molecular Weight Polysaccharide from *Enteromorpha prolifera* on RAW 264.7 Macrophages and Cyclophosphamide-Induced Immunosuppression Mouse Models. *Mar. Drugs* **2020**, *18*, 340. [CrossRef] [PubMed]

MDPI
St. Alban-Anlage 66
4052 Basel
Switzerland
Tel. +41 61 683 77 34
Fax +41 61 302 89 18
www.mdpi.com

Marine Drugs Editorial Office
E-mail: marinedrugs@mdpi.com
www.mdpi.com/journal/marinedrugs

www.ingramcontent.com/pod-product-compliance
Lightning Source LLC
LaVergne TN
LVHW070642100526
838202LV00013B/858
9783036583648